Mobile Health Applications for Quality Healthcare Delivery

Anastasius Moumtzoglou
P&A Kyriakou Children's Hospital, Greece

A volume in the Advances in Healthcare Information Systems and Administration (AHISA) Book Series

IGI Global
DISSEMINATOR OF KNOWLEDGE

Published in the United States of America by
IGI Global
Medical Information Science Reference (an imprint of IGI Global)
701 E. Chocolate Avenue
Hershey PA, USA 17033
Tel: 717-533-8845
Fax: 717-533-8661
E-mail: cust@igi-global.com
Web site: http://www.igi-global.com

Copyright © 2019 by IGI Global. All rights reserved. No part of this publication may be reproduced, stored or distributed in any form or by any means, electronic or mechanical, including photocopying, without written permission from the publisher. Product or company names used in this set are for identification purposes only. Inclusion of the names of the products or companies does not indicate a claim of ownership by IGI Global of the trademark or registered trademark.

Library of Congress Cataloging-in-Publication Data

Names: Moumtzoglou, Anastasius, 1959- editor.
Title: Mobile health applications for quality healthcare delivery / Anastasius Moumtzoglou, editor.
Description: Hershey, PA : Medical Information Science Reference, [2019] | Includes bibliographical references.
Identifiers: LCCN 2018042644| ISBN 9781522580218 (hardcover) | ISBN 9781522580225 (ebook)
Subjects: | MESH: Telemedicine | Medical Informatics Applications | Quality Assurance, Health Care--methods | Delivery of Health Care
Classification: LCC R858 | NLM W 83.1 | DDC 610.285--dc23 LC record available at https://lccn.loc.gov/2018042644

This book is published in the IGI Global book series Advances in Healthcare Information Systems and Administration (AHISA) (ISSN: 2328-1243; eISSN: 2328-126X)

British Cataloguing in Publication Data
A Cataloguing in Publication record for this book is available from the British Library.

The views expressed in this book are those of the authors, but not necessarily of the publisher.

For electronic access to this publication, please contact: eresources@igi-global.com.

Advances in Healthcare Information Systems and Administration (AHISA) Book Series

Anastasius Moumtzoglou
Hellenic Society for Quality & Safety in Healthcare and P. & A. Kyriakou Children's Hospital, Greece

ISSN:2328-1243
EISSN:2328-126X

Mission

The **Advances in Healthcare Information Systems and Administration (AHISA) Book Series** aims to provide a channel for international researchers to progress the field of study on technology and its implications on healthcare and health information systems. With the growing focus on healthcare and the importance of enhancing this industry to tend to the expanding population, the book series seeks to accelerate the awareness of technological advancements of health information systems and expand awareness and implementation.

Driven by advancing technologies and their clinical applications, the emerging field of health information systems and informatics is still searching for coherent directing frameworks to advance health care and clinical practices and research. Conducting research in these areas is both promising and challenging due to a host of factors, including rapidly evolving technologies and their application complexity. At the same time, organizational issues, including technology adoption, diffusion and acceptance as well as cost benefits and cost effectiveness of advancing health information systems and informatics applications as innovative forms of investment in healthcare are gaining attention as well. **AHISA** addresses these concepts and critical issues.

Coverage

- Pharmaceutical and Home Healthcare Informatics
- E-Health and M-Health
- IT Applications in Health Organizations and Practices
- Virtual health technologies
- IS in Healthcare
- Measurements and Impact of HISA on Public and Social Policy
- Nursing Expert Systems
- Rehabilitative Technologies
- IT Applications in Physical Therapeutic Treatments
- IT security and privacy issues

IGI Global is currently accepting manuscripts for publication within this series. To submit a proposal for a volume in this series, please contact our Acquisition Editors at Acquisitions@igi-global.com or visit: http://www.igi-global.com/publish/.

The Advances in Healthcare Information Systems and Administration (AHISA) Book Series (ISSN 2328-1243) is published by IGI Global, 701 E. Chocolate Avenue, Hershey, PA 17033-1240, USA, www.igi-global.com. This series is composed of titles available for purchase individually; each title is edited to be contextually exclusive from any other title within the series. For pricing and ordering information please visit http://www.igi-global.com/book-series/advances-healthcare-information-systems-administration/37156. Postmaster: Send all address changes to above address. ©© 2019 IGI Global. All rights, including translation in other languages reserved by the publisher. No part of this series may be reproduced or used in any form or by any means – graphics, electronic, or mechanical, including photocopying, recording, taping, or information and retrieval systems – without written permission from the publisher, except for non commercial, educational use, including classroom teaching purposes. The views expressed in this series are those of the authors, but not necessarily of IGI Global.

Titles in this Series

For a list of additional titles in this series, please visit: www.igi-global.com/book-series

Contemporary Applications of Mobile Computing in Healthcare Settings
R. Rajkumar (VIT University, India)
Medical Information Science Reference • ©2018 • 259pp • H/C (ISBN: 9781522550365) • US $205.00

Handbook of Research on Emerging Perspectives on Healthcare Information Systems and Informatics
Joseph Tan (McMaster University, Canada)
Medical Information Science Reference • ©2018 • 641pp • H/C (ISBN: 9781522554608) • US $355.00

Big Data Analytics in HIV/AIDS Research
Ali Al Mazari (Alfaisal University, Saudi Arabia)
Medical Information Science Reference • ©2018 • 294pp • H/C (ISBN: 9781522532033) • US $215.00

Advanced Systems for Improved Public Healthcare and Disease Prevention Emerging Research and Opportunities
Thierry Oscar Edoh (Technical University of Munich, Germany)
Medical Information Science Reference • ©2018 • 262pp • H/C (ISBN: 9781522555285) • US $185.00

Global Perspectives on Health Communication in the Age of Social Media
Seif Sekalala (Kean University, USA) and Brandon C. Niezgoda (Drexel University, USA)
Medical Information Science Reference • ©2018 • 348pp • H/C (ISBN: 9781522537168) • US $225.00

Healthcare Administration for Patient Safety and Engagement
Aleksandra Rosiek-Kryszewska (Nicolaus Copernicus University, Poland) and Krzysztof Leksowski (Military Clinical Hospital, Poland & Nicolaus Copernicus University, Poland)
Medical Information Science Reference • ©2018 • 343pp • H/C (ISBN: 9781522539469) • US $235.00

Big Data Management and the Internet of Things for Improved Health Systems
Brojo Kishore Mishra (C. V. Raman College of Engineering, India) and Raghvendra Kumar (LNCT Group of Colleges, India)
Medical Information Science Reference • ©2018 • 312pp • H/C (ISBN: 9781522552222) • US $255.00

Novel Applications of Virtual Communities in Healthcare Settings
Christo El Morr (York University, Canada)
Medical Information Science Reference • ©2018 • 247pp • H/C (ISBN: 9781522529583) • US $235.00

IGI Global
DISSEMINATOR OF KNOWLEDGE

701 East Chocolate Avenue, Hershey, PA 17033, USA
Tel: 717-533-8845 x100 • Fax: 717-533-8661
E-Mail: cust@igi-global.com • www.igi-global.com

In memory of my uncle George Birtachas

Table of Contents

Detailed Table of Contents

Angelina Kouroubali, Lefteris Koumakis, Haridimos Kondylakis, and Dimitrios G. Katehakis analyze the clinical and technological characteristics of mobile apps enabling cancer patients to record, manage, and share their information online securely. They discuss issues relevant to increasing patient experience and acceptance, improving adherence to treatment, and effective support of coordinated care. Outcomes of recent research projects, relevant to end digital user engagement, trust, interoperability, and usability/adaptability, lead to an integrated approach towards developing quality mobile health apps. Improving the quality of life and wellbeing seems to be the critical challenge. Regulation, standardization, and interoperability together with the existence of useful, accurate, and reliable tools for active patient engagement are imperative for efficient cancer disease management.

Elpis Vlachopapadopoulou, Eleni I. Georga, and Dimitrios I. Fotiadis present state-of-the-art m-health solutions for monitoring and treatment of children suffering from obesity. M-health solutions are used for self-management, remote monitoring, and counseling of several chronic conditions, including diabetes mellitus, heart failure, Parkinson's disease, etc. Concerning childhood obesity, those solutions can combine targeted games and motivational approaches towards both physical activity and diet, which could help in addressing this serious and global health issue, in the direction of minimizing co-morbidities and eventually preventing serious, life-threatening events.

Chinmay Chakraborty describes the implementation of tele-wound monitoring (TWM) for a patient's chronic wound using a smartphone and highlights the smartphone-enabled tele-wound monitoring (TWM) framework which is used for remote wound monitoring. The TWM is useful for both rural as well as urban people, as it provides good performance regarding wound monitoring and diagnosis.

Bibiana Metelmann and Camilla Metelmann argue that m-health can assist in prehospital emergency medicine in multiple ways. They provide insights into emergency medicine and present three different forms of m-health in this field. One is the retrieval of medical data (e.g., with the aid of smartphone applications). A second one uses uncrewed aerial vehicles. Moreover, the third one establishes real-time communication with medical experts.

Abraham Pouliakis, Effrosyni Karakitsou, and Niki Margari expect that the applications for the mobile device targeting cytopathology would flourish. There is potential for applications into various activities of the laboratory including but not limited to training, reporting of results, diagnosis and consultation, management of the laboratory, whole slide imaging and still image capture, quality control and assurance, and numerous channels for interactions between patient-doctor or among medical specialists.

Stavros Archondakis, Eleftherios Vavoulidis, Maria Nasioutziki, Ourania Oustampasidou, Angelos Daniilidis, Anastasia Vatopoulou, Alexios Papanikolaou, and Konstantinos Dinas present thorough research of mobile applications related to cytopathology and try to foresee applications that may benefit modern cytopathology. Furthermore, they examine the feasibility of such applications for inter-laboratory comparisons, proficiency testing, and diagnostic accuracy validation. Finally, the role of mobile applications for providing or/and enhancing the laboratory capabilities through educational training and other research activities is studied.

Stelios Zimeras analyzes various epidemic models under differential mathematical systems. Epidemic models assume that individuals go through a series of states at a specific, constant set of rates while different epidemic models have been proposed based on the characteristics of the systems and the topology of the network.

Preface

Person-centeredness is widely recognized as a multidimensional concept that advocates patients' informed decisions, successful management of their own health and care, and choice when to invite others to act on their behalf (Silva, 2014). It is a conception that comprehends patients as peer partners in planning, developing and assessing care. In other words, person-centered care is about co-production rather than consumerism. Moreover, the Institute of Medicine prioritizes six dimensions of patient-centeredness as decisive to supporting quality healthcare. These are (US Institute of Medicine, 2001):

- Being respectful of patients' values, preferences, and expressed needs
- Being coordinated and integrated
- Providing information, communication and education
- Ensuring physical comfort
- Providing emotional support and easing fear and anxiety, and
- Involving family and friends

However, reviewers have argued that the model of person-centered care is somewhat rhetorical and equates to 'consumer-based' model rather than a psychosocial approach. Moreover, they also contend that there is no unopposed definition of person-centered care in the empirical literature (Silva, 2014). As a result, the complexity of the theory raises the need to articulate its shared meaning and explicate how it can be put into use.

Additionally, the term 'patient-centered care' which is more frequently used than person-centered care and tends to describe a much wider range of disease areas has often been analyzed as a multifaceted construct (Ishikawa, Hashimoto, Kiuchi, 2013) with no single theory that can sufficiently define the whole idea or lacking a unified definition and operationalized measurement (Silva, 2014).

On the other hand, notwithstanding patient-centered care may be considered of modern origin, its essence can unquestionably be found in the Hippocratic Oath. Respect and broad-mindedness to the patient needs, relevant ethics, and concern for community well-being are prominently evident in Hippocrates. However, this inclination to the origins of medicine has been long discontinued. Beneficence as a bioethical teaching has lost part of its radiance, dominated by the belief of autonomy and by the current emphasis on defending the medical commonality. As a consequence, medicine has missed its holistic focal point, which patient-centered philosophy aims to regenerate for patients.

The holistic notion upholds that each aspect of patient's needs including corporeal, social and mental should be taken into account and perceived as a whole.

How exactly, do you do that? What does 'emotional, spiritual and mental needs' look like in a doctor-patient encounter?

The doctor-patient relationship can be seen as a social mechanism for salubrious impact on the patient's well-being (Benedetti, 2011). The important point is to realize why this social interplay is necessary to stimulate the endogenous mechanisms that handle expectation and placebo outcomes. However, the reason a social mechanism of that kind surfaced in the course of evolution appears to be considerably reasonable. There are numerous benefits of altruism and social partnership. Suppression of psychological uneasiness by human interactions warrants a robust mechanism to recover, at least in part. In this context, following evolutionary theory, the healthcare system can be more complicated and can acquire the qualities of an actual endogenous system. According to Humphrey (2002), the ability to stimulate expectation in addition to placebo mechanisms following the doctor-patient encounter is an emergent issue and essential feature of the 'natural healthcare service'. Humphrey (2002) claims that patient's body together with the brain have a considerable role in healing themselves but that capacity for self-cure is not revealed spontaneously, but can be triggered by the influence of the doctor. Therefore, the pivotal point is to realize why the patient-doctor encounter is needed to initiate the self-cure mechanisms.

The conceptualization of an endogenous healthcare system by Humphrey (2002) is extremely useful to know why the doctor-patient encounter is necessary in order to trigger expectation in addition to placebo mechanisms in the patient's brain. Doctors and health professionals represent environmental variables that act on the patient's brain by inducing expectancies of benefit and hope. Health professionals are crucial actors in this process, as they promise treatment and induce expectations and hope for the patient's future well-being. The patient's expectations also play a key role. If the patient wants to consult a physician, this is because of his beliefs about the doctor's healing skills. Therefore, the 'healer' is the environmental variable that triggers endogenous mechanisms of self-cure. From both an evolutionary, neuroscientific and patient-centered care perspective, it is obvious that the therapist belongs to the system and has a pivotal role in triggering all mechanisms that take place in the patient's brain.

Conclusively, patient-centered care should be defined as the symmetry of the artful and the perfunctory element that is represented by the Ancient Greek word 'techne'. As a result, patient-centered care is the competence to produce a preconceived outcome using consciously controlled and directed action, which involves (Moumtzoglou, 2014):

- The undivided completeness and universality of human health defined as the state of being free of physical or psychological malfunction
- The rational and ethical principles used by health professionals to distinguish between different procedures, and observe the correct diagnosis and action in each case
- The environmental variables that act on the patient's brain by inducing expectancies of benefit and hope

THE CHALLENGES

The health care environment is currently changing to meet technology and societal trends which converge to bring into being new communication patterns that connect and coordinate the roles of healthcare stakeholders. At the same time, the healthcare industry is steering inexorably toward a distributed-service design in which essential decision-making occurs at the point of care. One of the central engines of this shift towards decentralization and reorientation of healthcare services is mobile healthcare (mHealth). mHealth describes the use of a broad range of telecommunication and multimedia technologies within a wireless care delivery design and can be broadly defined as the delivery of healthcare services via mobile communication devices. mHealth establishes healthcare communities in which every stakeholder can participate. However, it disrupts the traditional service model where healthcare information, security and access is centrally managed, maintained and limited, transforming the healthcare sector and destroying components that are slow to adapt.

mHealth interventions range from simple to complex applications and systems that remotely coordinate and actively manage patient care. In this context, it offers an elegant solution to the problem of accessing the right information where and when it is needed within highly fluid, distributed organizations. Moreover, it removes geography and time as barriers to care by establishing connectivity with remote locations and remote workers, creates new points of contact with patients, and changes the frequency and intensity of healthcare delivery. It also establishes effective new treatment modalities like telehealth, remote patient monitoring, self-care and home health while it blurs the boundaries between professional medical advice and self-care. Overall, mHealth blends three bodies of knowledge: high technology, life sciences, and human factors.

On current trends, mHealth embraces medical and public health practice sustained by mobile phones, patient monitoring devices, personal digital assistants (PDAs), and tablet PCs. The spread of 3G and 4G networks has boosted the use of mobile applications offering healthcare services. 4G is a mobile network, IP-based, providing a connection via the best network using seamless roaming and independent radio access technologies. In 4G mobile systems, different access technologies are combined in the best possible way for different radio environments and service requirements. They promise much larger data rates supporting full mobility while enabling wireless connection and access to multimedia services with high-quality voice and high-definition video. In addition, the availability of satellite navigation technologies in mobile devices supports safety and autonomy of patients. Through sensors and mobile applications, mHealth permits the accumulation of extensive medical, physiological, lifestyle, daily activity and environmental data.

Consequently, mHealth serves evidence-driven care practice and research activities while expediting patients' access to health information and accommodating lifestyle and wellbeing applications, counseling systems, health information and medication reminders. However, beyond clinical connectivity, mHealth is a field that came to light holding the promise of quality improvement, cost reduction, wholesale gains in population health, access to care and better allocation of health-delivery resources. With mHealth, healthcare professionals can continuously monitor and manage health conditions. As a result, mHealth becomes embedded in some care delivery strategies, including the medical home, a health information exchange, the care team and patient-centric healthcare.

In its fullest flowering, mHealth it is expected to address the most intractable problems of healthcare quality and cost, chronic disease management, public health, wellness, and prevention. However, the impact of mHealth is just beginning to be felt as it results in more personalized medication and treatment and contributes to patient-centered care.

SEARCHING FOR A SOLUTION

There is no standardized definition of mHealth. However, in most cases, mobile health or mHealth is defined as medical and public health practice supported by mobile devices involving:

- The use and capitalization on a mobile phone's core utility of voice and short messaging service
- Applications including general packet radio service (GPRS), third and fourth generation mobile telecommunications (3G and 4G systems), global positioning system (GPS), and Bluetooth technology

Mobile health became functional in biomedical engineering and started with looking at wireless and sensor technologies that could be incorporated to monitor people's health at a distance. mHealth implementation came out in developing countries out of access necessity. Moreover, mobile phones had been around for years, but it was not until 1976 that mobile phones first appeared in Japan. However, a lot of work happened predominantly in the early millennium when mHealth started to develop mobile health applications for cellphones. The early days there were things like remote cardiac monitors that evolved to look at diabetes monitoring and other types of sensor technologies. The early programs provided support tools for supply chain management while mobile communications gave access to areas that people never had using fixed line telephones. More recently, mHealth evolvement provided access to emergency medical transportation services, facilitated patient-doctor encounter, and there was a movement to personal digital assistants use.

mHealth is increasingly being used in the healthcare field since its use is becoming a cost-effective method of identifying and monitoring health issues, as well as guiding the formulation of health policies. Programs to support the professional development of people in the health field, using mHealth technology, are becoming readily available. mHealth also provides health professionals with access to patient data as well as access to various information sources, both of which provide valuable assistance in the diagnosis and formulation of treatment. Individuals can use mHealth to access resource materials on health issues. Patients can self-monitor and transmit information to their health care provider making mHealth particularly important to people living in remote areas or those who are physically impaired.

While the timely emergence of mHealth did not resolve the myriad problems, it offers unique opportunities to reduce cost, increase efficiencies and improve the quality and access to care. Home-based monitoring helps hospitals track patient recovery and compliance, thereby minimizing costly episodes of re-admission. Coordination between departments and providers reduces wasteful spending and improves the quality of care. Moreover, with rapid consumer adoption of smartphones, physicians can perform two-way videoconferencing while patients and physicians have access to medical records and vital signs. Finally, wireless technology allows physicians to serve more patients despite geographical limitations.

In this context, the book explores the emergence of mHealth in the healthcare setting by:

- Focusing on the broad range of technologies available
- Tackling the effects of mHealth on the industry and stakeholders exploring the infrastructure and architecture needed to support these technologies
- Discussing the evolvement of various stakeholders and the impact of mHealth on existing technology
- Analyzing the transformation of the business model

Looking forward, it explores how mHealth reshapes access, quality, and treatment and demystifies the impact of mHealth on patient-centered care. Conclusively, it intends to:

- Support students understand the effect of mHealth technologies on quality in healthcare
- Help healthcare professionals better understand the needs of their patients
- Act as an assistant for patients to derive more benefits from their healthcare
- Encourage e-health systems designers and managers to ground everyday practice on mHealth technologies

The prospective audience includes undergraduate and extended degree programs students, graduate students of health care quality and health services management, executive education and continuing education, health care managers and health professionals.

ORGANIZATION OF THE BOOK

In Chapter 1, Yiannis Koumpouros and Aggelos provide the readers with a macroscopic analysis of the European mhealth related funded activities of the last decade. The study examines the current situation and future trends in three main axes (innovation, the areas of application and adoption) to assess whether the provided mhealth solutions are positioned to have a fundamental impact on healthcare domain. The mhealth research is accelerating fast and holds great promise, improving both patient outcomes while lowering the healthcare costs.

In Chapter 2, Adusumalli Sai Manoj, Mohammed Ali Hussain, argue that a mobile care system can be designed with the help of a wireless sensor network using IoT. That can be done by integrating different sensors to sense physiological data from the human body and then transmit the data to a healthcare cloud through a smartphone.

In Chapter 3, Angelina Kouroubali, Lefteris Koumakis, Haridimos Kondylakis, and Dimitrios G. Katehakis, analyze the clinical and technological characteristics of mobile apps enabling cancer patients to record, manage and share their information online securely. They discuss issues relevant to increasing patient experience and acceptance, improving adherence to treatment, and effective support of coordinated care. Outcomes of recent research projects, relevant to end digital user engagement, trust, interoperability, and usability/ adaptability, lead to an integrated approach towards developing quality mobile health apps. Improving the quality of life and well-being seems to be the critical challenge. Regulation, standardization and interoperability together with the existence of useful, accurate, and reliable tools for active patient engagement are imperative for efficient cancer disease management.

In Chapter 4, Elpis Vlachopapadopoulou, Eleni I. Georga, and Dimitrios I. Fotiadis, present state of the art mHealth solutions for monitoring and treatment of children suffering from obesity. mHealth solutions are used for self-management, remote monitoring and counseling of several chronic conditions, including diabetes mellitus, heart failure, Parkinson's disease, etc. Concerning childhood obesity, those solutions can combine targeted games and motivational approaches towards both physical activity and diet, which could help in addressing this serious and global health issue, in the direction of minimizing co-morbidities and eventually preventing serious, life-threatening events.

In Chapter 5, Chinmay Chakraborty describes the implementation of tele-wound monitoring (TWM) for a patient's chronic wound using a smartphone and highlights the smartphone-enabled tele-wound monitoring (TWM) framework which is used for remote wound monitoring. The TWM is useful for both rural as well as urban people, as it provides good performance regarding wound monitoring and diagnosis.

In Chapter 6, Bibiana Metelmann, and Camilla Metelmann argue that mHealth can assist in prehospital emergency medicine in multiple ways. They provide insights into emergency medicine and present three different forms of mHealth in this field. One is the retrieval of medical data, e.g. with the aid of smartphone applications. A second one uses uncrewed aerial vehicles. Moreover, the third one establishes real-time communication with medical experts.

In Chapter 7, Abraham Pouliakis, Effrosyni Karakitsou, and Niki Margari expect that the applications for the mobile device targeting cytopathology would flourish. There is potential for applications into various activities of the laboratory, including and not limited to: training, reporting of results, diagnosis and consultation, management of the laboratory, whole slide imaging and still image capture, quality control and assurance and numerous channels for interactions between patient-doctor or among medical specialists.

In Chapter 8, Stavros Archondakis, Eleftherios Vavoulidis, Maria Nasioutziki, Ourania Oustampasidou, Angelos Daniilidis, Anastasia Vatopoulou, Alexios Papanikolaou, and Konstantinos Dinas present thorough research of mobile applications related to cytopathology and try to foresee applications that may benefit modern Cytopathology. Furthermore, they examine the feasibility of such applications for inter-laboratory comparisons, proficiency testing and diagnostic accuracy validation. Finally, the role of mobile applications for providing or/and enhancing the laboratory capabilities through educational training and other research activities is studied.

In Chapter 9, Stelios Zimeras analyzes various epidemic models under differential mathematical systems. Epidemic models assume that individuals go through a series of states at a specific, constant set of rates while different epidemic models have been proposed based on the characteristics of the systems and the topology of the network.

In Chapter 10, Anastasius S Moumtzoglou envisions tailored M-Health communication in the context of the science of individuality, emphasizing the variability, stability and centrality of the individual. Reasons and evidence are cited regarding the promise of the science of individuality which promises to recognize the uniqueness of the individual fully. On the other hand, emerging M-Health technologies provide fundamentally different ways of looking at tailored communication technology. As a result, tailored communications research is poised at a crossroads. It needs to both build on and break away from existing frameworks into new territory, realizing the necessary commitment to theory-driven research at basic, methodological, clinical, and applied levels.

In Chapter 11, Anastasius S Moumtzoglou argues that self-care emerged from the concept of health promotion in the 1970s while from 2000 onwards the term 'self-management' gained popularity, with a greater focus on long-term conditions and the trend towards more holistic models of care. Although 'self-management' and 'self-care' are often used interchangeably, a distinction between the two concepts can be made. Both can be considered in terms of a continuum, with self-care at one end as 'normal activity' and self-management an extension of this. Self-management support is the assistance given to patients in order to encourage daily decisions that improve health-related behaviors and clinical outcomes. These concepts are envisioned on a continuum with one pole representing mobile health and the other self-care, and self-management support is thought as the nexus of mobile health and self-care.

P&A Kyriakou Children's Hospital, Greece

REFERENCES

Benedetti, F. (2011). *The Patient's Brain: The neuroscience behind the doctor-patient relationship*. Oxford, UK: Oxford University Press.

Humphrey, N. (2002). *The mind made flesh*. Oxford, UK: Oxford University Press.

Ishikawa, H., Hashimoto, H., & Kiuchi, T. (2013). The evolving concept of 'patient-centeredness' in patient-physician communication research. *Social Science & Medicine*, *96*, 147–153. doi:10.1016/j.socscimed.2013.07.026 PMID:24034962

Moumtzoglou, A. (2014). Redefining Patient-Centered Care. *International Journal of Reliable and Quality E-Healthcare*, *3*(2), iv–v.

Silva, D. (2014). *Helping measure person-centred care: A review of evidence about commonly used approaches and tools used to help measure person-centred care*. London: The Health Foundation.

US Institute of Medicine. (2001). *Crossing The Quality Chasm: A New Health System For The 21st Century*. Washington, DC: National Academy Press.

Acknowledgment

I would like to thank the reviewers for the care with which they reviewed the manuscripts and all the authors for their diverse and outstanding contributions to this book.

Chapter 1
The Rise of mHealth Research in Europe:
A Macroscopic Analysis of EC-Funded Projects of the Last Decade

Yiannis Koumpouros
University of West Attica, Greece

Aggelos Georgoulas
University of West Attica, Greece

ABSTRACT

The proliferation of mhealth holds great promise for improving human health. The mhealth industry has developed into a vivid ecosystem, growing steadily over the last years with the adoption of new technologies and business models that are transforming healthcare. To this end, the European Commission launched several initiatives offering great funding opportunities for researchers and organizations. The purpose of this chapter is to provide the readers with a macroscopic analysis of the European mhealth-related funded activities of the last decade. The study examines the current situation and future trends in three main axes (innovation, area of application, and adoption) to assess whether the provided mhealth solutions are positioned to have a fundamental impact on healthcare domain. The mhealth research is accelerating fast and holds great promise, improving both patient outcomes while lowering the healthcare costs.

INTRODUCTION

Health care is the industry that leads the technological developments while adopting the first the Information and Communication Technologies (ICTs) innovations (Koumpouros I., 2012). The complexity and inherent multiple healthcare system components enforce technological innovation in order to overcome impediments and failures which slow or inhibit progress in the healthcare sector. The challenges faced are numerous, i.e. the exponential growth of data produced, the financial viability of the system, security and privacy issues, the ageing of the population, and similar (OECD, 2018) (UN, 2017), (Koumpouros Y., 2014). There is a great need for well-established solutions able to manage the flow of information

DOI: 10.4018/978-1-5225-8021-8.ch001

Copyright © 2019, IGI Global. Copying or distributing in print or electronic forms without written permission of IGI Global is prohibited.

between the different parties and actors in the healthcare industry effectively. The explosion of new technological solutions, along with the appearance of the net generation, forced to find new ways to provide the health care services (PWC, 2012), (Jones & Shao, 2011), (Bayne & Ross, 2007).

The health care industry is one of the domains that are penetrated by many mobile technology solutions. For example, mobile technology is having a dramatic impact on the way health care is delivered to both urban and rural communities in developing countries (e.g. the African Region). The use of the term mHealth is widely used the past years for such a purpose. To date, there are several definitions of mHealth:

- The Global Observatory for eHealth - GOe (WHO, mHealth. New horizons for health through mobile technologies: Based on the findings of the second global survey on eHealth, 2011) and the European Commission (EC, COM(2014) 219 final, 2014) defined mHealth as *"medical and public health practice supported by mobile devices, such as mobile phones, patient monitoring devices, personal digital assistants (PDAs), and other wireless devices"*.
- The World Health Organization -WHO (Youssef, MacCallum, McDonald, Crane, & Jackman, 2012) refers to mHealth as *"the spread of mobile technologies as well as advancements in their innovative application to address health priorities"*.
- HIMSS - Healthcare Information and Management Systems Society (HIMSS, Healtcare Information and Management Systems Society, 2015) supports that *"mHealth is the generation, aggregation, and dissemination of health information via mobile and wireless devices."*
- The National Institutes of Health (NIH, n.d.) defines mHealth as *"the use of mobile and wireless technologies along with wearable and fixed sensors for the improvement of health outcomes, healthcare services, and health research"*.
- United Nations Foundation (VitalWaveConsulting, 2009) refers to mHealth as *"the provision of health-related services via mobile communications"*.

The chapter adopts the Global Observatory for eHealth (GOe) definition of mHealth (WHO, mHealth. New horizons for health through mobile technologies: Based on the findings of the second global survey on eHealth, 2011).

Integration of mobile technology into healthcare services has allowed consumers to manage their daily activities effectively. mHealth applications propose solutions to the emerging needs in the health care industry (e.g. the rising of chronic diseases and conditions, the ageing of population, the changes in societal behaviour which are contributing to a steady increase in costly long-term health problems, global pandemics, etc.), which contribute to reduce healthcare expenditure by limiting the number of hospital visits, while reducing readmissions. It is critical that such implementations focus on the public health goals underlying mHealth initiatives, rather than on specific technologies (Fraser, Bailey, Sinha, Mehl, & Labrique, 2011), (WHO, mHealth. New horizons for health through mobile technologies: Based on the findings of the second global survey on eHealth, 2011).

Koumpouros & Georgoulas presented the several challenges in the health care industry and the need for innovative technological applications (Koumpouros & Georgoulas, 2016). Mobile technology has expanded significantly across the globe in recent years. With almost 103.5 mobile cellular telephone subscriptions per 100 inhabitants (7.74 billion subscriptions in total) (ITU Statistics, 2018), the number of mobile phone users in the world is expected to pass five billion by 2019 (Statista, The Statistics Portal, 2016). Moreover, the number of active mobile broadband subscriptions reached 4.22 billion worldwide

(ITU Statistics, 2018). Mobile traffic has increased four-fold in recent years, and it is expected to grow exponentially shortly (due to advances in 3G and 4G network that has enabled utilization of mobile devices in several fields).

Globally, the health market is expected to grow at 36.5% CAGR (2017-2022) (Statista, 2018). This market is one of the fastest growing industries. The tremendous progress shown in the last few years can be justified due to patient's involvement in personal healthcare, implementation of smartphones and wearable devices into the healthcare industry, integration of wireless technologies with healthcare devices that are portable, etc.

The European Commission (EC, COM(2014) 219 final, 2014) strives to the direction of mobile solutions in order to:

- Increase prevention and improve quality of life by promoting healthy behaviours.
- Help in the direction of more efficient and sustainable practices in health care by reducing unnecessary visits and consultations, etc.
- Empower patients and enhance their responsibility for their health.

Research and innovation are pillars of the Europe 2020 Strategy to put Europe back on the path to smart, sustainable and inclusive growth. For example, Horizon 2020 is the latest EU's funding programme for research and innovation that provides support from basic research through to innovation with almost €80 billion of funding from 2014 to 2020. The emphasis under Horizon 2020 is to assess its impact on Europe's scientific and technological performance and research capacity and more widely on the European economy and society.

The main objective of this chapter is to provide an updated review of the European funded research efforts in the mHealth domain with a time span that reaches 2017. This will provide the reader with the latest technological solutions, their focus, the level of adoption, the funding opportunities, their impact, and other critical parameters.

At least to the knowledge of the authors, there is no other review on the specific domain. The current study is intended to provide researchers and decision-makers with a systematically organized knowledge base in order to better plan new mHealth research initiatives. The reader, after studying the chapter, will have a clear view on the challenges faced and opportunities are given by mHealth, the potential of the specific market, while recognizing the key players and the latest approaches in the specific domain.

PROJECTS AND TECHNOLOGY ANALYSIS

Over the last years, the EU has funded various projects involving the use of smartphones and other mobile devices in the healthcare industry in order to support the different stakeholders (patients, healthcare professionals, healthcare systems, etc.).

HORIZON 2020 is the current programme, under which the latest activities are funded, mainly under PHC-12-2014-1 – Clinical research for the validation of biomarkers and/or diagnostic medical devices, and independent living, PHC-26-2014 – Self management of health and disease: citizen engagement and mHealth subprogrammes. Previous programmes include FP7-ICT (EU FP7-ICT, 2014), and especially subprogrammes ICT-2007.5.1 - Personal health systems for monitoring and point-of-care diagnostics, ICT-2009.5.1 - Personal Health Systems, ICT-2011.5.1 - Personal Health Systems (PHS), ICT-2011.5.3

- Patient Guidance Services (PGS), safety and healthcare record information reuse, ICT-2013.5.1 - Personalised health, active ageing, HEALTH.2012.2.3.2-4 – Low-cost interventions for disease control in poor resource settings, and others.

Within the following paragraphs, we attempt an overview of the most current (on-going or recently finished) European funded projects in the field of mHealth. A thorough review of the two official EU databases was conducted to identify these projects:

- **CORDIS:** EU research projects under FP7 (2007-2013) (CORDIS, European Community - Community Research and Development Infromation, n.d.): This dataset contains projects funded by the European Union under the seventh framework programme for research and technological development from 2007 to 2013. Grant information is provided for each project, including reference, acronym, dates, funding, programmes, participant countries, subjects and objectives.
- **CORDIS:** EU research projects under Horizon 2020 (2014-2020) (CORDIS, European Community - Community Research and Development Infromation, n.d.): This dataset contains projects funded by the European Union under the Horizon 2020 framework programme for research and innovation from 2014 to 2020. Grant information is provided for each project, including Rcn (CORDIS record number), Reference, Acronym, Status, Programme, Topic, Title, Start Date, End Date, Objective, Total Cost, EC Max Contribution, Call Id, Funding Scheme, Coordinator, Coordinator Country, Participants, Participant Countries.

The search results were limited from the year 2008 and afterwards in order to study mHealth projects of the last decade, exploiting the latest technologies and mobile devices. The projects were selected by the following criteria:

1. research and development projects involving mobile solutions for delivering or supporting healthcare;
2. projects that utilize sensor or wearable technologies to support monitoring and evaluation;
3. technologies and devices that are in small size (even nano-) and are applied to patients to support their health status from a distance;
4. applications that use cell phones, tablets, etc., and/or wireless technologies to promote healthy living and adherence to therapies;
5. other small-sized devices that can fit a person's day to day life for general health purposes;
6. projects funded by the EU.

Table 1 presents the basic features of the studied projects.

The analysis of the presented projects reveals the distribution of partners and coordinators per country (Table 2), as well as the type of partner (i.e. University, Research Centre, Small Medium Enterprise-SME, Public organization, Other) (Figure 1). The budget distribution is depicted in Figure 2.

The majority of the projects (47%) was funded under the Horizon 2020 programme, while the rest of them (53%) belonged to the FP7 one (ICT, HEALTH and PEOPLE), and only two of the studied projects were funded under the Marie Curie initiative.

The health issues addressed by the projects are presented in Table 3 and Figure 3.

The number of pilots per project and the targeted end users is presented in Figure 4 and 5 accordingly.

The EU projects studied dealt with ten main categories, as presented in Figure 6.

A variety of technologies were applied to the frames of the projects (Figure 7).

Table 1. Characteristics of the reviewed mHealth projects

Project Name	Participating countries[1,2]	Programme / Topic	Budget (€)	Start date	End date	Condition(s) addressed	Technologies employed	Target groups / Pilots (no. of users)	Project scope
METABO (METABO, 2008)	**ES**(5); CZ(4); DE(2); FI(3); FR; EL(4); IT(5); LU; MT; SK	ICT-2007.5.1[3]	11.419.530	01/01/08	30/06/11	Diabetes	Sensors; App; Smartphone	Patients; HCP[4] / 1	Monitoring; Treatment; Self-Management
CHRONIOUS (CHRONIOUS, 2008)	**IT**(4); AT(2); CH; CY(2); CZ; DE(3); ES; EL(4); HU; PT; SI; UK(2)	ICT-2007.5.1	10.284.963	01/02/08	31/05/12	Chronic Diseases (COPD[5], CKD[6], Renal Insufficiency)	Sensors; Wearables; Smartphone; DSS	Patients; HCP / 1 (100)	Monitoring; Treatment; Self-Management
ICT4Depression (ICT4Depression, 2015)	**NL**(4); CH; IE; PT(3); SE	ICT-2009.5.1[7]	3.706.506	01/01/10	30/04/13	Depression	Sensors; Smartphone; App; Web; AI[8]	HCP; Patients / 1	Monitoring; Treatment; Self-Management; Drug Compliance
PSYCHE (PSYCHE, 2010)	**IT**(3); CH(2); DE; ES; FR(4); IE	ICT-2009.5.1	3.903.007	01/01/10	31/12/13	Bipolar Disorder	Sensors; Wearables; Smartphone; App; Data Mining	HCP; Patients / 1	Monitoring; Treatment; Self-Management
MONARCA (MONARCA, 2010)	**IT**; AT(3); CH(2); DE(4); DK(2)	ICT-2009.5.1	5.134.929	01/02/10	31/07/13	Bipolar Disorder	Sensors; Smartphone; App; DSS[9]	HCP; Patients / 1	Monitoring; Self-Assessment; Treatment
BRAVEHEALTH (BRAVEHEALTH, 2016)	**IT**(9); BE; CN_X_HK; FI; NL; PT(2); UK(3)	ICT-2009.5.1	10.382.905	01/03/10	31/07/12	CVD[10]	Sensors; Wearables; Smartphone; App; AI	Patients / 1	Monitoring; Treatment
INTERSTRESS (INTERSTRESS, 2010)	**IT**(6); BE; DE; ES; EL	ICT-2009.5.1	4.438.842	01/03/10	30/11/13	Psychological Stress	Wearables; Sensors; Smartphone; App; DSS; 3D; Virtual World	HCP; Patients / 1	Monitoring; Assessment; Treatment
REACTION (REACTION, 2010)	**ES**; AT(2); BE; DE(2); DK(2); EL(2); HU; SE; UK(2)	ICT-2009.5.1	16.318.147	01/03/10	28/02/14	Diabetes	Sensors; Smartphone; App; ePatch; DSS; BAN[11]	HCP; Patients / 3	Monitoring; Treatment; Self-Management
Nephron+ (Nephron+, 2010)	**EL**; AT; CH; DE(2); FR; NL(4)	ICT-2009.5.1	6.931.031	01/04/10	31/12/14	Renal Insufficiency	Sensors; Artificial Organs; Smartphone; App	Patients / 1 (animals)	Monitoring; Treatment; Self-Management
Help4mood (Help4Mood, 2011)	**UK**(5); ES(3); IT; RO	ICT-2009.5.1	3.599.074	01/01/11	30/06/14	Depression	Sensors; Smartphone; App; DSS; Avatar	HCP; Patients / 1	Monitoring; Treatment; Self-Management
MovingLife (Moving Life, 2011)	**ES**; BE; DK(2); IT;UK	ICT-2011.5.1[12]	584.415	01/09/11	30/04/13	Lifestyle; Diseases	Roadmaps		mHealth Solutions and Technologies
Commodity12 (Commodity12, 2011)	**DE**(2); CH; FR(2); IT; NL; PT; SI; UK(2)	ICT-2011.5.1	5.478.076	01/10/11	31/12/14	Diabetes	Sensors; Smartphone; DSS; AI; BAN	HCP; Patients / 1	Monitoring; Treatment

continued on following page

Table 1. Continued

Project Name	Participating countries[1,2]	Programme / Topic	Budget (€)	Start date	End date	Condition(s) addressed	Technologies employed	Target groups / Pilots (no. of users)	Project scope
MobiGuide (MobiGuide, 2011)	**IL**(3); AT; ES(4); IT(2); NL(3)	ICT-2011.5.3[13]	7.068.682	01/11/11	31/10/15	Chronic Diseases (Atrial Fibrillation, Gestational Diabetes, Gestational Hypertension)	Wearables; Smartphone; App; DSS; AI; BAN	HCP; Patients / 3	Monitoring; Treatment; Self-Management
RemPark (RemPark, 2011)	**ES**(3); BE; DE; IE(2); IL; IT; PT; SE	ICT-2011.5.1	4.735.804	01/11/11	30/04/15	Parkinson	Sensors; Wearables; Smartphone; App; BAN; AI	HCP; Patients / 4 (60)	Monitoring; Self-Management
Empower (Empower, 2011)	**AT**; CH; DE(2); EL; TR(2)	ICT-2011.5.3	4.276.946	01/02/12	31/01/15	Diabetes	Smartphone; App; Bluetooth; Sensors	HCP; Patients / 2	Self-Management; Monitoring
Decipher PCP (Decipher PCP, 2013)	**ES**(4); FI(3); IT(2); UK(2)	ICT-2011.5.3	3.551.931	01/02/12	31/05/16	mHealth; Procurement	PCP[14]	Admin; HCP; Patients / 1	Secure Cross-Border Access to Existing Patient Healthcare Portals
Supporting LIFE (Supporting LIFE, 2017)	**UK**(2); SE; NO; MW(2); CH; US; TW; IE	HEALTH.2012.2.3.2-4[15]	3.795.877	01/05/13	30/04/17	Malaria; Infantile Diarrhoea	Sensors; Smartphone; App; DSS	HCP / 2 (100)	Monitoring; Treatment; Diagnosis
Splendid (Splendid, 2013)	**EL**; CH; ES; NL; SE(3)	ICT-2013.5.1[16]	3.597.959	01/10/13	30/09/16	Obesity; Eating Disorder	Sensors; Smartphone; App	Patients; Citizens / 1	Self-Management; Monitoring; Prevention; Health Promotion
Welcome (Welcome, 2013)	**EL**(2); CH; DE(3); IE; IT; NL; PT; UK(3)	ICT-2013.5.1	8.272.080	01/11/13	31/10/17	COPD (With Comorbidities Chronic Heart Failure, Diabetes, Anxiety and Depression)	Sensors; Wearables; Smartphone; DSS	Patients / 5	Self-Management
Pegasof4f (Pegasof4f, 2014)	**IT**(8); CH(2); DE; ES(7); RO; UK(4)	ICT-2013.5.1	11.639.121	01/12/13	31/05/17	Obesity; Lifestyle; Food Awareness	Wearables; Smartphone; App; Serious Games	Citizens / 3 (300)	Self-Management; Health Promotion; Prevention
NYMPHA-MD (NYMPHA-MD, 2014)	**IT**(2); DK; ES(2)	ICT-2013.5.1	2.589.981	01/01/14	30/06/17	Bipolar Disorder	PCP	Admin / 3	Health Services
Unwired Health (UnwiredHealth, 2014)	**ES**(2); BE(2); DK; UK(3)	ICT-2013.5.1	3.842.262	01/01/14	31/12/16	Heart Failure	PCP	Patients; HCP; Admin / 3	Health Services; Monitoring
PERSONA (PERSONA, 2016)	**UK**	FP7-PEOPLE-2012-IOF	294.693	05/05/14	27/06/17	Depression	Sensors; Smartphone; BAN; Affective Computing	Patients / 0	Monitoring; Diagnosis
Health on the Move (Health on the Move, 2017)	**UK**	FP7-PEOPLE-2013-IEF[17]	221.606	08/09/14	07/09/16	mHealth Sociological and Ethical Issues	-		
MONILET (MONILET, 2015)	**IL**	PHC-12-2014-1[18]	71.429	01/11/14	30/04/15	Heart Disease; Pulmonary Disease; Sleep	Wearables; Cloud; Smartphone; App	Patients / 0	Monitoring; Self-Management

continued on following page

Table 1. Continued

Project Name	Participating countries[1,2]	Programme / Topic	Budget (€)	Start date	End date	Condition(s) addressed	Technologies employed	Target groups / Pilots (no. of users)	Project scope
HEARTEN (HEARTEN, 2015)	**FR**(2); IT(4); ES(3); EL(2); DE; PT	PHC-26-2014[19]	4.589.507	01/01/15	31/12/17	Heart Failure	Sensors; Wearables; Smartphone; App; Cloud	Patients; HCP; Carers; Others / 1	Monitoring; Self-Management; Prevention
m-Resist (m-Resist, 2015)	**ES**(5); BE(2); IL; FI; EL(2); HU; IT;	PHC-26-2014	4.034.222	01/01/15	31/12/17	Schizophrenia	Smartphone; App	Patients; HCP / 1	Self-Management; Monitoring
myAirCoach (myAirCoach, 2015)	**EL**(3); UK(3); DE; NL(2); SE(2); BE	PHC-26-2014	4.581.378	01/01/15	31/12/17	Asthma	Sensors; Smartphone; App; BAN; AI; Fi-Ware	Patients; HCP / 3	Self-Management; Monitoring
PD_Manager (PD_Manager, 2015)	**SI**(2); IT(3); EL(2); UK(2); ES; DE	PHC-26-2014	4.345.500	01/01/15	31/12/17	Parkinson	Sensors; Wearables; Smartphone; App; DSS; Data Mining; Games	Patients; HCP; Carers / 1 (230)	Monitoring; Self-Management; Assessment; Drug Adherence
MyCyFAPP (MyCyFAPP, 20115)	**ES**(4); DE(2); IT(2); NO; BE; PT; NL	PHC-26-2014	5.087.508	01/01/15	31/12/18	Cystic Fibrosis	Smartphone; App; DSS	Patients; HCP; Citizens / 1	Monitoring; Self-Management; Prevention
Sound of Vision (Sound of Vision, 2015)	**IS**(2); RO(3); HU; IT; PT(2)	PHC-26-2014	3.960.709	01/01/15	31/12/17	Visually Impaired	Smartphone; App; Serious Game; 3D; Haptic	Patients / 1	Self-Management
Do CHANGE (Do CHANGE, 2015)	**NL**(4); ES(3); UK(2); BE; TW(2)	PHC-26-2014	5.768.500	01/02/15	31/01/18	High Blood Pressure; Ischemic Heart Disease; Heart Failure	Wearables; Sensors; Smartphone; App	Patients; HCP / 3	Self-Management; Monitoring; Diagnosis; Health Promotion
iManageCancer (iManageCancer, 2015)	**DE**(4); EL; NL; UK(4); IT	PHC-26-2014	4.856.174	01/02/15	31/07/18	Cancer	Smartphone; App; Avatar; Serious Games; AI	Patients; HCP / 3	Self-Management; Monitoring; Adherence to Therapy
PATHway (PATHway, 2017)	**IE**; EL; UK(2); NL; DE; IT; BE	PHC-26-2014	4.899.080	01/02/15	30/09/18	CVD	Wearables; Sensors	Patients / 1	Self-Management; Health Promotion
WOMEN-UP (WOMEN-UP, 2015)	**ES**(3); FI(2); CZ; RO; CH; NL	PHC-26-2014	3.470.258	01/02/15	31/07/18	Urinary Incontinence	Smartphone; App; Wearables; Sensors; DSS	Patients / 3	Self-Management; Monitoring; Treatment
PAL (PAL, 2015)	**NL**(6); IT(3); UK; DE	PHC-26-2014	4.515.460	01/03/15	28/02/19	Diabetes	Smartphone; App; DSS; Robot; Avatar; Cloud	Patients; HCP; Carers / 3	Self-Management; Treatment; Monitoring; Health Promotion
NoHoW (NoHoW, 2015)	**DK**(2); UK(7); PT(3); FI(2); IE	PHC-26-2014	4.949.337	01/03/15	29/02/20	Obesity	Sensors; Smartphone; App	Patients / 3	Monitoring; Health Promotion
SMART4MD (SMART4MD, 2015)	**UK**(4); LU; IL; ES(3); CZ; SE; BE;	PHC-20-2014	4.363.280	01/04/15	31/03/19	Dementia	Smartphone; App	Patients; HCP; Carers / 4 (1100)	Monitoring; Treatment Compliance
eKuore (eKuore, 2017)	**ES**	PHC-12-2014-1	71.429	01/05/15	31/10/15	Pulmonary; Cardiac; Heart	Sensors; Smartphone; App	Patients; HCP / 0	Monitoring; Diagnosis

continued on following page

Table 1. Continued

Project Name	Participating countries[1,2]	Programme / Topic	Budget (€)	Start date	End date	Condition(s) addressed	Technologies employed	Target groups / Pilots (no. of users)	Project scope
EmERGE (EmERGE, 2015)	**UK**(7); DE; BE; ES(2); PT; HR	PHC-26-2014	5.457.480	01/05/15	30/04/20	HIV[20]	Smartphone; App	Patients / 5 (3900)	Monitoring
ScoliosisManager (ScoliosisManager, 2016)	**IT**	ICT-37-2015-1	71.429	01/06/15	30/11/15	Scoliosis	Wearable; Sensors; Smartphone; App	Patients; Carers; HCP / 0	Monitoring; Treatment; Self-Management
mHealth4Afrika (mHealth4Africa, 2015)	**IE**; ZA; KE; ET; MW(2); NO; UK	ICT-39-2015	1.999.995	01/11/15	31/10/18	Maternal Care; Newborn Care	Sensors; Smartphone; App	HCP / 4	Monitoring; Diagnosis
CAREGIVERSPRO-MMD (CAREGIVERSPRO-MMD, 2016)	**ES**(3); UK; EL(2); IT; FR	PHC-25-2015	4.087.199	01/01/16	31/12/18	Dementia	Smartphone; App; Gamification	HCP; Patients; Carers / 4 (550 Patients + 550 Carers)	Monitoring; Treatment Compliance
PreventIT (PreventIT, 2016)	**NO**; IT(4); NL(2); DE; UK; CH;	PHC-21-2015	4.607.950	01/01/16	31/12/18	Ageing	Wearables; Sensors; Cloud; Smartphone	Citizens / 1	Health Promotion; Prevention
Nutrigen Service (Nutrigen Service, 2016)	**ES**	SMEInst-06-2016-2017	71.429	01/08/16	31/12/16	Obesity	Smartphone; App; AI	Citizens / 0	Monitoring; Prevention

continued on following page

FUTURE RESEARCH DIRECTIONS AND ISSUES

An unprecedented growth is observed nowadays in the mhealth market. The increasing adoption of smart and wearable healthcare devices is expected to contribute heavily in this direction. Every day, more vendors are considering investing in mHealth apps.

The combination of new diagnostic and monitoring devices along with smart mobile devices has enabled to render seamless healthcare services. This is expected to lead to better lifestyle management, identification of cost and convenience factors, and other initiatives that will alleviate the government's healthcare burden.

According to the latest reports (Grand View Research, 2017), the mhealth applications can be broadly classified into eight major categories:

1. Fitness
2. Nutrition and diet
3. Women's health
4. Healthcare Providers / Payors
5. Lifestyle management
6. Disease management
7. Medication adherence
8. Others

The above classification can be easily mapped to the categories presented in the examined projects (Figure 6). This reveals that the commercial applications and the research activities are in the same direction. However, as expected, the commercial apps were targeting more general population, thus, were related to fitness and wellness. PwC (PriceWaterhouseCoopers, 2014) estimated an increase in

Table 2. Distribution of participants per country

COUNTRIES	CODES	PARTNERS		COORDINATORS	
		COUNT	%	COUNT	%
Belgium	BE	15	3,58%	0	0,00%
Czech Republic	CZ	7	1,67%	0	0,00%
Denmark	DK	9	2,15%	1	2,22%
Germany	DE	35	8,35%	2	4,44%
Ireland	IE	7	1,67%	2	4,44%
Greece	EL	25	5,97%	4	8,89%
Spain	ES	53	12,65%	12	26,67%
France	FR	10	2,39%	1	2,22%
Croatia	HR	1	0,24%	0	0,00%
Italy	IT	61	14,56%	8	17,78%
Cyprus	CY	2	0,48%	0	0,00%
Luxembourg	LU	2	0,48%	0	0,00%
Hungary	HU	4	0,95%	0	0,00%
Malta	MT	1	0,24%	0	0,00%
Netherlands	NL	30	7,16%	3	6,67%
Austria	AT	9	2,15%	1	2,22%
Portugal	PT	17	4,06%	0	0,00%
Romania	RO	6	1,43%	0	0,00%
Slovenia	SI	3	0,72%	1	2,22%
Slovakia	SK	1	0,24%	0	0,00%
Finland	FI	12	2,86%	0	0,00%
Sweden	SE	10	2,39%	0	0,00%
United Kingdom	UK	60	14,32%	6	13,33%
Iceland	IS	1	0,24%	1	2,22%
Norway	NO	3	0,72%	1	2,22%
Switzerland	CH	16	3,82%	0	0,00%
Turkey	TR	2	0,48%	0	0,00%
Israel	IL	5	1,19%	2	4,44%
China (except Hong Kong)	CN_X_HK	1	0,24%	0	0,00%
South Africa	ZA	1	0,24%	0	0,00%
Taiwan	TW	3	0,72%	0	0,00%
United States	US	1	0,24%	0	0,00%
Malawi	MW	4	0,95%	0	0,00%
Kenya	KE	1	0,24%	0	0,00%
Ethiopia	ET	1	0,24%	0	0,00%
TOTAL:		**419**	*100,00%*	**45**	*100,00%*

Figure 1. Type of partner

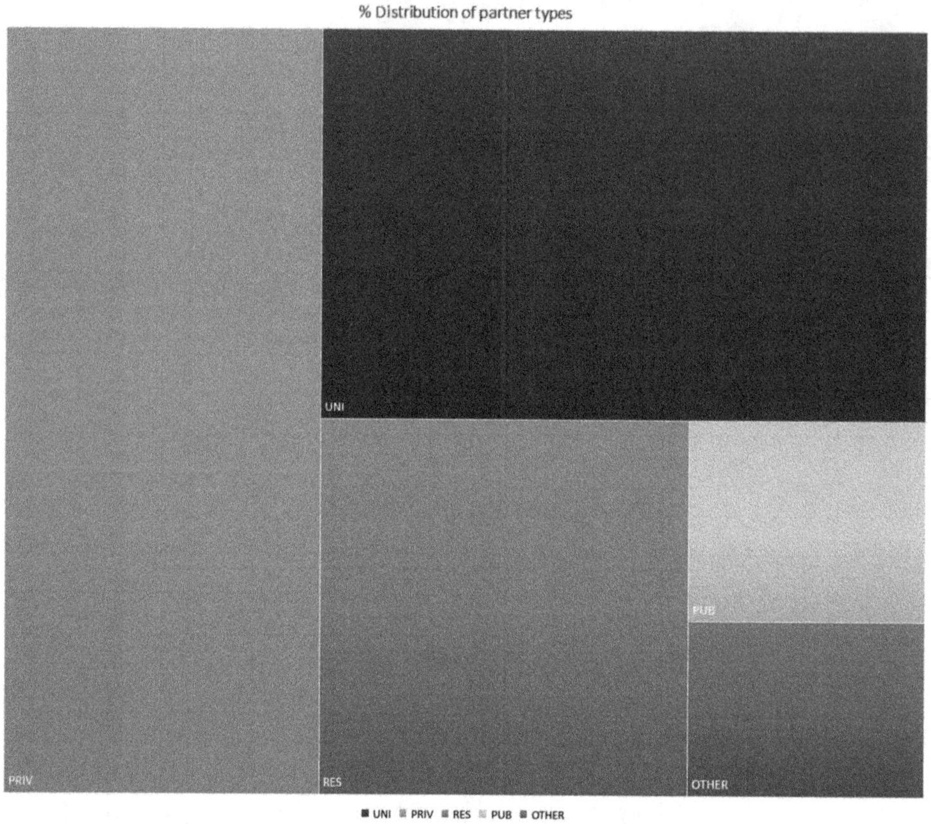

Figure 2. Budget distribution

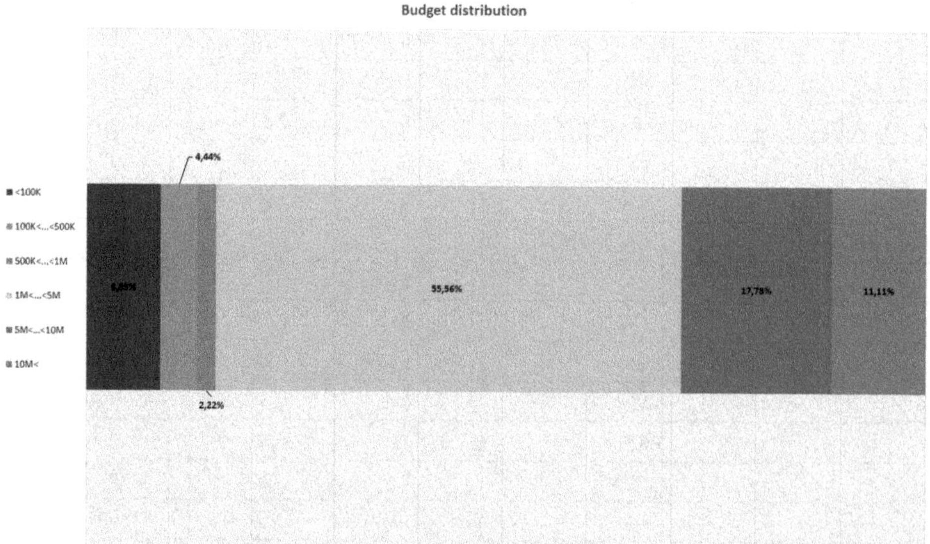

Table 3. Health issues addressed

HEATH ISSUE	# of projects	%
WEIGHT MANAGEMENT & HEALTHY DIET	**6**	**13,33%**
Diabetes	5	11,11%
Eating disorder	1	2,22%
Food awareness	1	2,22%
Obesity	4	8,89%
MENTAL DISORDERS	**8**	**17,78%**
Schizofrenia	1	2,22%
Psychological stress	1	2,22%
Depression	3	6,67%
Bipolar disorder	3	6,67%
NEUROLOGICAL DISEASES	**4**	**8,89%**
Dementia	2	4,44%
Parkinson	2	4,44%
MONITORING OF HEART AND CVD RELATED CONDITIONS	**11**	**24,45%**
Heart disease	3	6,67%
Heart failure	3	6,67%
CVD	2	4,44%
Chronic diseases (atrial fibrillation, gestational diabetes, gestational hypertension)	1	2,22%
CHRONIC DISEASES (COPD, CKD, RENAL INSUFFICIENCY)	1	2,22%
COPD (with comorbidities Chronic Heart Failure, Diabetes, Anxiety and Depression)	1	2,22%
OTHER	**14**	**31,11%**
Asthma	1	2,22%
Cancer	1	2,22%
Cystic fibrosis	1	2,22%
HIV	1	2,22%
Infantile diarrhoea	1	2,22%
Malaria	1	2,22%
Maternal care	1	2,22%
Scoliosis	1	2,22%
Urinary incontinence	1	2,22%
Visually impaired	1	2,22%
Renal insufficiency	2	4,44%
Pulmonary	2	4,44%

downloads of fitness and wellness apps from 40 million (2012) to 250 million (2016). Nowadays, the number of mHealth apps available in the market was doubled, in comparison to 2015, reaching almost 318,000 worldwide. More than 200 apps are being added every day (IQVIA Institute for Human and Data Science, 2017). According to recent studies (KSI - Knowledge Sourcing Intelligence LLP, 2017)

Figure 3. Conditions addressed

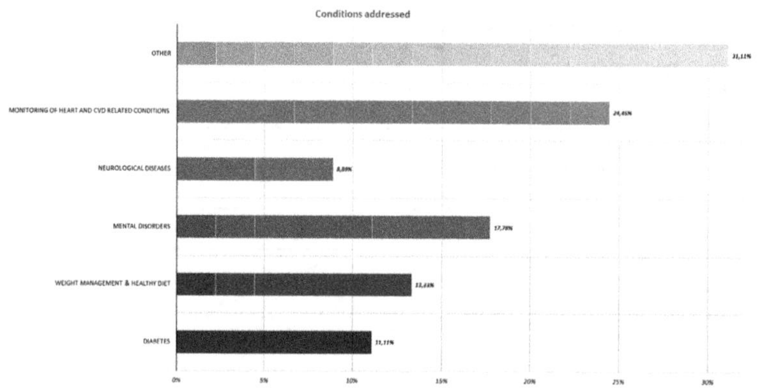

Figure 4. Number of pilots per project

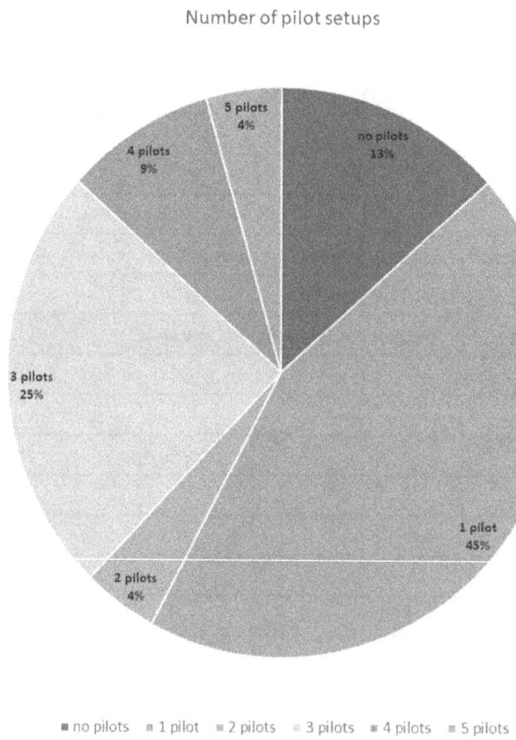

the global mHealth app market is projected to be valued at US$28.320 billion in 2018 and is expected to reach up to US$102.35 billion by 2023.

On the contrary, since the action lines of eligible research activities are given by the European Commission, the research efforts are focused on major diseases and health concerns with significant societal and economic impact. As seen in Table 3, the majority of the projects targeted the heart and CVD related conditions (24.45%), followed by with mental disorders (17.78%), weight management and healthy diet (13.33%), diabetes (11.11%) and neurological diseases (8.89%). Other conditions, including for example

Figure 5. Targeted end users

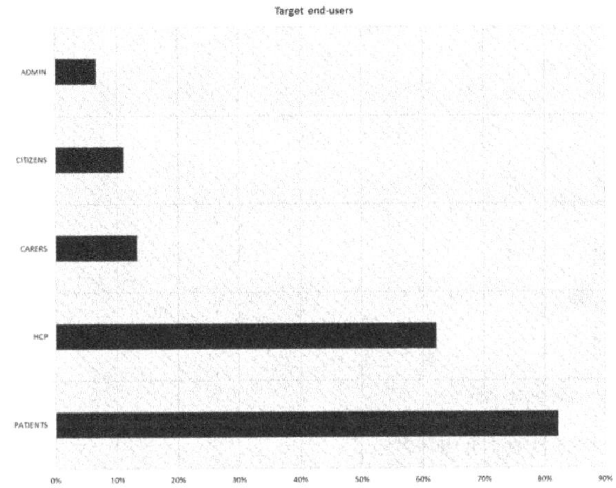

Figure 6. Categories addressed by the projects

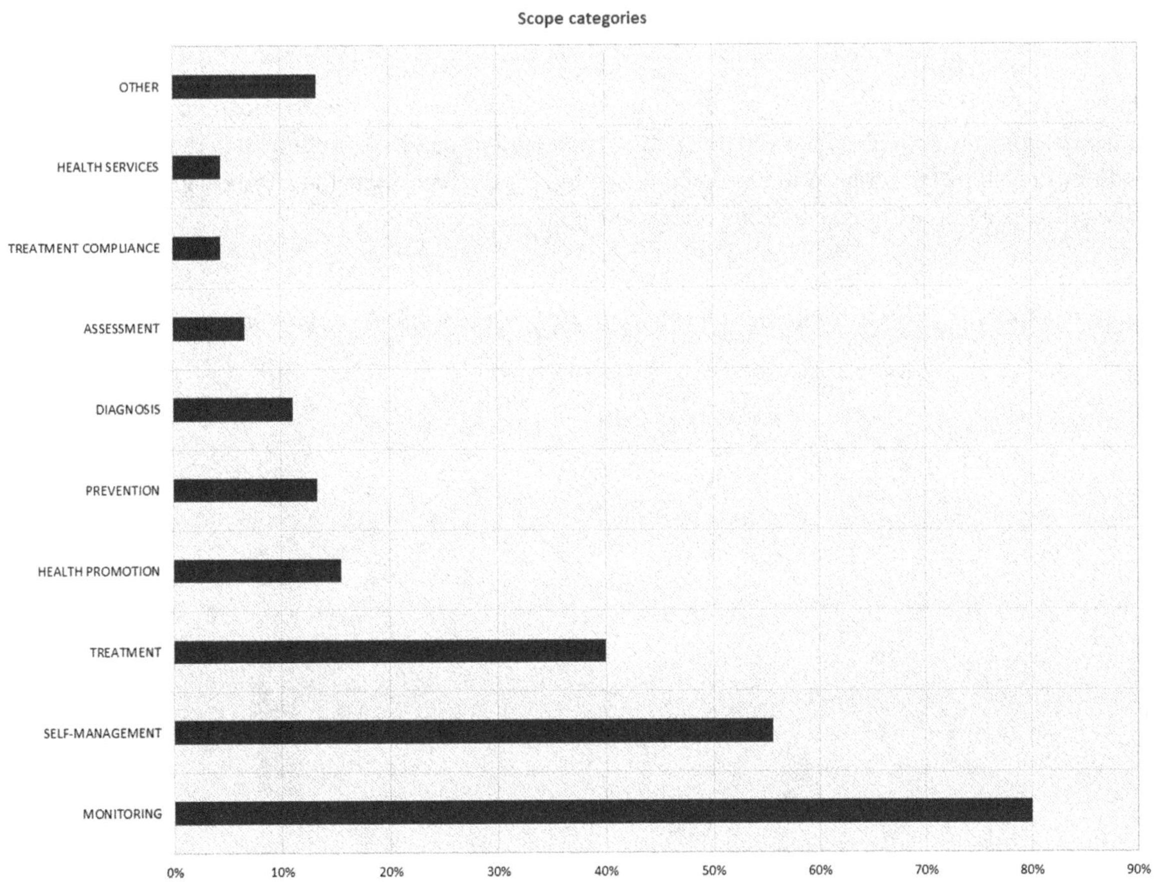

Figure 7. Technologies applied

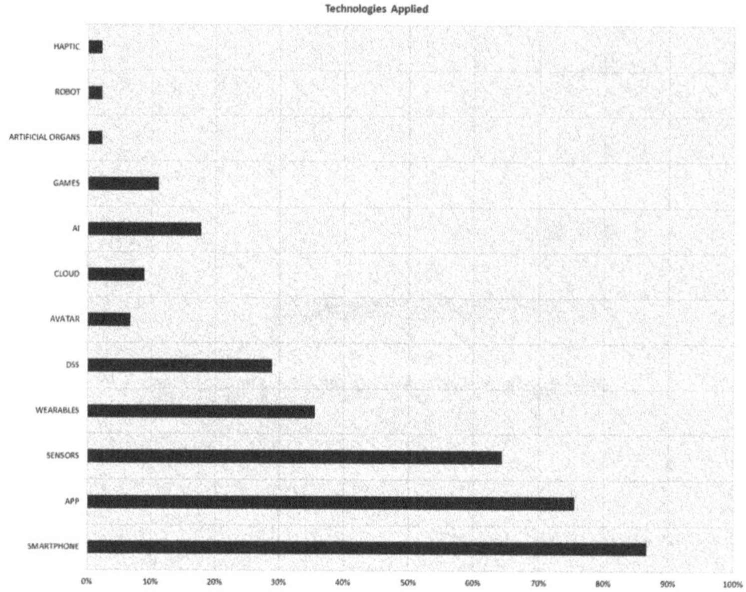

asthma, cancer, HIV, malaria, scoliosis, have limited representation, covering in total the 31,11%. Chronic medical conditions have also received the focus of mHealth research. As anticipated, most of the health conditions faced by the projects were related to ageing. Figure 8 presents the chronological distribution of the projects along with the condition addressed.

Figure 8. Chronological distribution of mHealth projects vs conditions addressed

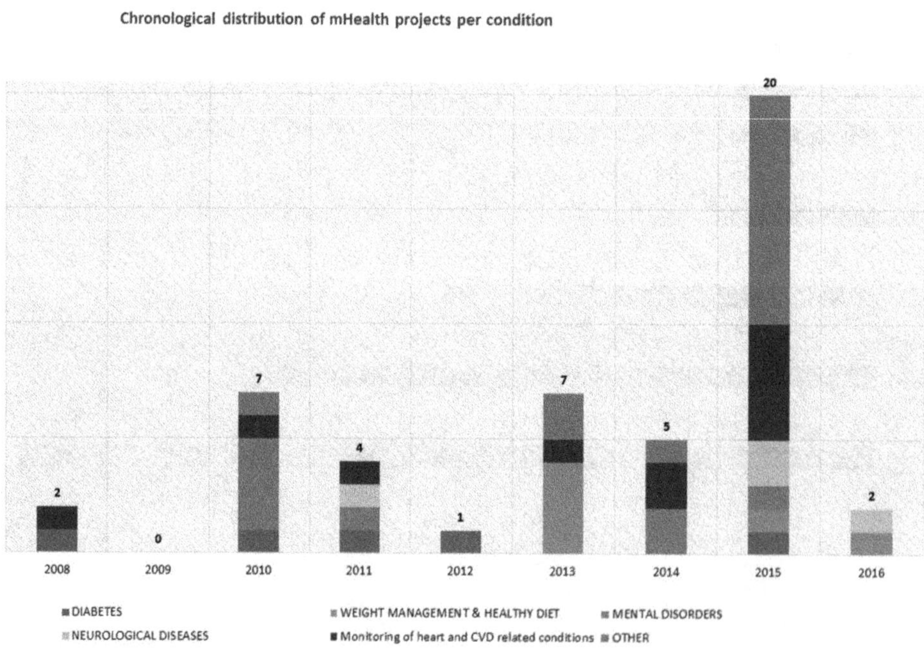

A significant stepping-stone towards more innovations always remains the available funding. In the case of the European Union, obtaining funding for research has always been a very challenging and extremely competitive task. Nowadays, Horizon 2020 is the main component of research funding on a European scale. All proposals are evaluated on the basis of three criteria (EC Horizon 2020):

- **Excellence**

Excellence refers to the quality of the project (soundness of the concept), the people and the partner organisations (including trans-disciplinary considerations) and to the extent that the proposed work is ambitious, has innovation potential, and is beyond state of the art (e.g. groundbreaking objectives, novel concepts and approaches).

- **Impact**

The impact depends on the type of proposal being funded. For example, in the case of Research and Innovation actions, impact is measured in relation to how the outputs of the project contribute towards four main axes: enhancing innovation capacity and integration of new knowledge; strengthening the competitiveness and growth of companies by developing innovations meeting the needs of European and global markets; other environmental and socially important impacts; exploitation of the project results.

- **Quality and Efficiency of the Implementation**

The quality and efficiency of the implementation are evaluated on the basis of the coherence and effectiveness of the work plan, the complementarity of the participants within the consortium, and the appropriateness of the management structures and procedures, including risk and innovation management.

Apart from the growth presented in the market, several issues still delay the adoption of mhealth applications in real life situations. For example, the weak reimbursement policies, the lack of accuracy, the uncertainty in government regulations, the lack of insurance coverage, are some of the barriers expected to hinder the growth rate. A critical issue related to the funded research activities is the fact that their sustainability is not guaranteed most of the times beyond the end of the project lifecycle. Thus, the expected societal and economic impact that drives EU related initiatives has still not been achieved.

The insights from the collected data (Table 2) reveal that the three countries dominate the mhealth research domain in EU (Italy, UK and Spain), with Spain keeping the reins of the project coordinator. It is really interesting that the public sector contributes the only to 6.68% of the examined consortia, whereas the private one dominates the research arena (34.48%). This contradicts the fact that the majority of the health care sector is public and may be the reason why there is no further adoption of the outcomes of the projects in the long run.

Even though there is no standard, it seems that the limited number of pilots and subjects participating in the study may have a negative impact on the project's sustainability and further success. Most of the projects have only one pilot site, which does not guarantee the required multicultural and multilingual dimension of the results (see Table 1). According to the available data, only seven projects employed a significant number of end users (more than 60). Any research activity should employee a statistically significant number of subjects in order to conclude in satisfactory results regarding usage, user subjective and objective satisfaction, using already existed valid and reliable instruments able to capture the users' satisfaction in an early research stage (Koumpouros Y., 2016). Moreover, an advanced Technology Readiness Level (TRL) would drive to a close to market product/service.

Even though an interdisciplinary approach seems to be mandatory for any research effort nowadays, only 15.56% of the projects followed it. However, this could lead to better adoption rates of the final solutions by the end users. Behavioral intervention technologies (BITs) is also another area of application of mHealth solutions exploiting interdisciplinary teams. Self-assessment, self-monitoring, psychoeducation, goal setting, and feedback are some of the interventions addressed by BITs (Mohr, Burns, Schueller, Clarke, & Klinkman, 2013).

The successful commercialization of the developed solutions is still an issue for EU. According to the study, an extremely limited number of products has the potential to be further commercialized. This is the case where a private organization is a partner in the consortium, and the final solution was based on further enhancement of one of the existing product of this SME. However, even in cases were several SMEs participate in the research project, there is still no guarantee for a marketable result. Maybe a large-scale implementation of the proposed intervention could facilitate the marketability of the projects' outcomes.

As far as the technological approach is concerned, most of the projects employed a smartphone using ZigBee, Bluetooth and other wireless protocols. Algorithms and Decision Support Systems are also utilized to help the different target groups. Availability of sensors is also driving the mHealth research activities. Wearables, mobile sensors, body weight scales, food weight scales and chewing sensors were used in most of the cases to monitor patients' biosignals and physical activity. Only a limited number of systems employed artificial organs (i.e. kidney). The low reliability of the collected data due to sensors' low accuracy is considered critical for future research activities. The last Horizon 2020 call encourages projects to exploit open source frameworks and platforms, such as FiWare and UniversAAL. However, this was not the case in the studied projects.

Big data and cloud computing have become state-of-the-art technologies nowadays. Valuable insights can be gained exploiting such technologies (Koumpouros Y., 2014). The "Health, Demographic Change and Well-being" (European Commission, 2016) and "Information and Communication Technologies" (European Commission, 2016) work programmes have recognized the value of these technologies and launched related calls. However, none of the reviewed research projects utilized big data, while only four of them exploited cloud computing technologies and services. Future projects should, therefore, exploit the possibilities of these technologies. It is also impressive that affective computing was mentioned in only one project related to depression.

Finally, ethical and legal challenges are main concerns in mHealth projects. These are related to (i) privacy protection and confidentiality, (ii) ethics approval and informed consent, (iii) transparency of the collected data management by the final system and during pilots and validation studies, (iv) IT-security and identity management. Data security and privacy are areas that require legal and policy attention to ensure that mHealth users' data are properly protected. Even though privacy and security issues were a concern in the studied projects, the advance of both the technology and the regulations require more efforts. Protection of data, unwanted sharing of sensitive information with third parties (Bielecki, 2012), accidental exposure or leaking of health data are some of the critical security issues arising in any project. The European dimension of the research consortia obliges to careful considerations regarding data sharing that should comply with the relevant EU laws and Directives, i.e. General Data Protection Regulation (European Commission, 2012), Directive 95/46/EC (European Parliament and the Council of 24 October 1995, 1995), Directive 2002/58/EC (European Parliament and the Council of 12 July 2002, 2002) and Charter of Fundamental Rights (European Parliament, 2000).

CONCLUSION

With the replacement of traditional healthcare delivery models by patient-centric care model, growth in adoption of mHealth solutions is expected. In addition, the growing penetration of smartphones is supporting this growth. By 2020, smartphone subscriptions would have exceeded the global population. This growth is mainly expected from less mature markets such as India, Egypt, Turkey, and the UAE. Untapped markets in developing economies provide a lot of growth opportunities for the mhealth due to increase adoption of related services to control the spread of communicable as well as non-communicable diseases.

The Communication on Digital Transformation of Health and Care in the Digital Single Market (European Commision, 2018) identifies three main pillars:

1. **Pillar 1: Secure Data Access and Sharing**

To facilitate greater cross-border healthcare access, the EC is building eHealth Digital Service Infrastructure which will allow e-prescriptions and patient summaries to be exchanged between healthcare providers. The first cross-border exchanges are due to take place during 2018, with the aim to have all other EU countries on board by 2020. In the longer term, the Commission is working towards a European electronic health record exchange format accessible to all EU citizens.

2. **Pillar 2: Connecting and Sharing Health Data for Research, Faster Diagnosis and Improved Health**

The decentralised European digital health infrastructure will facilitate tailored diagnosis and treatment, help health services to be better prepared to respond to cross-border health threats, and improve the development and surveillance of medical products. This will provide personalised medicine through a shared European data infrastructure, allowing researchers and other professionals to pool resources (data, expertise, computing processing and storage capacities) across the EU.

3. **Pillar 3: Strengthening citizen empowerment and individual care through digital services**

Digital services can improve the prevention and management of chronic conditions and allow patients to provide feedback to healthcare providers. Health systems will also benefit from innovative care models that use telehealth and mHealth to address the rising demand for healthcare. Digital tools will empower people to look after their health, stimulate prevention and enable feedback and interaction between users and healthcare providers.

The chapter reviewed the European funded projects in the mHealth domain in order to reveal the valuable benefits that derive from the capitalization of the mobile technologies; the challenges faced and opportunities given by mHealth, and the potential of the specific market. Several issues seem to delay the wider adoption of mhealth solutions (security, privacy, interoperability concerns, etc.). Additionally, many innovations have not achieved their initial targets.

By using the powerful analytics, healthcare apps can provide patients with digitally enabled care. The tech-savvy population supports such transformation. Mhealth solutions present unique opportunities with the ability to log information related to personal health at the touch of a screen. Initially, the mhealth industry was dominated by health and fitness apps, while the growth now is in remote consultation and monitoring. Asthma, cancer and diabetes management are only some of the numerous applications addressed by the mhealth platforms. Europe is expected to be the largest mobile health market in the world.

The total valuation of the wearable device and mhealth markets is expected to grow due to accelerated adoption of these tools by providers, hospitals, and patients, according to several market reports. mhealth solutions that improve the delivery care also help with the associated costs of healthcare by saving millions of euros for healthcare organizations. Software and data applications will be the largest drivers of market growth compared to hardware that hosts mhealth-related technology. Major drivers for the wearable device market growth are based on the fact that these devices are non-invasive for consumers, and are highly intuitive, and that healthcare consumers are starting to become more conscious of their fitness and health-related lifestyles. These devices can also deliver patient-generated data that can inform healthcare decision making and allow providers to implement them into healthcare tactics that enhance communication with patients from remote locations.

The growth of the mhealth solutions market can be attributed to the penetration of smart gadgets, increasing utilization of connected medical devices for remote monitoring and mhealth apps in the management of chronic diseases. Also, factors such as the advent of advanced connectivity and network technologies, robust penetration of 3G, 4G and 5G networks to provide uninterrupted healthcare services, and rising focus on patient-centric healthcare are expected to drive the growth of the mhealth platforms.

Based on product and service, the connected medical device segment dominated the mhealth product and service market in 2016. The mhealth solutions market growth can be attributed to the shifting consumer preferences towards a healthier lifestyle, need for continuous monitoring of various chronic health conditions of patients, and the need to overcome the financial burden on the caregivers.

The mhealth industry is expected to dominate the healthcare arena in the near future providing valuable support to patients, healthcare professionals and healthcare systems. However, several issues still need to be addressed more carefully in order to penetrate the market in even higher growth. Nowadays, the population is ready for such innovations. Interdisciplinary design and solutions that take into account the real-life behaviors of each participant are critical to achieve the objective.

ACKNOWLEDGMENT

This research received no specific grant from any funding agency in the public, commercial, or not-for-profit sectors.

REFERENCES

Bayne, S., & Ross, J. (2007). The ‘digital native’ and ‘digital immigrant’: a dangerous opposition. *Annual Conference of the Society for Research into Higher Education.*

Bhargave, R., & Johnmar, F. (n.d.). *ePatient 2015. 15 Surprising Trends Changing Health Care.* Retrieved 5 10, 2015, from epatient2015: www.epatient2015.com

Bielecki, M. (2012). *Leveraging Mobile Health Technology for Patient Recruitment: An Emerging Opportunity.* Northbrook, IL: Blue Chip Patient Recruitment.

BRAVEHEALTH. (2016). *Patient Centric Approach for an Integrated, Adaptive, Context Aware Remote Diagnosis and Management of Cardiovascular Diseases* (European Commission, CORDIS, Projects & Results Service). Retrieved Dec 2, 2016, from http://cordis.europa.eu/project/rcn/102204_en.html

Burns, M., Begale, M., Duffecy, J., Gergle, D., Karr, C., Giangrande, E., & DC., M. (2011). Harnessing context sensing to develop a mobile intervention for depression. *J Med Internet Res, 13*(3).

Burns, M., & Mohr, D. (in press). eHealth, telehealth, and Telemedicine. In Encyclopedia of Behavioral Medicine. Springer.

Canale, S. (2013). *The Bravehealth Software Architecture for the Monitoring of Patients Affected by CVD.* Fifth International Conference on eHealth, Telemedicine, and Social Medicine (eTELEMED 2013).

CAREGIVERSPRO-MMD. (2016). *Self-management interventions and mutual assistance community services, helping patients with dementia and caregivers connect with others for evaluation, support and inspiration to improve the care experience* (EU Project Official web site). Retrieved Jan 18, 2017, from caregiversprommd-project.eu/

CDC. (2009). *The power of prevention: Chronic disease...the public health challenge of the 21st century.* National Center for Chronic Disease Prevention and Health Promotion. National Center for Chronic Disease Prevention and Health Promotion.

CHRONIOUS. (2008). *An Open, Ubiquitous and Adaptive Chronic Disease Management Platform for COPD and Renal Insufficiency.* Retrieved from www.chronious.eu

Commodity12. (2011). *Continuous multi-parametric and multi-layered analysis of diabetes type 1 & 2.* Retrieved from www.commodity12.eu

CORDIS, European Community - Community Research and Development Information. (n.d.). *EC CORDIS Projects & Results Service.* Retrieved December 3, 2016, from http://data.europa.eu/euodp/en/data

Decipher, P. C. P. (2013). *Mobile health for European citizens.* Retrieved from www.decipherpcp.eu

Deloitte. (2014a). *Healthcare and Life Sciences Predictions 2020: A bold future?* Deloitte Centre for Health Solutions.

Deloitte. (2014b). *The four dimensions of effective health: People, places, payment, purpose.* Deloitte.

Deloitte Consulting. (2013). *European Interoperability Framework for eHealth.* ISA. doi:10.2759/14325

Department of Economic and Social Affairs, Population Division. (2001). World Population Ageing: 1950-2050. New York: United Nations.

Department of Economic and Social Affairs, Population Division. (2007). World Population Ageing 2007. New York: United Nations.

Dhukaram A. V. (2011). *End-User Perception Towards Pervasive Cardiac Healthcare Services: Benefits, Acceptance, Adoption, Risks, Security, Privacy and Trust.* Dublin, Ireland: PervasiveHealth.

Do C. H. A. N. G. E. (2015). *Do CHANGE: Do Cardiac Health Advanced New Generation Ecosystem.* Retrieved Jan 11, 2017, from www.do-change.eu

EC. (2014). *Green Paper on mobile Health.* Brussels: European Commission.

EC. (2015). *European Commission, Digital Agenda for Europe. A Europe 2020 Initiative.* Retrieved 5 15, 2015, from European Commission: http://ec.europa.eu/digital-agenda/en/connected-continent-legislative-package

EC. (2015). *Horizon 2020. The EU Framework Programme for Research and Innovation.* Retrieved 5 15, 2015, from European Commission: https://ec.europa.eu/programmes/horizon2020/

EC Horizon 2020. (n.d.). *Workprogramme 2018-2020 Evaluation Rules.* Retrieved from Research & Innovation Participant Portal: http://ec.europa.eu/research/participants/data/ref/h2020/other/wp/2018-2020/annexes/h2020-wp1820-annex-h-esacrit_en.pdf

eHGI. (2012). *Discussion Paper on Semantic and Technical Interoperability.* eHealth Governance Initiative (eHGI).

eKuore. (2017). *eKuore Pro: electronic stethoscope for health professionals.* Retrieved Feb 4, 2017, from www.ekuore.com/en/

EmERGE. (2015). *Creating mHealth solutions to facilitate remote access to health care providers and increase adherence for People Living with HIV (PLHIV).* Retrieved Jan 14, 2017, from www.emerge-project.eu

Empower. (2011). *Support of Patient Empowerment by an intelligent self-management pathway for patients.* Retrieved from www.empower-fp7.eu

EU FP7-ICT. (2014). *EU FP7-ICT (Information and Communication Technologies) Workprogramme.* Retrieved April 7, 2015, from http://cordis.europa.eu/fp7/ict/home_en.html

European Commision. (2018, April 25). *EC - Digital Single Market.* Retrieved from Communication on enabling the digital transformation of health and care in the Digital Single Market; empowering citizens and building a healthier society: https://ec.europa.eu/digital-single-market/en/news/communication-enabling-digital-transformation-health-and-care-digital-single-market-empowering

European Commission. (2012). *General Data Protection Regulation: Proposal for a Regulation of the European Parliament and of the Council.* Retrieved Dec 9, 2016, from EC Justice, Data protection: ec.europa.eu/justice/data-protection/document/review2012/com_2012_11_en.pdf

European Commission. (2016). *Horizon 2020, Work Programme 2016 - 2017, 5.i. Information and Communication Technologies.* Retrieved Jan 8, 2017, from ec.europa.eu/research/participants/data/ref/h2020/wp/2016_2017/main/h2020-wp1617-leit-ict_en.pdf

European Commission. (2016). *Horizon 2020, Work Programme 2016 - 2017, 8. Health, demographic change and well-being.* Retrieved Jan 6, 2017, from ec.europa.eu/research/participants/data/ref/h2020/wp/2016_2017/main/h2020-wp1617-health_en.pdf

European Parliament. (2000). *Charter of Fundamental Rights Of The European Union (2000/C 364/01).* Retrieved Jan 8, 2017, from Official Journal of the European Communities: www.europarl.europa.eu/charter/pdf/text_en.pdf

European Parliament and the Council of 12 July 2002. (2002). *Directive 2002/58/EC: Processing of personal data and the protection of privacy in the electronic communications sector.* Retrieved Jan 12, 2017, from eur-lex.europa.eu/eli/dir/2002/58/oj

European Parliament and the Council of 24 October 1995. (1995). *Directive 95/46/EC: Protection of individuals with regard to the processing of personal data and the free movement of such data.* Retrieved Jan 8, 2017, from data.europa.eu/eli/dir/1995/46/oj

Fagerberg, J., & Kurkinen, L. (n.d.). *mHealth and Home Monitoring.* Berg Insight. Gothenburg: M2M Research Series. *Berg Insight AB.*

Fiordelli, M., Diviani, N., & Schulz, P. J. (2013). Mapping mHealth research: a decade of evolution. *J Med Internet Res, 15*(5). doi:10.2196/jmir.2430

Fraser, H., Bailey, C., Sinha, C., Mehl, G., & Labrique, A. (2011). *Call to action on global eHealth evaluation: consensus statement of the WHO Global eHealth Evaluation Meeting, Bellagio, September 2011.* The Bellagio eHealth Evaluation Group.

Frost & Sullivan. (2012). *U.S. Hospital Health Data Analytics Market: Growing EHR Adoption Fuels A New Era in Analytics.* Retrieved 11 18, 2013, from Frost & Sullivan: http://www.frost.com/c/10046/sublib/display-report.do?id=NA03-01-00-00-00

FTC. (2013). *Mobile Privacy Disclosures. Building Trust Through Transparency.* Federal Trade Commission.

FTC. (2015). *Privacy and Security.* Retrieved 5 15, 2015, from Federal trade Commission. Protecting America's Consumers: http://business.ftc.gov/privacy-and-security

Gens, F. (2011). *Top 10 Predictions. IDC Predictions 2012: Competing for 2020.* IDC. Retrieved December 5, 2013, from IDC: http://cdn.idc.com/research/Predictions12/Main/downloads/IDCTOP10Predictions2012.pdf

Grand View Research. (2017). *mHealth App Market By Type (Fitness, Lifestyle Management, Nutrition & Diet, Women's Health, Healthcare Providers, Disease Management) And Segment Forecasts, 2018 - 2025.* Grand View Research.

Grunerbl A. (2014). Smartphone Based Recognition of States and State Changes in Bipolar Disorder Patients. *IEEE Journal of Biomedical and Health Informatics, 19*(1), 140-148.

GSMA & PwC. (2012). *Touching lives through mobile health - Assessment of the global market opportunity.* PriceWaterhouseCoopers.

Health on the Move. (2017). *Health on the move: Exploring the ethical, social, and political underpinnings of portable devices for healthcare and lifestyle.* Retrieved Feb 3, 2017, from http://cordis.europa.eu/project/rcn/187888_en.html

HEARTEN. (2015). *A co-operative mHEALTH environment targeting adherence and management of patients suffering from Heart Failure Table of Content.* Retrieved from www.hearten.eu

Help4Mood. (2011). *A Computational Distributed System to Support the Treatment of Patients with Major Depression*. Retrieved from help4mood.info

Higgins, J. P., & Green, S. (2006). Cohrane handbook for systematic reviews of interventions 4.2.6. In *The Cochrane Library, Issue 4*. Chichester, UK: JohnWiley & Sons, Ltd.

HIMSS. (2014). *3rd Annual HIMSS Analytics Mobile Survey*. HIMSS Analytics.

HIMSS. (2015). *Healtcare Information and Management Systems Society*. Retrieved 5 13, 2015, from HIMSS transforming health through IT: http://www.himss.org/

ICT4Depression. (2015). *User-friendly ICT Tools to Enhance Self-Management and Effective*. Retrieved from www.ICT4DEPRESSION.eu

iManageCancer. (2015). *Empowering patients and strengthening self-management in cancer diseases*. Retrieved Jan 10, 2017, from imanagecancer.eu

IMS. (2013). *Patient Apps for Improved Healthcare: From Novelty to Mainstream*. IMS Institute for Healthcare Informatics.

International Telecommunication Union (ITU). (2014). *The World in 2014. ICT facts and Figures*. Geneva: International Telecommunication Union.

INTERSTRESS. (2010). *Interreality in the Management and Treatment of Stress-Related Disorders*. Retrieved from www.interstress.eu

IQVIA Institute for Human and Data Science. (2017). *The Growing Value of Digital Health: Evidence and Impact on Human Health and the Healthcare System*. Institute Report.

ISA. (n.d.). *eHealth European Interoperability Framework*. Interoperability Solutions for European Pyblic Administration.

ITU Statistics. (2018). Retrieved from Global and regional ICT data (2005-2017): www.itu.int/en/ITU-D/Statistics/Pages/stat/default.aspx

Jones, C., & Shao, B. (2011). *The Net Generation and Digital Natives. Implications for Higher Education*. The Open University.

Kafalı, Ö. (2013). COMMODITY12: A smart e-health environment for diabetes management. *Journal of Ambient Intelligence and Smart Environments*, *5*, 479–502.

Koumpouros, I. (2012). Information and Communication Technologies & Society. Athens: New Technologies Publications.

Koumpouros, Y. (2014). Big Data in Healthcare. In A. Moumtzoglou & A. Kastania (Eds.), *Cloud Computing Applications for Quality Health care Delivery. A volume in the Advances in Healthcare Information Systems and Administration Book Series* (pp. 35–59). IGI Global.

Koumpouros, Y. (2016). A Systematic Review on Existing Measures for the Subjective Assessment of Rehabilitation and Assistive Robot Devices. *Journal of Healthcare Engineering*, 10. doi:10.1155/2016/1048964

Koumpouros, Y., & Georgoulas, A. (2016). mHealth R&D activities in Europe. In E. A. Moumtzoglou (Ed.), M-Health Innovations for Patient-Centered Care (pp. 22-27). IGI Global.

Krohn, R., & Metcalf, D. (2012). *mHealth: From Smartphones to Smart Systems.* HIMSS.

KSI - Knowledge Sourcing Intelligence LLP. (2017). *Mobile Health (mHealth) App Market - Industry Trends, Opportunities and Forecasts to 2023.* Author.

Labrique, A., Vasudevan, L., Kochi, E., & Mehl, G. (2013). mHealth innovations as health system strengthening tools: 12 common applications and visual framework. *Global Health, Science and Practice, 1*(2), 160–171. doi:10.9745/GHSP-D-13-00031 PMID:25276529

m-Resist. (2015). *Mobile Therapeutic Attention for Patients with Treatment Resistant Schizophrenia.* Retrieved from www.mresist.eu

Marcos, C. (2015, Apr 15). Solving the interoperability challenge of a distributed complex patient guidance system: A data integrator based on HL7's Virtual Medical Record standard. *J Am Med Inform Assoc.*

McKinsey & GSMA. (2010). *mHealth: A new vision for healthcare.* McKinsey & Company, Inc. and GSMA.

McKnight, J., Babineau, B., & Gahm, J. (2011). *North American Health Care Provider Information Market Size & Forecast.* ESG-Enterprise Strategy Group.

METABO. (2008). *Controlling Chronic Diseases related to Metabolic Disorders.* Retrieved from www.metabo-eu.org

mHealth4Africa. (2015). *Community-based ICT for Maternal Healthcare in Africa.* Retrieved Jan 21, 2017, from www.mhealth4afrika.eu

mHealthAlliance & VitalWaveConsulting. (2013). *Sustainable Financing for Mobile Health (mHealth): Options and opportunities for mHealth financial models in low and middle-income countries.* mHealth Alliance.

mHealthAlliance. (2012). *Baseline Evaluation of the mHealth Ecosystem and the Performance of the mHealth Alliance.* mHealth Alliance.

mHealthCompetenceCentre. (2014). *News.* Retrieved 5 10, 2015, from mHealth Competence Centre: http://www.mobilehealthglobal.com/in-the-news/news/41/the-mhealth-app-market-will-reach-26-bilion-usd-revenue-by-2017-says-himss-europe-report

Miluzzo, E., Lane, N., Fodor, K., Peterson, R., Lu, H., Musolesi, M., . . . Campbell, A. (2008). Sensing meets mobile social networks: The design, implementation and evaluation of the CenceMe application. In *SenSys '08 Proceedings of the 6th ACM conference on Embedded network sensor systems* (pp. 337-350). ACM.

MobiGuide. (2011). *Guiding Patients Anytime, Everywhere.* Retrieved from www.mobiguide-project.eu

Mohr, D., Burns, M., Schueller, S., Clarke, G., & Klinkman, M. (2013). Behavioral Intervention Technologies: Evidence review and recommendations for future research in mental health. *General Hospital Psychiatry, Special Section: Health Information Technology and Mental Health Services Research: A Path Forward, 35*, 332-338.

MONARCA. (2010). *MONitoring, treAtment and pRediCtion of bipolAr Disorder Episodes*. Retrieved from www.monarca-project.eu

MONILET. (2015). *Monitoring Bracelet for Health Use*. Retrieved Jan 12, 2017, from http://cordis.europa.eu/project/rcn/194665_en.html

Moore, G. E. (1965). Cramming more components onto integrated circuits. *Electronics Magazine*, 4.

Morris, M., & Guilak, F. (2009). Mobile heart health: Project highlight. *IEEE Pervasive Computing, 8*(2), 57–61. doi:10.1109/MPRV.2009.31

Moving Life. (2011). *MObile eHealth for the VINdication of Global LIFEstyle change and disease management solutions*. Retrieved from www.moving-life.eu

myAirCoach. (2015). *Analysis, modelling and sensing of both physiological and environmental factors for the customized and predictive self-management of Asthma*. Retrieved Jan 14, 2017, from http://www.myaircoach.eu

MyCyFAPP. (2015). *My App for Cystic Fibrosis*. Retrieved Jan 14, 2017, from http://www.mycyfapp.eu

Nephron+. (2010). *ICT enabled Wearable Artificial Kidney and Personal Renal Care System*. Retrieved from www.nephronplus.eu

NIH. (n.d.). *National Institutes of Health. Office of Behavioral and Social Sciences Research*. Retrieved 5 14, 2015, from NIH. Office of Behavioral and Social Sciences Research: http://obssr.od.nih.gov/scientific_areas/methodology/mhealth/

NoHoW. (2015). *Evidence-based tools for weight loss maintenance*. Retrieved Jan 8, 2017, from nohow.eu/

Nutrigen Service. (2016). *Nutrigen service: Managing health through dietary needs, virtual consultations, and genetics*. Retrieved Jan 16, 2017, from cordis.europa.eu/project/rcn/205147_en.html

NYMPHA-MD. (2014). *Next Generation Mobile Platforms for HeAlth, in Mental Disorders*. Retrieved from www.nympha-md-project.eu

OECD. (2018). *Elderly population (indicator)*. OECD. doi:10.1787/8d805ea1-en

PAL. (2015). *Personal Assistant for a healthy Lifestyle*. Retrieved from www.pal4u.eu

PATHway. (2017). *Technology-enabled behavioural change as a pathway towards better self-management of CVD*. Retrieved Feb 1, 2017, from www.pathway2health.eu/

PD_Manager. (2015). *mHealth platform for Parkinson's Disease management*. Retrieved from www.parkinson-manager.eu

Pegasof4f. (2014). *Personalised Guidance Services for optimising lifestyle in teen-agers through awareness, motivation and engagement.* Retrieved from www.pegasof4f.eu

Peleg, M. (2013). Making healthcare more accessible, better, faster, and cheaper: the MobiGuide Project. *European Journal of ePractice: Issue on Mobile eHealth, 20*, 5-20.

PERSONA. (2016). *PERSONAlised Health Monitoring System.* Retrieved Feb 1, 2017, from http://cordis.europa.eu/project/rcn/108629_en.html

Philbrick, W. C. (2013). *mHealth and MNCH: State of the Evidence. Trends, Gaps, Stakeholder Needs, and Opportunities For Future Research on the Use of Mobile Technology to Improve Maternal, Newborn, and Child Health.* mHealth Alliance, UN Foundation. mHealth Alliance, UN Foundation.

Prevent, I. T. (2016). *The PreventIT Project: Improving health and active aging with mobile technology.* Retrieved Jan 16, 2017, from www.preventit.eu/

PriceWaterhouseCoopers. (2014). *Emerging mHealth: paths for growth.* PriceWaterhouseCoopers.

PSYCHE. (2010). *Personalised monitoring SYstems for Care in mental HEalth.* Retrieved from www.psyche-project.org

PWC. (2012). *The power of the net generation.* PWC.

Qiang, C., Yamamichi, M., Hausman, V., & Altman, D. (2011). *Mobile Applications for the Health Sector. ICT Sector Unit.* The World Bank.

REACTION. (2010). *Remote Accessibility to Diabetes Management and Therapy in Operational healthcare Networks.* Retrieved from www.reaction-project.eu

RemPark. (2011). *Personal Health Device for the Remote and Autonomous Management of Parkinson's Disease.* Retrieved from www.rempark.eu

research2guidance. (2012). *3rd mHealth Expert Survey.* research2guidance.

research2guidance. (2013). *Mobile Health Market Report 2013-2017. The commercialization of mHealth applications* (vol. 3). research2guidance.

research2guidance. (2015). *EU Countries' mHealth App Market Ranking 2015: Which EU countries are best for doing mHealth business.* research2guidance in partnership with mHealth Summit. research-2guidance.

ScoliosisManager. (2016). *Monitoring platform for scoliosis treatment to empower kids, parents, physicians and orthotists.* Retrieved Jan 15, 2017, from cordis.europa.eu/project/rcn/197418_en.html

Sharp, R. (2012). *Lacking regulation, many medical apps questionable at best.* Retrieved 5 15, 2015, from The New England Center for Investigative Reporting, Boston University: necir.org/2012/11/18/medical-apps/

SMART4MD. (2015). *(S) Support (M) Monitoring (A) And (R) Reminder (T) Technology (4) for (M) Mild (D) Dementia.* Retrieved Jan 13, 2017, from www.smart4md.eu/

Sound of Vision. (2015). *Sound of Vision: Natural sense of vision through acoustics and haptics*. Retrieved Jan 10, 2017, from www.soundofvision.net

Splendid. (2013). *Personalised Guide for Eating and Activity Behaviour for the Prevention of Obesity and Eating Disorders*. Retrieved from splendid-program.eu

Statista. (2015). *Smartphone penetration worldwide 2008-2014*. Retrieved Jan 10, 2017, from Statista, The Statistics Portal: www.statista.com/statistics/218532/global-smartphone-penetration-since-2008/

Statista. (2015). *Value of the global mHealth (mobile health) market 2012-2020 (fee-based)*. Retrieved 5 7, 2015, from Statista. The Statistics Portal: http://www.statista.com/statistics/295771/mhealth-global-market-size/

Statista. (2016). *The Statistics Portal*. Retrieved 1 8, 2017, from Number of smartphone users worldwide from 2014 to 2020 (in billions): www.statista.com/statistics/330695/number-of-smartphone-users-worldwide/

Statista. (2018). *The Statistics Portal*. Retrieved from mHealth (mobile health) industry market size projection from 2012 to 2020 (in billion U.S. dollars): https://www.statista.com/statistics/295771/mhealth-global-market-size

Statista. (2018). *The Statistics portal*. Retrieved from Mobile phone users worldwide 2015-2020: https://www.statista.com/statistics/274774/forecast-of-mobile-phone-users-worldwide/

Supporting, L. I. F. E. (2017). *Supporting LIFE: Fighting Child Mortality*. Retrieved Jan 5, 2017, from http://www.supportinglife.eu

TheWorldBank. (2012). 2012 Information and Communications for Development: Maximizing Mobile. The World Bank.

TheWorldBank. (2015). *Indicators*. Retrieved 5 11, 2015, from The World Bank. IBRD-IDA: http://data.worldbank.org/indicator?display=graph

Thomson, B. (n.d.). *FDA Regulation of Mobile Health* (2nd ed.). Chester Street Publishing, Inc.

Travis, P., Bennett, S., Haines, A., Pang, T., Butta, Z., Hyder, A., ... Evans, T. (2004). Overcoming health-systems constraints to achieve the Millennium Development Goals. *Lancet*, *364*(9437), 900–906. doi:10.1016/S0140-6736(04)16987-0 PMID:15351199

UN, D. o. (2017). The 2017 Revision, Key Findings and Advance Tables. *World Population Prospects*.

Union, P. O. (Ed.). (n.d.). *EU Open Data Portal*. Retrieved December 4, 2016, from European Union Open Data Portal: http://data.europa.eu/euodp/en/data

UnwiredHealth. (2014). *UnwiredHealth EU Project Official web page*. Retrieved from http://www.unwiredhealth.eu

van Heerden, A., Tomlinson, M., & Swartz, L. (2012). Point of care in your pocket: A research agenda for the field of m-health. *Bulletin of the World Health Organization*, *90*(5), 393–394. doi:10.2471/BLT.11.099788

VitalWaveConsulting. (2009). mHealth for Development: The Opportunity of Mobile Technology for Healthcare in the Developing World. UN Foundation-Vodafone Foundation Partnership.

Welcome. (2013). *Wearable Sensing and Smart Cloud Computing for Integrated Care to COPD Patients with Comorbidities*. Retrieved from www.welcome-project.eu

WHO & UNICEF. (2010). *Countdown to 2015: Taking stock of maternal, newborn and child survival. 2000-2010 Decade Report*. World Health Organization and UNICEF.

WHO. (2011). mHealth. New horizons for health through mobile technologies: Based on the findings of the second global survey on eHealth (Vol. 3). World Health Organization.

Witten, I., & Eibe, F. (2005). Data mining: Practical machine learning tools and techniques (2nd ed.). San Francisco, CA: Morgan Kaufmann Publishers Inc.

WOMEN-UP. (2015). *Cost effective self-management of Urinary Incontinence*. Retrieved Jan 22, 2017, from www.women-up.eu

Youssef, A., MacCallum, T., McDonald, D., Crane, R., & Jackman, M. S. (2012). *Healthcare Information and Management Systems Society*. Retrieved May 15, 2014, from HIMSS transforming health through IT: http://www.himss.org/ResourceLibrary/mHimssRoadmapContent.aspx?ItemNumber=30392

KEY TERMS AND DEFINITIONS

Behavioral Intervention Technologies (BITs): It includes mHealth and eHealth interventions to support people in changing behaviors and cognitions related to mental health, health and wellness. It is a multidisciplinary field, including psychologists, physicians, software engineers, human factors engineers, computer scientists, etc. BITs apply behavioral and psychological intervention strategies by using the latest ICTs.

Biosensor: It refers to an analytical device able to detect, record and transmit information regarding physiological/biological change or process (e.g., blood pressure, etc.). Some other indicative applications relate to the detection of body movement, temperature and fluid analysis, which are turned into electrical signals. In summary, it converts a biological response into an electrical signal. The biosensor is made up of a biological recognition element (e.g., an enzyme, a nucleic acid, or an antibody) and a transducer (to convert the recognition event into a measurable signal).

Body Area Network (BAN): A body area network (BAN) or a body sensor network (BSN) or a wireless body area network (WBAN) can be defined as a system of low power devices/sensors in close proximity to the body of the user that cooperate using a wireless network for the benefit of the subject/end user. The devices may be wearable, implants, etc., and through gateway devices, it is possible to connect them to the Internet and transmit data to a local base station and remote places. A WBAN system can use WPAN wireless technologies as gateways to reach longer ranges. In the medical sector, they are used to help medical professionals to monitor patients' data and activities remotely.

Chronic Care Management (CCM): The term is interchanged with disease management and is referred to activities (e.g., motivating patients to persist in therapies, etc.) carried out by health care professionals to help patients with chronic diseases (e.g., diabetes, high blood pressure, multiple sclerosis, etc.) learn and understand their condition and live with it having reasonable quality of life.

eHealth: Refers to the use of information and communication technologies for the support of healthcare practice. It covers electronic exchange of health-related data, while may be used for clinical, educational, research and administrative purposes.

Information and Communication Technologies (ICTs): The term is referred in the technologies used from the telecommunication and informatics sectors as well as any possible combination of them. It may include any communication device (e.g., telephone, tv, radio, cell phones, computers, satellite systems, wireless networks, etc.), as well as the software, applications and services associated with them which enable users to exchange information. The term covers also the audio-visual sector in combination with computer networks and telecommunication networks.

mHealth: The term is referred to the use of mobile technologies combined with wearable and fixed sensors to provide health-related services.

Patient-Centered: Patient-centered refers to any case (process, operation, system, etc.) that is focused, designed and developed based on the patient's needs and the patient's pathway, while trying to fulfill his/her expectations. The term is usually used in patient-centered care.

Personal Area Network (PAN): A personal area network (PAN) or a wireless personal network (WPAN) is a computer network for data transmission among devices (e.g., telephones, cell phones, computers, PDAs, wearable computer devices, etc.) organized around a person's workspace. When using wireless technologies (e.g., irDA, Bluetooth, ZigBee, etc.) for data transmission the term WPAN is used, while PAN can also use computer buses (e.g., USB or FireWire). PANs can cover a range of almost 10 meters.

Wearable Devices: The term can also be found as wearables, wearable technology, fashionable technology, etc. It refers to accessories that can be worn on the body and clothing incorporating electronic technologies and computer. The main idea behind wearables is the ability to connect to the Internet, thus enabling data exchange between the device and the network. Wearables can provide biofeedback and tracking of physiological function and transmit the information. Biosnesors are also used for wearables. Glasses, watches, headbands, bracelets, and others are some examples of wearable devices. Smart tattoos and implanted devices are a more invasive version of wearables.

ENDNOTES

1 In "Participating Countries" column, in bold is indicated the coordinator's country.

2 Country codes have been retrieved from Eurostat web page http://ec.europa.eu/eurostat/statistics-explained/index.php/Glossary:Country_codes.

3 ICT-2007.5.1 – Personal health systems for monitoring and point-of-care diagnostics.

4 HCP: Health Care Professionals.

5 COPD: Chronic Obstructive Pulmonary Disease.

6 CKD: Chronic Kidney Disease.

7 ICT-2009.5.1 – Personal Health Systems.

8 AI: Artificial Intelligence.

9 DSS: Decision Support System.

10 CVD: Cardiovascular disease.

11 BAN: Body Area Network.

12 ICT-2011.5.1 – Personal Health Systems (PHS).

13 ICT-2011.5.3 – Patient Guidance Services (PGS), safety and healthcare record information reuse.

14 PCP: Pre-Commercial Procurement.

15 HEALTH.2012.2.3.2-4 – Low-cost interventions for disease control in resource poor settings.

16 ICT-2013.5.1 – Personalised health, active ageing, and independent living.

17 FP7-PEOPLE-2013-IEF – Marie-Curie Action: "Intra-European fellowships for career development."

18 PHC-12-2014-1 – Clinical research for the validation of biomarkers and/or diagnostic medical devices.

19 PHC-26-2014 – Self management of health and disease: citizen engagement and mHealth.

20 HIV: Human Immunodeficiency Virus.

Chapter 2
Patient Health Monitoring Using IoT

Adusumalli Sai Manoj
Koneru Lakshmaiah Education Foundation, India

Mohammed Ali Hussain
Koneru Lakshmaiah Education Foundation, India

Paleti Surya Teja
Koneru Lakshmaiah Education Foundation, India

ABSTRACT

In today's world, health is one of the vital issues to solve through wireless communication technology. It should be efficient in terms of cost and reliable communication with suitable protocols. To monitor the health conditions of a patient, a mobile care system can be designed with the help of wireless sensor network using IoT. This can be done by integrating different sensors to sense physiological data from a human body and then transmit the data to a remote healthcare cloud through a smartphone as an interface. All the vital signs monitored are portable and will have the ability of short-range wireless communication. Then the data can be uploaded to the central server to keep track of the patient's health condition. In emergency, a notification will be sent to the nearest hospital by sending a warning message through mobile application.

INTRODUCTION

Internet Of Things (IoT) technology has attracted much attention in recent years for its potential to alleviate the strain on healthcare systems caused by an aging population and a rise in chronic illness. Patient monitoring has advanced over the years, from bedside monitors in the hospital to wearable devices that can monitor patients and communicate their data remotely to medical servers over wireless networks. It is a process that involves monitoring major vital signs of a patient, to check if their health is normal or deteriorating within a period. In a remote situation, vital signs information can help health care providers to easily send help to patients when their health is at immediate risk. E-Health technology can bring

DOI: 10.4018/978-1-5225-8021-8.ch002

Copyright © 2019, IGI Global. Copying or distributing in print or electronic forms without written permission of IGI Global is prohibited.

a variety of benefits to patients, caregivers, and health institutions, by facilitating improved healthcare services through the utilization of Information and Communication Technologies (ICTs). The forthcoming generation of healthcare services will require advances in computing and Wireless Sensor Networks (WSNs) to leverage truly intelligent and adaptive features for smarter health services. This is possible through Internet Of Things where the values of the vital signs will be monitored continuously, and if any of the vital-signs values are less than the threshold value, then the notification will be sent to the doctor in the nearby hospital. If the vital signs values are critical i.,e far beyond threshold value then precautions to be taken are sent to the patient's mobile which is discussed below. You can see the process of how the data about the patient will be transferred to the hospital in the Block diagram of Figure 1. This chapter discusses every block in detail.

BACKGROUND

Stephanie Baker et al. have discussed many challenges, technologies and opportunities where they deal with types of vital signs and sensors and their principles required for vital signs monitoring and about cloud technology and its importance in Internet Of Things. The authors have discussed the need for security measures in the cloud, and the main focus was on wearable sensors for healthcare Michelle Omoogun et al. developed a prototype of wearable sensors where patient's vital signs are monitored and if there is any deviation in the vital signs readings then message will be sent to the patient indication that there is a deviation in his vital signs readings. The patient can also view the location of the nearest hospital in case of an emergency.

PATIENT HEALTH MONITORING USING IoT

This chapter is mainly focused on designing a prototype for vital signs monitoring using IoT. This is used for patient's health monitoring without the need for doctor and intimating the doctor if the vital signs cross their threshold value through the mobile application. Initially, we will be focusing on the type of microcontroller used for sensors to be controlled, and then we will go to the vital signs that are to be monitored and a sensor for each vital sign and their position to be kept to the body. Then, the next focus is the cloud platform where data of a patient's vital signs are stored for future purposes. Finally, we end

Figure 1. Block diagram of patient health monitoring using internet of things

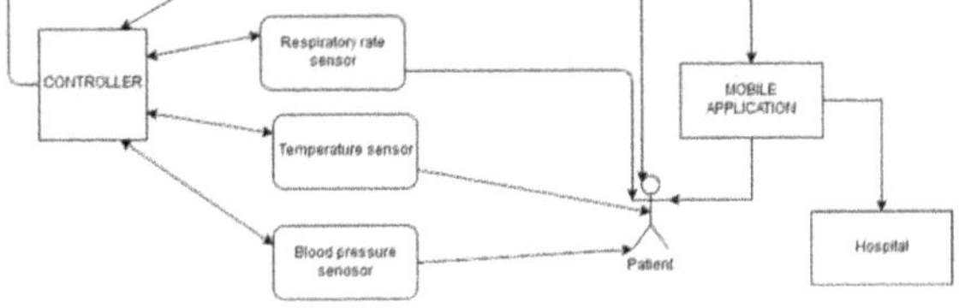

with the mobile application where the patient can keep track of his vital signs status, and this is used for intimating the doctor about his vital signs status if it goes beyond the threshold value and integrating all these as a prototype that can be developed for patient health monitoring using IoT.

Issues, Controversies, Problems

The problem with this kind of remote monitoring system is that most of the times the patients must be within a specified location to either monitor their health or receive emergency help. The drawbacks include the security risk that comes with having large amounts of sensitive data stored in a single database, the potential need to regularly have an individual's sensors recalibrated to ensure that they are monitoring accurately, and possible disconnections from healthcare services if the patient was out of the cellular range or their devices ran out of battery.

Microcontroller

The microcontroller is a mini computer on an integrated circuit which is dedicated for performing a task and execution of a specific application. It contains memory, Processor as well as programmable peripherals. The sensors are attached to the human body for sensing vital-signs which are controlled by a microcontroller, and this transfers the sensed data to the cloud.

There are different types of microcontrollers; this chapter proposes an ESP8266 microcontroller with which NodeMCU is made of. To this board, sensors are integrated measuring the vital-signs, and this has inbuilt Wi-Fi module where the data can be sent to the cloud without any other communicating module like GSM (Global System for Mobile Communications). GSM is also a type of wireless communication module for exchanging data over a network. So, GSM is not necessary if we use NodeMCU.

NodeMCU platform is like the Arduino platform, but the reason why this is selected is if we use Arduino board then we must use another module to connect the sensors over the Internet whereas NodeMCU does not need any module as it has inbuilt Wi-Fi module which can be seen in Figure 2. The normal way of powering NodeMCU is through the USB cable.

Figure 2. NodeMCU

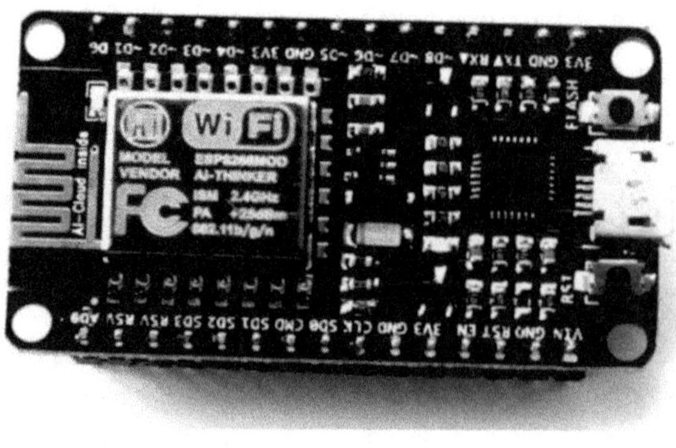

Interest Towards NodeMCU

The parameters that are good in NodeMCU when compared to other Microcontrollers are size and cost. Table 1 and Table 2 show variations of cost and size between different microcontrollers.

Advantages of NodeMCU

- The cost of NodeMCU is less than other microcontrollers.
- The size is also smaller compared to other controllers.
- It requires 3.3v of energy where others need 5v of energy.
- Inbuilt Wi-Fi module.

Disadvantages of NodeMCU

Reduced Pinout

NodeMCU has only one analog pin which might be the important disadvantage of this selection, but this can be changed using multiplexing of sensors connected to the board. If two analog sensors are connected to the microcontroller then first the value of sensor A will be read and then the value of sensor B alternatively by multiplexing. (Multiple analogue inputs on only one analogue pin, 2016). If vital signs that are to be monitored are more than two, then the Arduino microcontroller is best to choose.

Either you use Arduino or NodeMCU 9v battery is enough for power supply because Arduino needs 5v input power and NodeMCU needs 3.5v power for activation.

Software Platform

The software platform used in nodemcu is Arduino IDE. This is used to program NodeMCU. The language used in Arduino IDE is C language. More detailed information about Arduino IDE can be found at (Information about Arduino IDE, 2018).

Table 1. Cost

Microcontroller	Cost (Rs)
AtMega 328	500
PIC 18F4550	499
NodeMCU	300

Table 2. Size

Microcontroller	Size
NodeMCU	49 x 24.5 x 13mm
AtMega 328	68.6 mm × 53.3 mm

Vital Signs

Vital signs are used for measuring critical health such as pulse rate, respiratory rate, body temperature and blood pressure. These vital signs are measured with sensors which are connected to the human body as shown in Figure 3. These sensors are controlled by a controller which is connected at one end (Figure 1) and sends the data to the Cloud as shown in Figure 9.

Pulse Rate

This is also known as heart rate which is defined as the number of contractions of the heart per minute. It is denoted by BPM (Beats per minute). The ranges of pulse rate vary with different age groups in determining critical health. We are classifying age groups into two types: children and adults where children will have age less than 18 and adults with age 18 and above.

Table 3 and Table 4 listed below show the normal heart rate and threshold heart rate classification based on gender and age taken from (Heart rate statistics, 2015).

The maximum heart rate of a person can be calculated using this formula

220 - your age = predicted maximum heart rate

Example: A 50-year-old is predicted maximum heart rate is 170 beats/minute.

Table 3. Normal heart rate

Gender	Age	Heart rate (BPM)
Male	Children (<18)	70-75
	Adults (>18)	66-69
Female	Children (<18)	74-77
	Adults (>18)	69-72

Table 4. Maximum heart rate

Gender	Age	Heart rate (BPM)
Male	Children (<18)	145-150
	Adults (>18)	151-154
Female	Children (<18)	143-146
	Adults (>18)	148-151

Figure 3. Photoplethysmographic pulse sensor

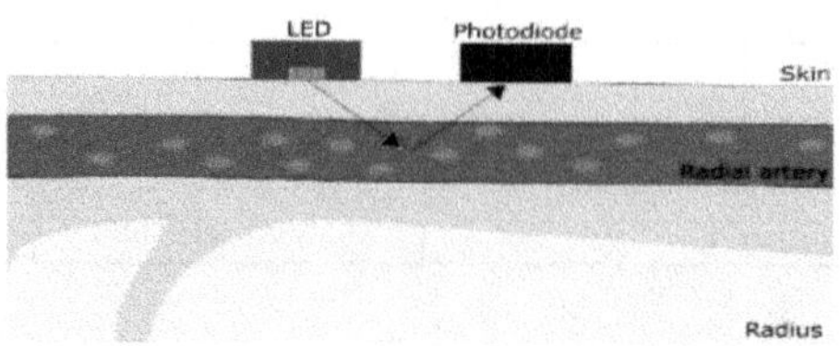

Pulse Sensor: PPG (Photoplethysmographic Pulse Sensor)

Pulse can be used to detect a wide range of emergency conditions such as cardiac arrest, pulmonary embolisms and vasovagal syncope. It is also used for fitness tracking.

The heartbeat rate can be read from various places in our body like chest, wrist, earlobe, finger-tip as discussed by (Guru et al., 2017). The best place to place this sensor is near the wrist which can be placed in a watch so, that it is very convenient to use without any discomfort (Baker et al., 2017). The Sensor placed to the human body is shown in Figure 3.

This sensor placed under the hand will be measuring the heart rate continuously, and the data will be uploaded to the cloud which will be used for future analysis, and as mentioned in the above table if the value of heart rate crosses the threshold value then information of the patient along with the location is sent to the doctor in the nearest hospital through the designed mobile application. The designing of the PPG circuit is shown in Figure 4.

Precautions for Heart Rate Abnormality

- Breathe deeply it will keep you relaxed.
- Splash your face with cold water. It stimulates a nerve that controls your heart rate.
- Don't panic, stress and anxiety will make your irregular heart rate worse.

If a patient with heart rate less or more than the values mentioned above message will be sent to the mobile of the patient with the above precautions to be taken before the doctor arrives at him from the nearest hospital. These precautions are recorded from (Heart rate precautions, 2018).

Design of PPG Conditioning Circuit

LED (Light Emitting Diode) of 575nm is used as source, and a light dependent resistor of 10kΩ is used as a detector. The output from the sensor is given to the high pass filter whose cut off frequency is set to 0.5Hz as the frequency of PPG signal is between 0.5Hz-35Hz. The output of the high pass filter is given to the instrumentation amplifier AD-620 for further amplification. The gain of AD-620 is given by (Laulkar et al., 2012).

Figure 4. PPG Signal conditioning circuit

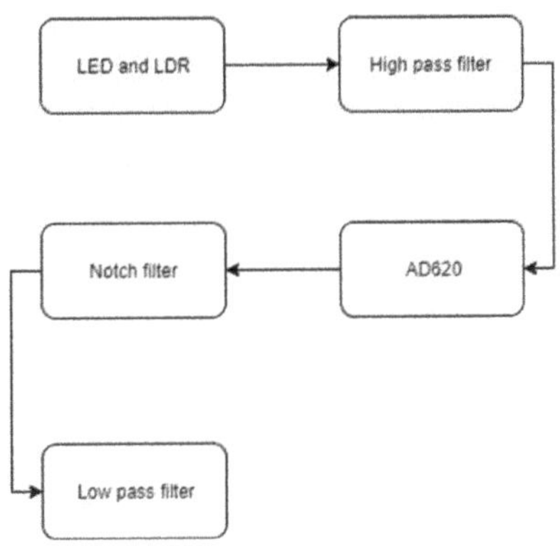

$$G = \left(\frac{49.4k\Omega}{RG}\right) + 1 \quad (1)$$

RG is the external resistor. In this circuit, the external resistor used is 1.5kΩ, so the gain of AD-620 becomes 34. After the amplification, the output is given to the notch filter. The notch filter is a combination of inverting adder and multiple feedback (MFB) bandpass filter. The gain of the bandpass filter is set by (2)

$$Av = -\left(\frac{R2}{R1}\right) \quad (2)$$

which comes out to be 5. FreqThe frequency bandpass filter is given as (3) -

$$fo = \frac{1}{2} * \pi * C * \sqrt{R1 \mid\mid R2 * R2} \quad (3)$$

which comes out to be 1124.85Hz. The notch filter is used to filter 50Hz frequency. The output of the notch filter is given to a low pass filter whose cut-off frequency is set to 35Hz. The total gain of the circuit is 1000 (Omoogun et al., 2017).

Respiratory Rate

A person's respiratory rate is determined by the number of breaths he takes per minute. It is measured by breath per minute. The ranges of respiratory rate vary with different age groups in determining critical health. We are classifying age groups into five types like an infant, toddler, pre-schooler, school age, adolescent. The statistics shown in Table 5 are recorded from (Respiratory rates statistics, 2018). These values are the threshold values for sending the notification to the doctor in the nearby hospital.

Table 5. Normal respiratory rate

Type	Age range	Respiratory rate (BPM)
Infant	1-12 months	30-60
Toddler	1-3 years	24-40
Pre-schooler	4-5 years	22-34
School-age	6-12 years	18-30
Adolescent	13-18 years	12-16
Adult	>18 years	12-18

Stretch Sensor

This sensor is used to measure the respiratory rate of a person. This sensor is attached to the jacket of the patient which is placed at the chest. The central part of the sensor is comprised of a piezoelectric transducer realized using polyvinylidene-fluoride (PVDF). The design of the Piezoelectric transducer is shown in Figure 5

This PVDF (Polyvinylidene Difluoride) as a respiratory sensor yields various advantages like the smaller size, quicker reaction time, higher precision, simpler integration capacity and lower power dissipation compared to other sensors. As a tensile force is applied to a PVDF transducer, the charge Q created due to the application of pressure can be represented as

$$Q = d\sigma A$$

where '*d*' is the piezoelectric strain coefficient and is applied in tensile stress, and '*A*' is an area of the electrode. This sensor produces charge in response to the applied pressure caused by respiration. This is the common method as done in (Mahbub et al., 2017) and (Atalay et al., 2015).

This sensor placed in the jacket will keep on monitoring the respiratory rate of the patient and upload the data to the cloud and as mentioned in the above table if the value increases or decreases then information is sent to the mobile of the patient and the doctor in the nearest hospital with patient information and location of the patient through mobile application.

Figure 5. An equivalent model of the piezoelectric transducer

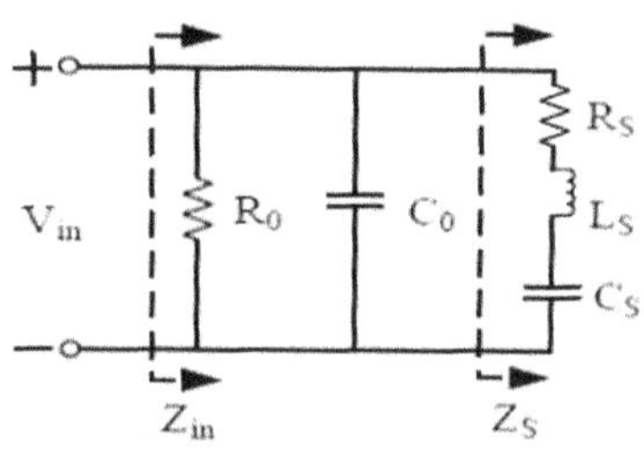

Figure 6. Placement of stretch sensor for a patient

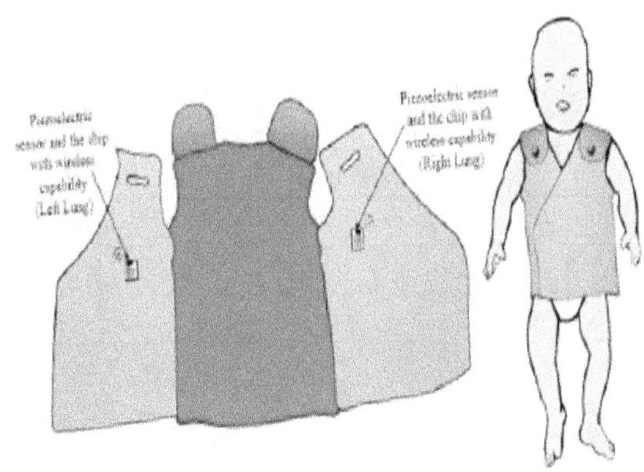

Precautions for Respiratory Rate Abnormality

- Loosen if any tight clothing.
- If there are any open wounds in the neck or chest, they must be closed immediately, Bandage the wounds at once.
- Do not take any food or drink.
- Try to avoid crowded places or closed places; ventilated places are ideal.

If the respiratory rate of the patient falls than the value in the table mentioned above, it would be treated as abnormality condition, and the precautions will be sent to the patient's mobile which are to be followed by the patient before he is taken to the doctor.

Body Temperature

The body temperature is used to detect hypothermia, heat stroke, fever and many more. The range of body temperature varies with different age groups. We are classifying the age group into three types as children, adults, older as shown in Table 6. The sensor to make it wearable is made with a polymer as shown in (Nakamura et al., 2016).

Thermistor Sensor

Human body temperature can be measured using a thermistor sensor. The sensor is attached to the human skin, and the measurement is performed with the assumptions that the temperature of the thermistor and skin are same. This sensor works on the principle of the negative temperature coefficient(NTC) as discussed by (Narczyk et al., 2016).

Measuring human body temperature in the range between 25 °C and 45 °C means that resistance of the thermistor changes from about 980 Ω to about 2250 Ω. This sensor can be effectively used for measuring when embedded in textiles.

This sensor continuously monitors the body temperature and will upload the data to the cloud, and if the value is less or more than the threshold value as indicated in the above table, then the indication is sent to the mobile phone of the patient and the doctor in the nearest hospital along with the location of the patient. This sensor can be placed on the body as discussed by (Aqueveque et al., 2017).

Table 6. Normal body temperature

Type	Age group	Temperature (°F)
Children	1-17years	97.9-99
Adults	18-65years	97-99
Older	>65years	<98.6

Temperature in °F = Temperature in °C * (9/5) + 32

Figure 7. Thermistor curve

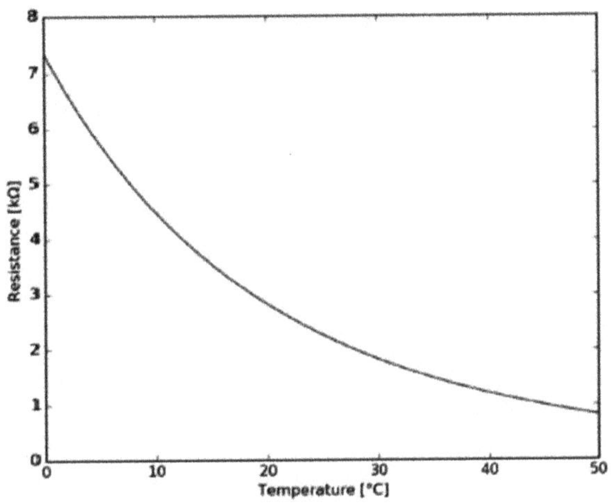

Precautions for Body Temperature Abnormality

- Drink plenty of fluids such as soup and water but avoid fruit juices or sports drinks.
- Apply a cloth soaked in lukewarm water and salt on the forehead to lower your body temperature.
- Do not do forceful eating and avoid consuming spicy and oily food for a few days.
- It is better to bath with lukewarm water and stay away from cold baths or ice rubs.

If the body temperature of the patient increases, then the above precautions will be sent to the patient's mobile that before the doctor's arrival to the patient in case of an emergency.

Blood Pressure

It is the pressure of circulating blood on the walls of blood vessels. It can come in three forms low, normal and high. BP is certainly a valuable parameter in health care, and the ability to monitor it continuously would improve the quality of the health care system. The range of BP varies with different age groups and by gender. Table 7 is recorded from (Blood pressure statistics, 2018).

PPG Sensor (Photoelectric Plethysmograph Sensor)

The amount of blood pressure can be calculated using PAT (Pulse arrival time) i.,e two PPG sensors, one at the earlobe and one on the wrist is used to estimate pulse arrival time between these locations and thus estimates the blood pressures.

This sensor monitors the blood pressure and sends the readings to the cloud and if the value increases or decreases than the threshold value as mentioned above a notification will be sent through a mobile application to the doctor in the nearby hospital about the patient's health condition along with the location of the patient.

Table 7. Normal blood pressure

Age	Female (mmHg)	Male (mmHg)
6-9	98-114	97-115
10-11	100-118	102-120
12-18	117/77	120/85
19-24	120/79	120/79
25-29	120/80	121/80
30-35	122/81	123/82
36-39	123/82	124/83
40-45	124/83	125/83
46-49	126/84	127/84
50-55	129/85	128/85
56-59	130/86	131/87
>60	134/84	135/88

Figure 8. PPG sensor for BP monitoring

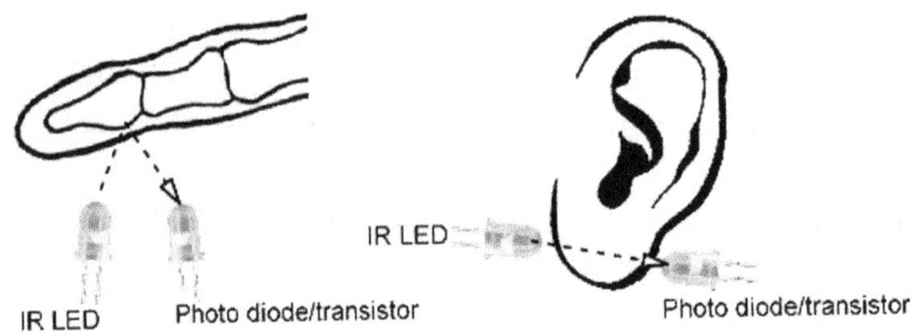

Precautions for Blood Pressure Abnormality

- Let them take the breath in from nose and out through nose at even slower pace.
- The patient can be given fruit juice because high potassium levels in the juice will reduce the blood pressure.
- If there is a nose bleeding, then do proper first aid.

The above precautions for high blood pressure will be sent to the patient's mobile if the BP content of the patient deviates from the values as mentioned above. So, the patient can take preventive measures before the doctor arrives at his location. These precautions are sent to the mobile as discussed by (Omoogun et al., 2017).

CLOUD PLATFORM: THINGSPEAK

The data collected from different sensors like Pulse sensor, Respiratory sensor, Thermistor sensor, PPG sensor which is used to measure the heart rate, respiratory rate, body temperature, and blood pressure respectively is stored in the cloud in the form of a graph showing daily analysis and can be retrieved for future analysis. This is similar as discussed by (Raskovic et al., 2017). However, this chapter's proposal is more effective than that method. Thingspeak is an open source platform which can be understood very easily (Thingspeak, 2018). Vital signs readings that are taken from a patient's body are the inputs to the Thingspeak which are stored in a graph manner, and these values are stored in Thingspeak through the write API key provided by the Thingspeak. In the mobile application, the read API key is accessed to know the deviation in the vital sign values of the patient. Then the notification will be sent to the doctor about the patient health status along with the patient location and to the patient about his status and the doctor's information.

In this way, the data is stored in thingsspeak each vital sign reading is taken individually as shown in Figure 9.

Mobile Application: MIT

Any intimation in deviation of any parameter or alert to the doctor in the nearest hospital is sent from a mobile application designed in MIT. This is very effective in sending accurate information without making any delay and with correct information to the doctor. The monitoring through a mobile application is also discussed by (Daou et al., 2015). Figure 10 shows the home screen interface of the smart health application.

In case of any abnormal issue, the information of the patient along with his location is sent to the doctor in the nearest hospital from the patient's location. As shown in Figure 11 patients are allotted with nearest hospitals.

Figure 9. Data stored in thingspeak

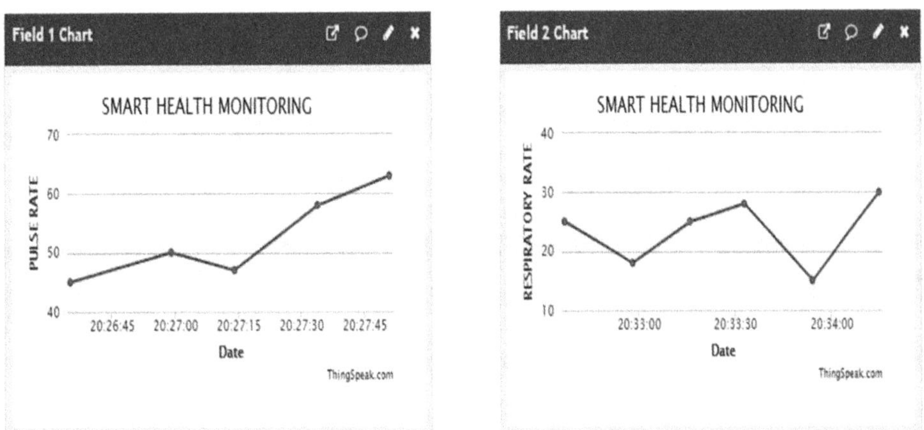

Figure 10. MIT application

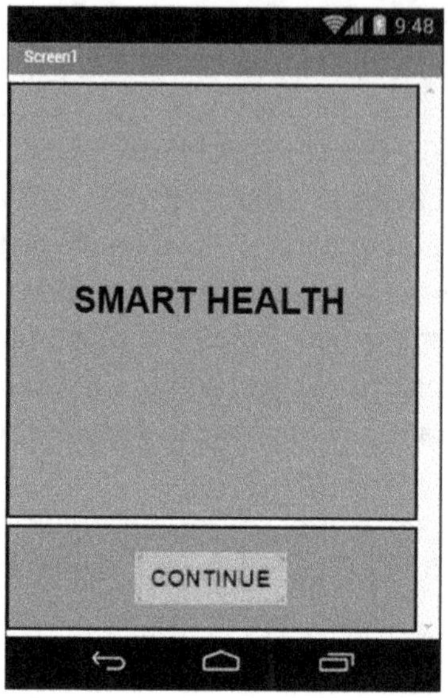

Pseudo Code for Patient Assigning to the Hospital

Step 1: Monitoring of sensors' reading on vital signs.
Step 2: Checking of any deviation in the values of vital signs.
Step 3: If there is a deviation then check for hospitals nearby.
Step 4: Find the doctor on duty in the nearby hospital and send the patients' health condition along with his location.
Step 5: If there are two patients with health abnormality then check for higher priority based on the condition and assign them to the nearby hospital.
Step 6: Doctor discharges the patient after the recording of normal parameters.

DISCUSSION

The assigning of a doctor to a patient is shown clearly in Figure 11. If a patient has got some health problem, i.e. any deviation in the threshold value of the vital signs, then based on the patient's location. The doctor who is having no appointments in the nearest hospital is assigned to the patient. Based on the critical level of his health, a notification will be sent to the doctor to take the necessary steps before he arrives at the hospital and precautions are also sent to the patient to look after. Until the patient is cured, he will be under that doctor's surveillance. Once a patient's vital signs are normal then a doctor's appointment will get open, and another patient if available will be assigned to him.

Figure 11. Assigning the hospital to the patient

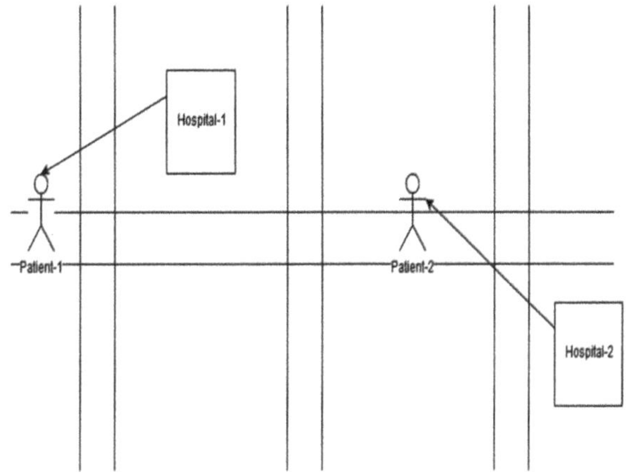

CONCLUSION

The proposed model is a novel design methodology for health monitoring using remote sensing by Internet Of Things. These vital signs have proven to be important in finding health abnormalities of a person. The placement of sensors to the body which is proposed above is a comfortable way of wearable sensors without any discomfort for the patient during his daily activities. Finally, this method produces accurate results which are less cost-effective.

REFERENCES

Aqueveque, P., Gutierrez, C., Saavedra, F., & Pino, E. J. (2017). Monitoring Physiological Variables of Mining Workers at High Altitude. *IEEE Transactions on Industry Applications*, *53*(3), 2628–2634. doi:10.1109/TIA.2017.2675360

ArduinoI. D. E. (2018). Retrieved from https://www.arduino.cc/

Atalay, O., Kennon, W. R., & Demirok, E. (2015). Weft- Knitted Strain Sensor for Monitoring Respiratory Rate and Its Electro-Mechanical Modelling. *IEEE Sensors Journal*, *15*(1), 110–122. doi:10.1109/JSEN.2014.2339739

Baker, S., Wei Xiang and Atkinson, I. (2017). Internet Of things for smart Healthcare: Technologies, Challenges and Opportunities. *Journal of IEEE ACCESS.*

Blood pressure statistics. (2018). Retrieved from https://www.belmarrahealth.com/understanding-blood-pressure-readings-is-key-to-overall-well-being/

Daou, R. A. Z., Aad, E., Nakhle, F., Hayek, A., & Horscok, J. (2015). Patient Vital Signs Monitoring via Android Application. *Proceedings of International Conference on Advances in Biomedical Engineering (ICABME)*. 10.1109/ICABME.2015.7323278

Eshkeiti, A. M., Joyce, B. B., Narakathu, S., Emamian, S. G. R., Avuthu, J., & Atashbar, M. Z. (2014). A novel self-supported printed flexible strain sensor for monitoring body movement and temperature. Proceedings of IEEE SENSORS.

Guru, M., & Ragib, H., & Khan, R. (2017). Towards Non-Intrusive Continuous Healthcare Monitoring with the smart Hospital growth. *Proceedings of 14th IEEE Annual Consumer Communications & Networking Conference (CCNC).*

Heart rate precautions. (2018). Retrieved from https://www.webmd.com/heart-disease/what-to-do-heart-races#1

Heart rate statistics. (2015). Retrieved from http://www.statcan.gc.ca/pub/82-626-x/2013001/t004-eng.html

Laulkar, R., & Daimiwal, N. (2012). Acquisition of PPG signal for diagnosis of parameters related to heart. *Proceedings of 1st international symposium on physics and technology of sensors(ISPTS).*

Mahbub, I., Pullano, S. A., Wang, H., Islam, S. K., Fiorillo, S., To, G., & Mahfouz, M. R. (2017). A Low- Power Wireless Piezoelectric Sensor-Based Respiration Monitoring System Realized in CMOS Process. *IEEE Sensors Journal, 17*(6), 1858–1864. doi:10.1109/JSEN.2017.2651073

Multiple analog inputs on only one analog pin. (2016). Retrieved from http://www.instructables.com/id/Multiple-Analog-Inputs-on-Only-One-Analoge-Pin/

Nakamura, T., Yokota, Y., Terakawa, J., Reeder, W., Voit, T., Someya, & Sekino, M. (2016). Development of flexible and wide-range polymer-based temperature sensor for human bodies. *Proceedings of IEEE-EMBS International Conference on Biomedical and Health Informatics (BHI).*

Narczyk, P., Siwiec, K., & Pleskacz, W. A. (2016). Precision human body temperature measurement based on thermistor sensor. *Proceedings of IEEE 19th International Symposium on Design and Diagnostics of Electronic Circuits& Systems (DDECS).* 10.1109/DDECS.2016.7482451

Omoogun, Ramsurram, Guness, Seeam, Bellekens, & Seeam. (2017). Critical Patient eHealth Monitoring System using wearable sensors. *Proceedings of 1st International Conference on Next Generation Computing Applications.*

Raskovic, V., Denkovski, D., Atanasovski, V., & Gavrilovska, L. (2017). Cloud based solution for vital signs tracing. *Proceedings of 17th International conference on smart technologies.*

Respiratory rates statistics. (2018). Retrieved from https://www.aclsmedicaltraining.com/normal-values-in-children

Thingspeak. (2018). Retrieved from https://thingspeak.com/

KEY TERMS AND DEFINITIONS

Cloud: Accessing computer and software applications through a network connection.

E-Health: Usage of information and communications technologies in healthcare.

Mobile Application: Type of application software to run on a mobile device, such as a smartphone or tablet.

Sensors: A device which detects physical property and responds to it.

Vital Signs: Important measurements that indicate the state of a patient's essential body functions.

WSN: Group of spatially dispersed and dedicated sensors for monitoring and recording the physical conditions of environment or humans and organizing the collected data at a central location.

Chapter 3
An Integrated Approach Towards Developing Quality Mobile Health Apps for Cancer

Angelina Kouroubali
FORTH-ICS, Greece

Lefteris Koumakis
FORTH-ICS, Greece

Haridimos Kondylakis
FORTH-ICS, Greece

Dimitrios G. Katehakis
FORTH-ICS, Greece

ABSTRACT

The ever-growing demand for acquiring, managing, and exploiting patient health-related information has led to the development of several mobile health apps to support cancer patients. This chapter analyzes the clinical and technological characteristics of mobile apps enabling cancer patients to securely record, manage, and share their information online. It discusses issues relevant to increasing patient experience and acceptance, improving adherence to treatment, and effective support of coordinated care. Outcomes of recent research projects relevant to end user digital engagement, trust, interoperability, and usability/adaptability lead to an integrated approach towards developing quality mobile health apps. Improving quality of life and wellbeing in a secure and safe manner that respects the patients' privacy seems to be the key challenge. Regulation, standardization, and interoperability together with the existence of useful, accurate, and reliable tools for active patient engagement are imperative for efficient cancer disease management.

DOI: 10.4018/978-1-5225-8021-8.ch003

Copyright © 2019, IGI Global. Copying or distributing in print or electronic forms without written permission of IGI Global is prohibited.

INTRODUCTION

Cancer is a generic term used to describe a large group of diseases that can affect any part of the body and is a leading cause of death worldwide (World Health Organization, 2018a). Cancer incidents have increased from 12.7 million in 2008 to 14.1 million in 2012, and this trend is projected to continue, with the number of new cases expected to rise a further 75%. This will bring the number of cancer cases close to 25 million over the next two decades (International Agency for Research on Cancer, 2015). The different phases in the cancer care continuum are prevention, early detection, diagnosis, treatment, survivorship, and end-of-life care. Many cancers can be prevented by not smoking, maintaining a healthy weight, not drinking too much alcohol, eating plenty of vegetables, fruits and whole grains, vaccination against certain infectious diseases, not eating too much processed and red meat and avoiding too much sunlight exposure (Kushi et al, 2012; Parkin et al., 2011). However despite prevention measures, some cancers do occur, while advances in medicine are helping patients increase their survival rate when cancer occurs. Cancer survivors live longer, following improved access to effective screening, diagnosis, and treatments. Individuals with cancer as a chronic condition need more complex, patient-centered quality of care across the entire cancer trajectory (Hewitt et al., 2005). As cancer is perceived as a chronic, rather than an acute, disease, concepts of patient empowerment and self-management become relevant also in the oncologic field (Kushi et al., 2012).

Cancer patients have supportive care needs during and after treatment. These relate to physical, emotional, and social needs that vary over time and between treatments. Cancer patients experience symptoms related to both the disease and the treatment, such as pain and fatigue. Care and support for patients with cancer should include early recognition of signs and symptoms, support for self-care, personalized care planning, and routine use of patient-reported outcome measures (Maher, 2013). Routine reporting of patient outcomes greatly facilitates the identification of present problems and impact of treatment. Patient reported outcomes also enhance patient-clinician communication that promote shared decision-making (Kotronoulas et al., 2014; Valderas et al., 2008). Reporting of outcomes and interacting with physicians over a digital application or app has been shown to lower overall symptoms of distress, improve quality of life (QoL), and result in fewer emergency visits and improved overall survival (Basch et al., 2016; Denis et al., 2017; Ruland et al., 2013).

Mobile devices are becoming an integral part of the healthcare industry, changing how care is delivered and received. Mobile health (mHealth) is a broad concept, used to describe a range of mobile technologies, most often consumer health care technologies, such as web-based information resources, remote monitoring, and telehealth. The World Health Organization describes mHealth as technologies like mobile phones, personal digital assistances, smartphones, patient monitoring devices, mp3 players for mobile learning and mobile computing (World Health Organization, 2011).

In recent years, Internet of Things (IoT) has emerged as a new computing paradigm, in which a continuum of devices and objects are interconnected with a variety of communication solutions (e.g. Bluetooth, WiFi, ZigBee, and GSM), enabling connectivity among heterogeneous IoT devices that can help improve the living standard of citizens. It is anticipated that more than 50 billion devices, ranging from smartphones, laptops, sensors, and game consoles, will be connected to the Internet through several heterogeneous access network technologies such as radio-frequency identification (RFID) and wireless sensor networks (Yaqoob et al., 2017). Future wireless systems will include myriad smart features and applications to make 5G the most intelligent and dominant wireless technology thus far (Al-Falahy & Alani, 2017).

Healthcare systems around the world are becoming increasingly interested in strengthening the role of patients in their own care. Empowerment occurs when patients increase their capacity to think critically and make autonomous, informed decisions. In that process, the role of healthcare providers, technology providers, citizens, and policy makers is of paramount importance. An increasing trend shows a shift of healthcare models towards early detection and home care monitoring. However, despite the fact that mHealth and IoT have the potential to improve the quality of care of patients, there are certain concerns about the accuracy and unregulated status of health apps.

This chapter aims to (i) analyze the clinical and technological characteristics of cancer mobile apps that enable patients to securely record, manage and share their information, (ii) propose an integrated approach towards developing quality mobile health apps for cancer, and (iii) discuss issues relevant to the increase of patient experience and acceptance, adherence to treatment, and effective support of coordinated care.

BACKGROUND

The field of mHealth has a central role to play in redefining existing healthcare models (Cucciniello et al., 2015). MHealth has been shown to improve communication and enhance the integration of care processes (Fife & Pereira, 2011). As a technology that goes beyond the boundaries of healthcare organizations, it can enhance transparency and increase the productivity and accountability of healthcare providers and systems (Cucciniello & Nasi, 2014), hence contributing to the quality of care. Within the care process, mHealth systems can empower patients, enhance quality of life and improve the appropriateness of care (Heinrich & Kuiper, 2012). During the last decade, mHealth has shifted its focus, from the technical development to how the use of apps can influence people and their health (Fiordelli et al., 2013). MHealth has been used in different phases of cancer treatment. It can play a significant role in empowering patients through self-management tools that help them with their condition and associated side effects in their own privacy (Heinrich & Kuiper, 2012).

Personal Health Management

MHealth has revolutionized the ability of citizens to manage their own health and personal health data. Personal health record (PHR) systems facilitate the collection of information about an individual's health and health care, stored in electronic format intended for use by consumers, patients or their informal caregivers. The electronic health record (EHR) is a more generic term and encompasses the PHR and the electronic medical record (EMR) concepts. Essentially, the term EHR describes the systematic collection of health information about an individual patient, that is provided by healthcare professionals or the patient himself and can be shared across multiple healthcare environments when it is required, through various network technologies (Katehakis & Tsiknakis, 2006). The aim of PHR systems is to address patients' evolving needs using specific methods to improve their care and foresee health issues. PHR systems that follow a modular architecture can be enhanced with additional disease specific modules that will assist patients based on their particular condition. The potential of personal health records (PHRs) to improve healthcare delivery and reduce costs has been recognized in many countries worldwide. In recent years, many regional and national healthcare networks based on PHRs have been established in Europe (Dogac, 2012), Australia, and America.

A PHR with cancer modules has been seen as a potentially useful tool for patients in cross-sectoral cancer care (Kondylakis et al., 2017a). It has the potential to support patients in managing their chronic illness and is conceptualized to facilitate information exchange between patients and their healthcare professionals as well as among healthcare professionals or institutions across health care sectors. The phases of the course of illness create a challenge for implementation (Baudendistel et al., 2015) and specific modules need to be oriented towards the long-term and episodic character of cancer as a chronic disease. PHR adoption and use in the context of cancer is not yet widespread (Wiljer et al., 2010), however, when it is implemented, PHR use is frequent and increasing (Gerber et al., 2014).

An EHR encompassing information from a PHR that is interoperable with an EMR reflects a holistic view of health care as it includes both health providers as well as patients. The EHR is transforming the health care field worldwide (Sheikh et al., 2017). Patients have the ability to control and interact with their data in addition to having access to information provided by their healthcare team. EMR data is combined with data gathered from sensors or other wearable computing devices. In addition, personal data entries such as self-reported outcomes add to an integrated overview of patient data that can be shared with providers. The possibility of patients interacting with their own health data gives them autonomy over decision-making processes that may positively affect their health (Roehrs et al., 2017).

MHealth for Cancer

Research has shown that cancer patients value the use of apps for health care management and feel comfortable using them (Girault et al., 2015). A recent survey of 375 cancer patients reported that about half of the patients (48.5%) were willing to send data via an app supporting their oncological treatment and follow-up, while two-thirds (68.7%) agreed to use these regularly sent data as an ideal complement to the standard follow-up. The most mentioned characteristics that should be included in a cancer-focused app were pseudonymizing, data protection, and feedback from a physician based on the patients' input (Kessel et al., 2017). A review by Nasi et al. has shown that most applications focus on supporting medical decision-making and much less on supporting patients during the entire care process of cancer care (Nasi et al., 2015). More studies concerning the use of apps are warranted as they are still in an initial phase of development (Wang et al., 2014) and their full potential is not used regarding evidence-based content, usability, security, and interactivity (Boulos et al., 2014; Wang et al., 2014).

Designing a user-centered, patient focused application or tool, tailored to the individual user needs, requires the early involvement of both patients and healthcare professionals in the development, implementation, and evaluation processes. User preferences and daily routines need to be taken into consideration in chronic illness management. In addition, adequate patient support and technical advice for users have to be provided. Health data needs to be collected, viewed and utilized in a patient accessible way. Customizable functionalities in apps that can be easily modified based on user needs are very important in order to manage care-related information (Klasnja et al., 2010). Apps should also be easy to use, tailored to the individual, and include social support. Different partnerships and an innovative approach to developing, reviewing and testing mobile apps for cancer survivors are needed. User involvement is very important and needs to be established from the application conception. An application with clear involvement of cancer survivors in its development and evaluation is more likely to address actual rather than hypothetical patient needs. User feedback from doctors and cancer patients will help determine which apps or types of apps are most effective, and among which groups of survivors.

Cancer applications may include features for the assessment of the occurrence, frequency and distress of symptoms, together with a connection to a monitoring web interface. They may also include a risk assessment model that sends alerts via text message to health care providers, continuous access to evidence-based, self-care advice, links to relevant websites for more information, and graphs for the patients and health care providers to view the history of symptom reporting. A good app should empower patients by providing useful information that enables them to manage the challenges of cancer treatment. Self-management apps play a crucial role in helping patients to both cope with illness and communicate with their healthcare professionals. In addition, cancer apps play an important role in raising awareness and providing information about disease. Other features need to include, the possibility to record questions addressed to healthcare providers, medications, symptom tracking, reminders and schedules as a calendar to keep track of appointments, contacts and an easy-to-use journal. Glossary of medical terms will facilitate understanding information often conveyed in medical terms. Cancer patients face particularly difficult situations during their treatment including brain fog and temporary memory issues. Some application features that can support patients with these symptoms include, (i) recording answers from doctors and nurses, (ii) dictating or writing notes regarding side effects, concerns, and issues to use them for follow-ups, (iii) recording conversations with doctors, and (iv) possibilities to email recorded messages to friends and family. Important features need also to focus on stress relief complimentary to standard care. Online health journals are also important because they can be shared with friends and family and inspire other patients around the globe.

Cancer Apps and Quality

The complexity of illness and the need for cross-sectoral health care require the shift towards a patient-centered care paradigm where patients have the opportunity to play an active role in their own healthcare. User adoption is crucial in order to achieve the potential benefits of health apps and PHR systems. User needs and requirements from both the patient and healthcare provider perspectives need to be addressed (Baudendistel et al., 2015).

Despite the existence of hundreds of studies involving cancer-focused mobile phone apps, there is a lack of collective efforts to determine cancer-focused apps that effectively represent useful, accurate, and reliable tools for cancer disease management (Rincon et al., 2017). Reporting of health apps evaluation is rare or non-existent (Bender et al., 2013). There is a lack of evidence base and medical professional involvement in the development of the majority of cancer apps (Collado-Borrell et al., 2016). Safety concerns highlight the need for regulation, full authorship disclosure and clinical trials. A robust framework for identifying high quality applications is necessary. This will address the current barrier pertaining to a lack of consumer confidence in their use and further aid to promote their widespread implementation within healthcare (Mobasheri et al., 2014). Applications should also undergo a thorough evaluation and quality labeling procedure to ensure quality and effective functionalities. Categories of criteria for apps evaluation include engagement, functionality, aesthetics, information quality, and subjective quality scale. Quality assessment scales of mobile health apps can also be used to provide a checklist for the design and development of new high quality health apps (Stoyanov et al., 2015).

Privacy, security and confidentiality of health data managed in mHealth apps are of pivotal importance. Users should be able to control access to their information at any moment. The app should present a privacy policy informing the patients who will use their data, how it will be used, the privacy methods implemented and their rights and contact information for support. Users need to explicitly accept the proposed policy and give their consent to data collection. Designers need to be able to certify that their policies satisfy the legal requisites in privacy and security (Martínez-Pérez, B. et al., 2015).

IMPLEMENTING MOBILE APPS FOR CANCER PATIENTS

Advances in early detection, diagnosis, and treatment of cancer has resulted in patients being cured of their cancer or managing it as a chronic illness. The shift from cancer as a terminal illness to cancer as a chronic illness requires that patients and their families assume a more central role in the management of the oncologic disease, healthcare professionals take a partnership with patients accepting to share responsibilities, and policymakers provide adequate support to the healthcare systems in implementing new models (McGuire, 2016). Therefore, new models and approaches arise in cancer care, increasing the need for a general paradigm shift that encompasses concepts of patient empowerment and self-management in cancer as a chronic condition (Hewitt et al., 2005).

Patient empowerment as a concept emerges from social sciences generally described as a "*social process of recognizing, promoting, and enhancing peoples' abilities to meet their own needs, solve their own problems, and mobilize necessary resources to take control of their own lives*" (Jones & Melei, 1993). The nature of malignant disease requires patients to learn about and comprehend the illness, make difficult decisions regarding ensuing treatment, and cope with the consequences of the illness. It has been found that having relevant information not only helps cancer patients to understand the disease, but also facilitates their decision-making and coping with the disease (Iconomou et al., 2002; Friis et al., 2003). Patients should be actively involved and participate in decision making on treatment, in order to promote decisions that are consistent with their values, preferences and daily life management possibilities. This shared decision making process empowers patients and helps them make treatment choices based on well-discussed and well-informed options (Elwyn et al., 2015).

In a patient empowerment framework, importance should be given to mutual participation between patient and caregiver, and in improving how well the caregiver and patient can communicate with each other. Barnato et al. noted that, "*In an ideal world [...] patients would come to a cancer consultation armed with sufficient knowledge, clarity about their personal value, and the ability to engage in a thoughtful discussion about the pros and cons of treatment options. Providers, in turn, would be prepared to support their patients, armed with an understanding of the patient's knowledge gaps, personal values about possible outcomes and treatment preferences*" (Barnato et al., 2007). Therefore, it appears critical to develop tools, which can increase the quality of communication, eliciting the emergence of the patient perspective as an individual, while being also time efficient and thus more easily integrated with the current clinical routine.

However, one should keep in mind that focusing on the patient's perspective and beliefs can also reveal patients who, depending on their condition and situation, cannot or do not desire to play an active role in decisions regarding their healthcare. Indeed, some patients do not even prefer a patient-centered or a patient empowerment approach (DeHaes & Koedoot, 2003; Aujoulat et al., 2007). For instance, many patients in palliative cancer treatment have no wish to take part in decision making when their health conditions worsen (DeHaes & Koedoot, 2003). Therefore patient empowerment should not come at the cost of a patient centered approach (Kvåle & Bondevik, 2008), respectful of the extent to which individuals want to participate in decisions on their own health, but rather offer individuals with opportunities, skills and tools to become "empowered". Hospitals often provide patients and families with standard leaflets, which are useful in gaining more knowledge about the disease, available treatment option or side effects of treatments but this is not always enough (Holmstrom & Roing, 2010). Health-care professionals can teach self-management and increase patient's problem solving skills, in order to develop patients' understanding of their situations, and consequently, eliciting actual change and leading to self-management of their disease (Bodenheimer et al., 2002; McCorkle et al., 2011).

Self-management support has been defined by the Institute of Medicine as "*the systematic provision of education and supportive interventions by health care staff to increase patients' skills and confidence in managing their health problems, including regular assessment of progress and problems, goal setting and problem-solving support*" (Adams & Corrigan, 2003). The prioritization of self-management support for cancer survivors not only builds on the evidence that patients want to be involved in healthcare decisions, but it is also grounded on a shift towards a more personalized and tailored approach to care, following cancer treatment. Therefore, there is a greater need for planned supported self-management, so that patients are confident and informed in terms of self-management and the support available to them (Hibbard & Cunningham, 2008). This holds in particular for those forms of cancer, which can be considered more as "chronic". Self-management support should include systematic information and education provision, regular assessment of progress and problem, progressive goal setting as well as problem-solving support and training. Attitudes toward self-management, from the perspective of both the patient and the family, shall be taken into account. Eliciting preferences regarding involvement in healthcare from patients and their families is therefore a pre-requisite to implement self-management interventions, which should be followed by actions that take into account their preferences and their abilities (McCorkle et al., 2011).

Integrating technological self-management support into standard follow-up is fundamental in providing cancer survivors with the knowledge, skills, and confidence to manage the long-term implications of cancer treatment and initiate their own aftercare, when necessary. MHealth technologies provide the opportunity to customize communication, rapidly extract relevant information, and deliver different tools, integrated in a single platform.

Relevant European Union Projects

Several European Union (EU) projects have been implemented for the design and development of personalized health applications for the management of chronic diseases for patient empowerment and self-management. These projects offer the background of implementing health apps for cancer patients. Some of them are briefly presented below:

- **MyHealthAvatar:** "A Demonstration of 4D Digital Avatar Infrastructure for Access of Complete Patient Information" (http://www.myhealthavatar.eu/, 2013-2016) created a graphical representation of the user, acting as a mediator between the end-users and health related data collections, focusing on the interoperability and the data integration aspects. MyHealthAvatar was designed as a lifetime companion for individual citizens to facilitate the collection, the access and the sustainability of health information.
- **ESMART:** The "Electronic Symptom Management System Remote Technology" (https://www.strath.ac.uk/science/computerinformationsciences/esmart/, 2014-2019) demonstrates the effects

of a real-time, mobile phone based, remote patient monitoring intervention on key patient outcomes, and delivery of care provided to people with cancer during and after chemotherapy.

- **DESIREE:** The "Decision Support and Information Management System for Breast Cancer" (http://desiree-project.eu/, 2015-2018) provides a web-based software ecosystem for the personalized, collaborative and multidisciplinary management of primary breast cancer by specialized breast units, from diagnosis to therapy and follow-up.
- **iManageCancer:** "Empowering patients and strengthening self-management in cancer diseases" (http://imanagecancer.eu/, 2015-2018) provided a cancer specific self-management platform designed according to the needs of patient groups. It focused on the wellbeing of cancer patient with special emphasis on avoiding, early detecting and managing adverse events of cancer therapy, and, on the psycho-emotional evaluation and self-motivation goals. In this context, developed cancer specific apps allowed patients, through an easy-to-use interface for mobile devices, to keep track of their health and disease status and to keep a health diary on personal clinical observations such as side effects of therapies, which the patient can share with his healthcare providers. Health and disease status included therapies and results of clinical interventions or tests.
- **CATCH:** "Cancer: Activating Technology for Connected Health" (https://www.catchitn.eu/, 2016-2020) is a Marie Curie action that offers PhD positions in different institutions to research on connected health for patients with cancer. Considering some cancers as chronic disease rather than fatal illness moves the point of focus in the fight against cancer from sustaining life towards maximizing functional capacity and QoL.
- **BOUNCE:** "Predicting Effective Adaptation to Breast Cancer to Help Women to BOUNCE Back" (https://www.bounce-project.eu/, 2017-2021) delivers a unified clinical model of modifiable factors, associated with optimal disease outcomes and advanced computational tools, to be deployed for a prospective multi-centre clinical pilot at four major oncology centers. The overreaching goal of the project is to incorporate elements of a dynamic, predictive model of patient outcomes in building a decision-support system used in routine clinical practice to provide physicians and other health professionals with concrete, personalized recommendations regarding optimal psychosocial support strategies.

Integrated Architecture

In order to implement a mobile app focusing on empowering cancer patients, an integrated, modular and extensible architecture is required. A high-level, two-layer architecture facilitates the development of a multitude of interrelated apps, based on common modules that should be available. A data management layer is collecting and integrating all available data. The graphical user interface layer includes many individual apps offering three kinds of services, administration apps, core patient apps and cancer-specific apps. Generic services (admin and core patient apps), as well as cancer management services, are described first, followed by the description of the data layer that underlines them. The list of presented services is by no means complete. It can be extended with the addition of any relevant modules to support clinical and administrative needs (e.g. for insurance eligibility notification, etc.) not included here. The suggested modular architecture of a cancer mobile app is presented in Figure 1. The apps facilitate the communication and use of data among different supporters including patients, health providers, family, friends and social networks, researchers and policymakers.

Figure 1. Multiple modules required for cancer patient empowerment

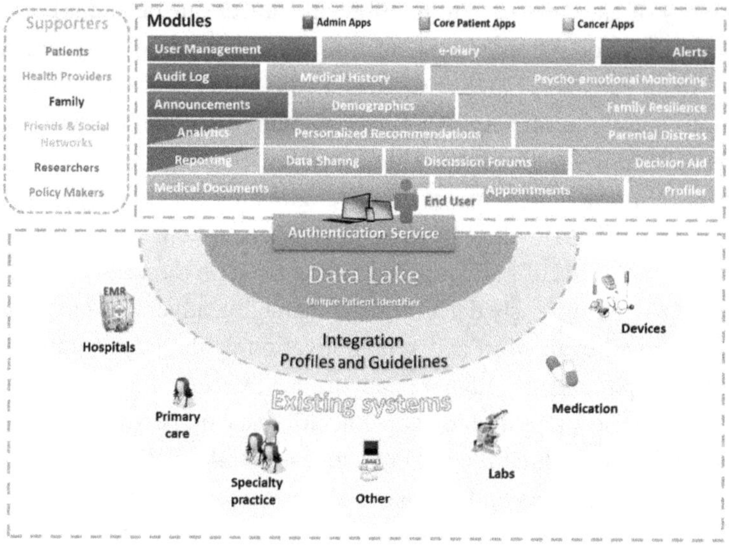

Generic Services

Generic services consist of basic health monitoring modules that should be available to support both admin and core patient services.

Admin services consist of apps enabling user management (registration, complete delete data, remind password etc.), auditing, platform announcements and alerts, and apps for analyzing the available data through data mining algorithms. Only doctors can analyze data that has been shared with them, whereas the administrators can see statistic information about the number of user accounts available, the usage of the platform etc. Individuals should be able to share securely and in compliance with all legal/ ethical national and international requirements their data with other persons and health care services providers. On the other hand, health care service providers should have the necessary modules for visualizing, analyzing and reporting on these data, being able to compare patient status and to communicate offline with patients.

Core patient services consist of apps for mostly capturing medical history such as allergies, problems, procedures, laboratory results, measurements and demographics. All medical documents such as discharge letters, laboratory results, imaging data and others should be able to be stored in one place that the individuals will be able to navigate, search and visualize. Clinical documents such as discharge letters, images and the results from clinical examinations/ admissions can be stored using the documents app. In addition, an app should allow users to share selected data with other users or doctors. A forum and connections to social media in a regulated manner are important for patients as they can discuss health topics of interest and receive a sense of uplifting enhancing the communication aspect of such a platform. An e-diary offers a graphical overview of all available information, based on the appropriate profile settings, enabling also the users to make and view appointments with their doctors. An intelligent personal health recommendation app enables patients to search for health information in a high quality document corpus selected by health experts. Intelligent alerts in case of drug interactions and other serious events detected are also part of such a module.

Cancer Specific Services

Besides generic modules, to support apps for admin and core patient services, there are available cancer specific apps. They provide for questionnaires recording the psycho-emotional status of cancer patients, tools measuring the resilience of the patient's family, and parental distress in case of children. A decision aid app assists patients in making informed decisions about their treatment options based on the individual patient's priorities. All collected information feeds a profiler app enabling the graphical representation of patient profile. These services are further described below:

- **Psycho-Emotional Monitoring:** As cancer highly affects the psycho-emotional status of the individuals, standardized, validated, psycho-behavioral questionnaires should be used in order to monitor psycho-emotional status of cancer patients and their individual resources in coping with cancer. This could feed interventions not only targeting at improving the health status of the patient but also her/ his ability to cope with this disease.
- **Family Resilience:** When a family member faces a potentially terminal illness, the prospect of death presents a crisis and a challenge to the entire family as a system. According to the family systems theory (Bateson, 1970), individuals cannot be understood in isolation from one another, but rather as a part of their family, as the family is an emotional unit (Kerr, 1988). Families are systems of interconnected and interdependent individuals: what happens to one family member affects the other members. To support a holistic management of cancer, tools to measure effectively the family resilience are very relevant. Such tools individuate critical areas that can deplete the patient's resources and help foster interventions that empower the entire family system as required. Those tools shall investigate areas concerning crucial psychological factors within a family such as low esteem/ self-efficacy, negative thinking, emotional reactions, personal sense of competence, self-reliance, health beliefs and other factors. These factors are directly related to interpersonal relationships such as communication and problem solving skills, family disharmony, instability or breakout and family attitudes and values.
- **Parental Distress:** Childhood cancer is one of most stressful situations parents can face (Schepers et al., 2018). Parents experience significant distress at diagnosis and during treatment. A considerable percentage of families develop psychosocial problems and are at risk of ongoing distress (Jantien Vrijmoet-Wiersma et al., 2008). In the same idea of holistic management as the family resilience tool, developing solutions to monitor parental distress is paramount in addressing it effectively. An example of such a tool is the Psychosocial Assessment Tool (PAT) (Pai et al., 2007) designed for families of children with cancer and distinguishes among families that are at universal, targeted or clinical risk for psychosocial problems. However, although such tools already exist, they are used in isolation, and are not combined with other information available for patients and their families.
- **Decision Aid:** These tools translate evidence into a patient-friendly form by providing, at a minimum, information on the options, benefits and risks, and implicit methods to clarify personal values. In addition, many decision aids also include information on the condition, probabilities of the outcomes of options (benefits/ harms), exercises to help patients explicitly clarify their values, and guidance in the steps of decision-making. A variety of decision aids has been developed and proved successful in increasing knowledge, enhance active involvement in decision-making by patients, and decrease patients' decisional anxiety (Gorini et al., 2016). These tools have the poten-

tial to facilitate patient empowerment in the decision-making process. However, there is the need to provide decision aids according to individual characteristics, such as the thinking and decision styles. All these aspects should be considered in order to optimize decision-making.

- **Profiler:** Having all information available from the patient profile, a module should be available to analyze patient answers to the psycho-emotional and family resilience questionnaires, patient choices and decisions in order to create a personal profile in real-time. Using this tool doctors will be able to easily search for a specific patient and visualize results, providing appropriate recommendations.

Data Layer

The bottom layer of the data management architecture is an instantiation of the data lake concept (Koumakis et al., 2018). A state of the art mobile health app for cancer management should have the capacity to connect with external applications, lifestyle sensors and devices. However, the vast amount of data currently generated and collected come in different streams and forms. These range from physician notes, personal health records, images from patient scans, health conversations in social media, continuous streaming information from wearables and other monitoring devices.

For enabling a common representation of knowledge across the continuum of care and across the different information sources, a platform needs to be in place to support information integration and semantic uplifting at runtime, complementing user profiles. Ontologies and semantics can play a key role and big data management infrastructures can help in efficiently processing big amounts of information (Kondylakis et al., 2018). Having a way to model all available information allows both the real-time access over the integrated information and the offline extract, transform, load (ETL) of the semantically transformed and integrated information to a triple store. The benefit of the first approach is that the latest information is always accessed, however at a cost of the execution time. On the other hand, accessing the already transformed information is faster.

Interoperability Issues

Technical challenges for the implementation and adoption of electronic health records (EHRs) and PHRs, have mostly to do with issues relevant to interoperability, device connectivity, security, compliance with national and international legislation regulation, as well as with local policies, usability and accessibility from different devices by users with different profiles (Katehakis, et al., 2017).

Interoperability enables two directional communication between systems and is based on commonly accepted data standards, ensuring accurate data transmission in a secure way. Interoperability between systems is an imperative need in order to better support both clinical work but also economic and social aspects of health care. Due to the continuous ageing of the population, organizations are pushed to make effective use of available clinical and administrative data originating from different sources. Data generated within an organization can be used for different purposes by another organization. For example, in order to provide effective care, clinicians need comprehensive longitudinal data sets, while researchers and policy makers need quality data, in order to support health planning. Innovative use of existing data is also essential for deeper understanding and effective clinical interventions, as in the case of bioinformatics and personalized or precision medicine. Both collaborators and competitors have recognized the need for greater data sharing. Exchange can occur within a small network or it can expand to regions, nations and cross-national initiatives (Sheikh et al., 2017).

Clinical data standards enable healthcare institutions to share clinical information. The permanent availability and accessibility of this information is essential. However, the conventional storage of the information in a proprietary format or database that is only accessible to a single commercial system or application does not suffice because this makes sharing the information across systems impractical. Standardization in medical informatics enables the interconnection and the interoperability between both care and research systems, as well as the alignment of local clinical systems for easier data integration. In other words, it is very important that the specific meaning is preserved across information systems. Semantic interoperability guarantees that both transmitter and recipient interpret the shared information identically. Indeed, clinical data standards should enable the transfer of data and its metadata between clinics in different geographical locations, with possibly different local languages, in such a way that continuity of medical care and aggregation of medical research is made possible.

Fully interoperable electronic medical record systems are not yet a wide reality. Some degree of standardized transmission has been achieved but true semantic interoperability exists only in limited settings including EHR components. Interoperability can advance only through sustained efforts to address clinical needs and financial constraints. A broader view of interoperability is required, as consumers move towards alternative approaches of care including mobile, wearable and home based technologies. Wide commercial availability of health care apps, sensor systems, and wearable technologies as well as the new home monitoring and communication systems technologies require viewing interoperability as an integration of entertainment, communication, home management and health. Interoperability is a primary consideration to achieve communication of applications, medical devices and health care providers. In addition, the growing demand to secondary use of clinical and administrative data renders the pressure towards solving interoperability challenges more imperative.

Efforts towards standardizing population-based cancer surveillance in the United States and Canada has led to the design of a document to guide EHR vendors and public health central cancer registries in the implementation of standardized electronic reporting (Kussaibi et al., 2010; National Center for Chronic Disease Prevention and Health Promotion, 2014; HL7 International, 2015). It includes both business rules and standardized specifications. Such a standard can be used with third party terminologies such as the Current Procedures Terminology (CPT) code set (American Medical Association, 2018), SNOMED CT (SNOMED International, 2018), Logical Observation Identifiers Names & Codes (LOINC) (Regenstrief Institute, 2018), and International Classification of Diseases (ICD) codes (World Health Organization, 2018b). In addition, several ontologies have been defined specifically for cancer, trying to integrate other existing biomedical ontologies such as the ACGT MO (Brochhausen et al., 2011) and the MHA Semantic Core Ontology (Kondylakis et al., 2015).

Organizations such as Health Level Seven International (HL7) (Health Level Seven International, 2018) and Personal Connected Health Alliance (PCHAlliance) Continua (Personal Connected Health Alliance, 2018) help towards the delivery of standards-based, open specifications that can support the flow of data from the point of capture into EHRs in the same format and coded content. Consensus on systems requirements is also important. Integrating the Healthcare Enterprise (IHE) (Integrating the Healthcare Enterprise, 2018) describes how standards may be used effectively.

In the context of HL7 and lightweight semantic interoperability, it is important to mention Fast Healthcare Interoperability Resources (FHIR) (pronounced 'fire'), which is a next generation standards framework created by HL7 (HL7 International, 2018). FHIR combines the best features of HL7's v2,

HL7 v3 and CDA (Boone, 2011) product lines while leveraging the latest web standards and applying a tight focus on implementability. FHIR defines a set of "resources" for health. These resources represent granular clinical concepts that can be exchanged in order to quickly and effectively solve problems in healthcare and related processes. The resources cover the basic elements of healthcare - patients, admissions, diagnostic reports, medications and problem lists - with their typical participants and support a range of richer and more complex clinical models. Several restricted message information models (RMIMs) are being represented into the resource description framework (RDF) in order to support semantic interoperability. FHIR resource definitions do not directly promise semantically consistent data out-of-the-box. Instead, to serve distinct contexts (e.g., EHRs, public health reporting workflows, wearable devices), FHIR resources might use specific data payloads with distinct terminologies.

SMART on FHIR is an example of a platform developed to support interoperable apps for EHRs (Mandel et al., 2016). Server implementers can create FHIR implementations with a small set of FHIR resources and incrementally expand coverage to address priorities. Implementation entails creating EHR-specific logic to transform internal data structures to corresponding FHIR resources and with SMART-specified profiles. SMART aimed to produce specifications that work for forward-thinking medical app developers and are implementable within today's evolving healthcare technology landscape (SMART, 2018).

Apps exploiting both SMART and FHIR, specifically for cancer, have already started to emerge. An example of such apps is SMART precision cancer medicine, a FHIR based app to provide cancer genomic information at the point of care (Warner et al., 2016). In addition, a proprietary version of SMART is also supported from a suite of tools designed for cancer management within the iManageCancer EU project (Kondylakis et al., 2017a).

Security Considerations

To ensure that privacy and personal data of patients are protected, the current EU General Data Protection Regulation (GDPR) obligates data controllers to adopt data protection by design and by default approach in developing systems that process personal data. The GDPR is a regulation of general application and is principles-based. It includes the principle that the protection of personal data shall be a default property of personal data information systems, which is captured in an obligation of data controllers to implement data protection by design and by default. This means that data controllers must implement the data protection principles, facilitate the enforcement of the data subjects' rights, as well as implement technical and organizational measures to secure the personal data under their care. Several options have been put forward regarding operationalization of privacy by design. Cavoukian, for example, notes that the broad concept of privacy by design encompasses many elements in practice (Cavoukian, 2011), and further develops seven fundamental privacy by design principles which suggests strategies for implementing privacy by design. The EU Agency for Network and Information Security (ENISA) has also published several documents on strategies and ways of implementing privacy by design (European Union Agency for Network and Information Security, 2018).

A fundamental principle of a personal health record is that the patient is the owner of his/ her own data and controls the access for others like healthcare professionals family, and friends. Apart from the data sharing issue, which rises due to this principle, a secure framework for the authorization, authentication, delegation, and auditing is mandatory for secure access and communication between services and patient interaction with the platform. Every patient registered to the platform can upload all kind of data into his/ her account. As these data are private and sensible, specific requirements for data protection have to be addressed. More specifically, apps should support:

- Roles and rights management to control access to the platform.
- Secure upload of data via a Hyper Text Transfer Protocol with Secure Sockets Layer (HTTPS).
- Data storage in an encrypted way.
- Patient full control over his/ her data. The patient can upload, edit and delete his/ her data at any time without giving a reason.
- Uploaded data belong to the patient.
- Secondary usage of data is only possible after anonymization of the data (Koumakis et al., 2018).
- Signing of contracts for secondary usage of anonymized data between the patient (data provider) and the data user (Kondylakis et al., 2017b).
- Patient capacity to sharing of data with other people at any time. These people are not allowed to download, edit or delete the data. They gain only the allowance to read the data after signing a contract with the patient.
- An audit trail system monitoring all the actions in the platform.

Based on the existing technologies, OAuth v2.0 is the de facto standard for authorization and communication with a web based or mobile application (OAuth 2.0, 2018). With OAuth users can revoke a specific application program interface (API) client without affect other API clients, nor does user need to change password (e.g. in case one API party's server is hacked). A new promising technology for information, communication and technology (ICT) security and especially for the auditing mechanism is blockchain. Blockchain is like a distributed ledger that has all the details for every transaction. Each transaction is validated and authenticated by protected digital signatures (cryptography). In blockchain, there is no central point of access and anyone can process transactions using the computing power. The fundamental strength of a blockchain system lies in its data integrity and networked immutability (write once and read only) digital events that can be applied in the healthcare domain (Kuo et al., 2017). Furthermore, blockchain may have significant potential to improve data interoperability in the healthcare domain (Linn & Koo, 2016).

Software Quality Assurance

Software quality assurance consists of a methods and tools to monitor the software engineering processes in order to ensure quality. Software validation and verification activities should be conducted throughout the entire software life cycle. The scope of verification is to check that a product, service, or system (or portion thereof, or set thereof) meets a set of initial design requirements, specifications, and regulations. In the development phase, verification procedures involve performing special tests to model or simulate a portion, or the entirety, of the application. Validation is the process of evaluating software during or at the end of the development process to assure the quality of desired outcome.

The design and evaluation of any app should adhere to certain principles of systems and software engineering, such as the ones defined by ISO 25000 series for systems and software quality requirements and evaluation (International Organization for Standardization, 2014). A set of functional and non-functional requirements have to be collected by the development team (based on the needs of the end users), implemented and validated (by the development team) and evaluated (by end users). Different requirements exist for different components such as the security mechanism, the application programming interfaces (mainly for the communication with the databases) and end user interface. ISO 25000 has organized the requirement into eight main categories, and its respective sub-categories, including functional suitability, performance efficiency, compatibility, usability, reliability, security maintainability and portability.

Common conformity assessment schemes for interoperability of health systems needs to be in place in order to promote the adoption and take-up of interoperability testing of eHealth solutions against identified eHealth standards and profiles. In addition, quality assurance through quality labeling is very important to promote the design, development and implementation of functional and effective applications.

SOLUTIONS AND RECOMMENDATIONS

Understanding factors that promote resilience may help people suffering chronic diseases to not only cope with unpredictable changes in health and abilities, but to thrive in spite of these changes. This should not be done at the expense of compromising patient security and safety, and this includes secondary use of data and appropriate management of information security issues related to biomedical research.

The continuous advancements in healthcare practice, the limitations of the traditional healthcare processes and the need for flexible access to health information, create a continuous demand for the retrieval, processing and exchange of EHR information among all relevant stakeholders. Patient empowerment benefits give incredible potential to all relevant stakeholder communities, including patients and their associations, caretakers, healthcare professionals, healthcare providers, policy makers, academia, public authorities, technology companies, and others. Patients expect to be in a position to access and share their own data, as well as to be in a position to provide feedback on quality of treatments. Technological advancements and better access of patients to digital tools are capable to support patient empowerment to combat chronic diseases, by allowing targeted and faster research, more secure access to health data and their exchange, and by enabling patients to interact with their doctors and caretakers more effectively.

Adequately informed patients, who share decision-making with their medical team, have been shown to have greater autonomy and physical well-being within randomized and prospective observational studies. Patients offered higher levels of information also tend to have improved compliance, and significantly reduced anxiety and depression (Davies et al., 2008). If they are not adequately informed, the anger and frustration associated with an inability to understand their treatment options can lead to anxiety, depression, poor compliance and cooperation with strategies to reduce treatment related side effects. Information is especially important in the area of lifestyle, since published evidence has highlighted that patients who decide to improve their lifestyle will have major benefits in terms of quality of life and physical outcomes. Figure 2 demonstrates a typical overview of an integration platform for the sharing of medical information between patients and healthcare professionals, within the context of a national health system.

National infrastructures in Europe provide for horizontal electronic Government (eGov) services (such as for electronic identification), as well as electronic services to support national health systems (e.g. for eConfirmation, eReimbursement, ePrescription, and others). Services are provided to both the public, as well as the private sector (i.e. primary care, hospitals, clinical centers, pharmacies, etc.). An integration platform, operating under specific interoperability agreements, may provide for (indicatively) certain home care, decision support, and research services.

Figure 2. Typical medical information integration platform to support coordinated care within a National Health System

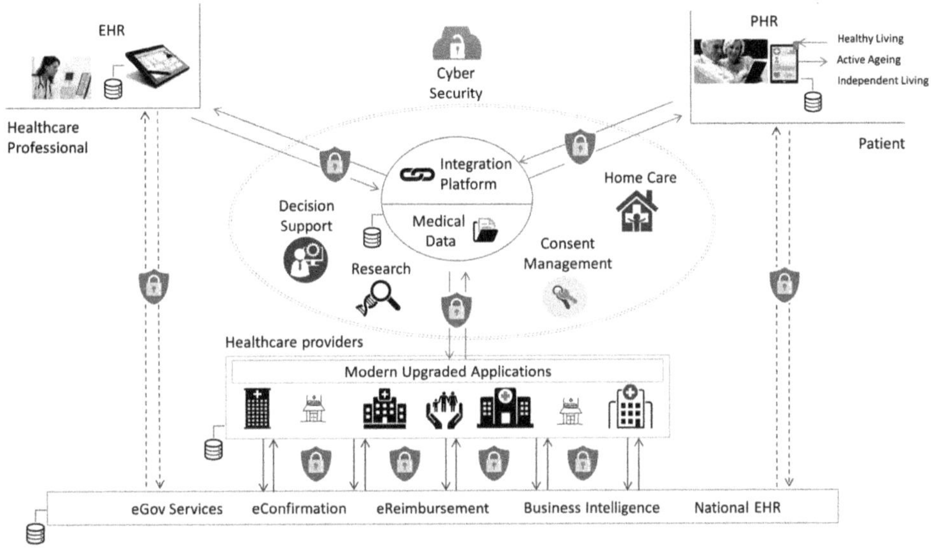

The widespread adoption of mobile technologies facilitates the introduction of new and innovative ways to improve health care delivery. Citizens can now use them to manage their own health and promote healthy living and active ageing by accessing useful information and linking to useful resources when needed; healthcare professionals and patients included.

Apps available cannot replace e.g. an oncologist, but they can provide the means to make the painful process easier for patients and their families during the treatment. Apps do not intend to diagnose or treat cancer by themselves. Still they can aid for early cancer diagnosis and treatment, provided they are tested and certified properly. For doing so, proper regulation is required and a framework to support interoperability at all levels (at home, at primary care, at the hospital, regionally, at a national or international level) for all relevant use cases (eHealth Network, 2015).

Screenshots of possible graphic interfaces of a cancer app are shown in Figure 3.

Limiting semantic fragmentation is a key challenge to address. Properly designed data (structure ad semantics) and authentication application program interfaces can successfully shield mobile app developers from complexity in integrating with proprietary vendor systems.

FUTURE RESEARCH DIRECTIONS

The proposed approach and integrated architecture for the development of high quality health apps for cancer does not replace medical practice but rather enhances and facilitates patient management. The platform, acting as a facilitator, supports a more effective management of cancer chronic conditions and their psycho-emotional aspects. Further work needs to be conducted, in order for the proposed architecture to be in a position to better fit available methodologies and treatments, as well as local configuration needs. Relevant challenges are relevant to the management of interoperability and security issues, as well

Figure 3. The graphical user interface of a mobile app for the citizen

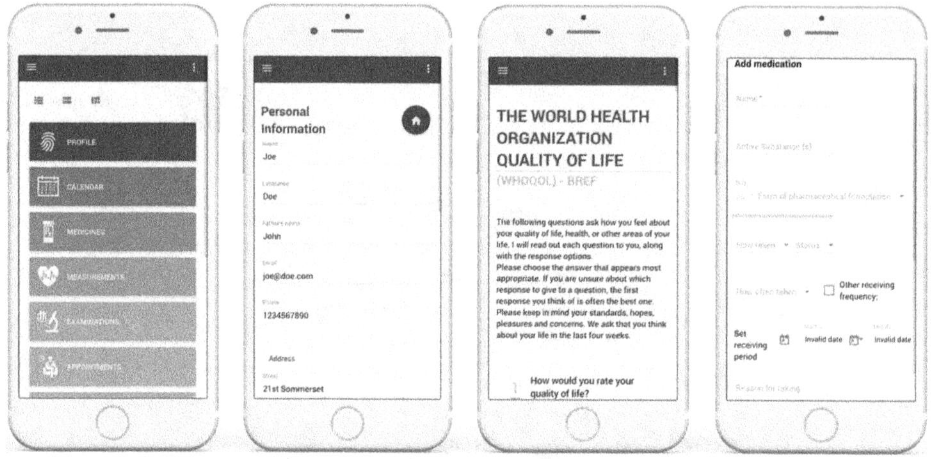

as patient motivation to introduce valuable data. Further issues under investigation include the provision of timely feedback, tailored educational material to patient needs and comprehension capabilities, patient guidance to relevant connections, effective communication support between patients and clinicians, filtering of relevant information, and usage of data for research purposes. Some of the indicated problems, as far as PHR adoption is concerned, include usability, privacy, security, and complexity of use. Main difficulties that remain are questionable quality of the data its interpretation (Roehrs et al., 2017).

Future research in apps for cancer patients need to focus on the challenges and issues related to security, privacy, and trust, and ways to help users gain confidence in adopting the PHR. Other aspects for future study involve the improvement of user experience looking at usability, personalization, familiarity, and comfort. In addition, it is important to envision an expanded PHR that will include wearable computing, IoT, and artificial intelligence. As these technologies mature and are applied to health, new frontiers will be open in the improvement of the user experience.

Evidence-based information and medical professional involvement in design and implementation of cancer apps need to become more common to better support behavior change, decision making following diagnosis, but also the difficult aspects of end-of-life decisions and care. Further research should explore expectations of users about usability features of applications related to cancer in general and to specific cancers.

Work relevant to EHR interoperability for data exchange is still ongoing. Standardization organizations such as HL7 already work towards the development of functional models to improve providers' workflows to support the timely transition of relevant clinical information at each point of care. This requires a systems engineering perspective, which considers all parts of the ecosystem and collaborative activity between care team members, where the patient and designated family caregivers are considered as members of the care team (Katehakis et al., 2017). Key issues include not matching semantic standards, quality needs and safe data exchange techniques. These limit the opportunities to reuse these data for research and better healthcare since they are usually kept in data silos.

CONCLUSION

The World Health Organization has set forth the global action plan for the prevention and control of noncommunicable diseases (NCDs) (World Health Organization, 2018c). This plan calls for six policy actions: (i) prevention and control of NCDs needs to become a priority in global, regional and national agendas; (ii) national response needs to be accelerated through leadership, governance and multisector action; (iii) risk factors and underlying social determinants need to be reduced through the creation of health-promoting environments; (iv) health systems need to be oriented and strengthened towards prevention and control through people centered health care and coverage; (v) national capacity for high-quality research and development needs to be promoted and supported; and (vi) trends and determinants of NCDs need to be monitored.

As cancer has been transformed into a chronic disease, cancer survival means living with a chronic and complex condition. As mobile technologies have become integral part of daily life, there is a great opportunity using effectively mobile applications for empowering cancer patients. As there is a vast number of parameters affecting the long-term management of the disease, fragmented approaches do not unleash the potential benefits of an integrated mobile app. A holistic integrated mobile app should focus on all areas of the cancer continuum, from prevention, surveillance, intervention for consequences of cancer and its treatment to coordination between specialists and care providers and rehabilitation. To the best of the authors' knowledge, such an app currently does not exist. This chapter has presented a holistic approach and a set of requirements for the design and implementation of state of the art patient centered mobile cancer applications focusing on patient empowerment and self-management.

REFERENCES

Adams, K., & Corrigan, J. M. (2003). *Priority Areas for National Action: Transforming Health Care Quality*. Washington, DC: National Academies Press.

Al-Falahy, N., & Alani, O. Y. (2017). Technologies for 5G Networks: Challenges and Opportunities. *IEEE IT Professional*, *19*(1), 12–20. doi:10.1109/MITP.2017.9

American Medical Association. (2018), *CPT® (Current Procedural Terminology)*. Retrieved from https://www.ama-assn.org/practice-management/cpt-current-procedural-terminology

Aujoulat, I., D' Hoore, W., & Deccache, A. (2007). Patient empowerment in theory and practice: Polysemy or cacophony? *Patient Education and Counseling*, *66*(1), 13–20. doi:10.1016/j.pec.2006.09.008 PMID:17084059

Barnato, A. E., Llewellyn-Thomas, H. A., Peters, E. M., Siminoff, L., Collins, E. D., & Barry, M. J. (2007). Communication and Decision Making in Cancer Care: Setting Research Priorities for Decision Support/ Patients' Decision Aids. *Medical Decision Making*, *27*(5), 626–634. doi:10.1177/0272989X07306788 PMID:17873249

Basch, E., Deal, A. M., Kris, M. G., Scher, H. I., Hudis, C. A., Sabbatini, P., ... Schrag, D. (2016). Symptom monitoring with patient-reported outcomes during routine cancer treatment: A randomized controlled trial. *Journal of Clinical Oncology*, *34*(6), 557–565. doi:10.1200/JCO.2015.63.0830 PMID:26644527

Bateson, G. (1970). A systems approach. *International Journal of Psychiatry*, *9*, 242–244. PMID:5482974

Baudendistel, I., Winkler, E., Kamradt, M., Brophy, S., Längst, G., Eckrich, F., ... Ose, D. (2015). The patients' active role in managing a personal electronic health record: A qualitative analysis. *Supportive Care in Cancer*, *23*(9), 2613–2621. doi:10.100700520-015-2620-1 PMID:25652149

Bender, J. L., Yue, R. Y. K., To, M. J., Deacken, L., & Jadad, A. R. (2013). A lot of action, but not in the right direction: Systematic review and content analysis of smartphone applications for the prevention, detection, and management of cancer. *Journal of Medical Internet Research*, *15*(12), e287. doi:10.2196/jmir.2661 PMID:24366061

Bodenheimer, T., Lorig, K., Holman, H., & Grumbach, K. (2002). Patient self-management of chronic disease in primary care. *Journal of the American Medical Association*, *288*(19), 2469–2475. doi:10.1001/jama.288.19.2469 PMID:12435261

Boone, K. W. (2011). *The CDA Tm Book*. Springer Science & Business Media. doi:10.1007/978-0-85729-336-7

Boulos, M. N. K., Brewer, A. C., Karimkhani, C., Buller, D. B., & Robert, P. (2014). Mobile medical and health apps : State of the art, concerns, regulatory control and certification. *Online Journal of Public Health Informatics*, *5*(3), 1–23. PMID:24683442

Brochhausen, M., Spear, A. D., Cocos, C., Weiler, G., Martín, L., Anguita, A., ... Sfakianakis, S. (2011). The ACGT Master Ontology and its applications–Towards an ontology-driven cancer research and management system. *Journal of Biomedical Informatics*, *44*(1), 8–25. doi:10.1016/j.jbi.2010.04.008 PMID:20438862

Cavoukian, A. (2011). *Privacy by design in law, policy and practice: a white paper for regulators, decision-makers and policy-makers*. Retrieved from http://www.ontla.on.ca/library/repository/mon/25008/312239.pdf

Collado-Borrell, R., Escudero-Vilaplana, V., Ribed-Sánchez, A., Ibáñez-García, S., Herranz-Alonso, A., & Sanjurjo-Sáez, M. (2016). Smartphone applications for cancer patients; what we know about them. *Farmacia Hospitalaria*, *40*(1), 25–35. PMID:26882831

Cucciniello, M., Guerrazzi, C., Nasi, G., & Ongaro, E. (2015). Coordination mechanisms for implementing Complex Innovations in the Health Care Sector. *Public Management Review*, *17*(7), 1040–1060. doi:10.1080/14719037.2015.1029348

Cucciniello, M., & Nasi, G. (2014). Transparency for trust in government: How effective is formal transparency? *International Journal of Public Administration*, *37*(13), 911–921. doi:10.1080/01900692.2014.949754

Davies, N. J., Kinman, G., Thomas, R. J., & Bailey, T. (2008). Information satisfaction in breast and prostate cancer patients: Implications for quality of life. *Psycho-Oncology*, *17*(10), 1048–1052. doi:10.1002/pon.1305 PMID:18203242

DeHaes, H., & Koedoot, N. (2003). Patient centred decision making in palliative cancer treatment: A world of paradoxes. *Patient Education and Counseling*, *50*(1), 43–49. doi:10.1016/S0738-3991(03)00079-X PMID:12767584

Denis, F., Lethrosne, C., Pourel, N., Molinier, O., Pointreau, Y., Domont, J., ... Letellier, C. (2017). Randomized trial comparing a web-mediated follow-up with routine surveillance in lung cancer patients. *JNCI. Journal of the National Cancer Institute*, *109*(9). doi:10.1093/jnci/djx029 PMID:28423407

Dogac, A. (2012). Interoperability in eHealth systems. *Proceedings of the VLDB Endowment International Conference on Very Large Data Bases*, *5*(12), 2026–2027. doi:10.14778/2367502.2367568

eHealth Network. (2015). *Refined eHealth European interoperability framework*. Retrieved from http://ec.europa.eu/health//sites/health/files/ehealth/docs/ev_20151123_co03_en.pdf

Elwyn, G., Frosch, D. L., & Kobrin, S. (2015). Implementing shared decision-making: Consider all the consequences. *Implementation Science; IS*, *11*(1), 114. doi:10.118613012-016-0480-9 PMID:27502770

European Union Agency for Network and Information Security. (2018). *Handbook on security of personal data processing*. Retrieved from https://www.enisa.europa.eu/publications/handbook-on-security-of-personal-data-processing

Fife, E., & Pereira, F. (2011). Digital home health and mHealth: prospects and challenges for adoption in the U.S. FITCE 50th Congress (FITCE), 1-11.

Fiordelli, M., Diviani, N., & Schulz, P. J. (2013). Mapping mhealth research: A decade of evolution. *Journal of Medical Internet Research*, *15*(5), e95. doi:10.2196/jmir.2430 PMID:23697600

Friis, L. S., Elverdam, B., & Schmidt, K. G. (2003). The patient's perspective. *Supportive Care in Cancer*, *11*(3), 162–170. PMID:12618926

Gerber, D. E., Laccetti, A. L., Chen, B., Yan, J., Cai, J., Gates, S., ... Lee, S. J. C. (2014). Predictors and intensity of online access to electronic medical records among patients with cancer. *Journal of Oncology Practice / American Society of Clinical Oncology*, *10*(5), e307–e312. doi:10.1200/JOP.2013.001347 PMID:25006222

Girault, A., Ferrua, M., Lalloué, B., Sicotte, C., Fourcade, A., Yatim, F., ... Minvielle, E. (2015). Internet-based technologies to improve cancer care coordination: Current use and attitudes among cancer patients. *European Journal of Cancer*, *51*(4), 551–557. doi:10.1016/j.ejca.2014.12.001 PMID:25661828

Gorini, A., Masiero, M., & Pravettoni, G. (2016). Patient decision aids for prevention and treatment of cancer diseases: Are they really personalised tools? *European Journal of Cancer Care*, *25*(6), 936–960. doi:10.1111/ecc.12451 PMID:26856816

HL7 International (2015). *HL7 CDA ® Release 2 Implementation Guide: Reporting to Public Health Cancer Registries from Ambulatory Healthcare Providers*. Release 1, DSTU Release 1.1 – US Realm.

HL7 International. (2018). *FHIR Release 3*. Retrieved from http://www.hl7.org/fhir/

Health Level Seven International. (2018). *Homepage*. Retrieved from http://www.hl7.org/

Heinrich, C., & Kuiper, R. A. (2012). Using handheld devices to promote medication adherence in chronic illness. *The Journal for Nurse Practitioners*, *8*(4), 288–293. doi:10.1016/j.nurpra.2011.10.010

Hewitt, M., Greenfield, S., & Stovall, E. (Eds.). (2005). *From cancer patient to cancer survivor: lost in transition*. National Academies Press.

Hibbard, J. H., & Cunningham, P. J. (2008). How engaged are consumers in their health and health care, and why does it matter? *Research Brief*, (8), 1–9.

Holmstrom, I., & Roing, M. (2010). The relation between patient-centredness and patient empowerment: A discussion on concepts. *Patient Education and Counseling*, *79*(2), 167–172. doi:10.1016/j.pec.2009.08.008 PMID:19748203

Iconomou, G., Viha, A., Koutras, A., Vagenakis, A. G., & Kalofonos, H. P. (2002). Information needs and awareness of diagnosis in patients with cancer receiving chemotherapy: A report from Greece. *Palliative Medicine*, *16*(4), 315–321. doi:10.1191/0269216302pm574oa PMID:12132544

Integrating the Healthcare Enterprise. (2018). *Homepage*. Retrieved from http://www.ihe.net/

International Agency for Research on Cancer. (2015). *World cancer report 2014*. Retrieved from https://www.iarc.fr/en/publications/pdfs-online/wcr/2003/WorldCancerReport.pdf

International Organization for Standardization. (2014). *ISO/ IEC 25000:2014, Systems and software engineering -- Systems and software Quality Requirements and Evaluation (SQuaRE) -- Guide to SQuaRE. ISO/ IEC JTC 1/ SC 7, Software and systems engineering*. Retrieved from https://www.iso.org/standard/64764.html

Jantien Vrijmoet-Wiersma, C. M., van Klink, J. M., Kolk, A. M., Koopman, H. M., Ball, L. M., & Maarten Egeler, R. (2008). Assessment of parental psychological stress in pediatric cancer: A review. *Journal of Pediatric Psychology*, *33*(7), 694–706. doi:10.1093/jpepsy/jsn007 PMID:18287109

Jones, P., & Melei, A. I. (1993). Health is empowerment. *Advances in Nursing Science*, *15*(3), 1–14. doi:10.1097/00012272-199303000-00003 PMID:8434899

Katehakis, D. G., Kondylakis, H., Koumakis, L., Kouroubali, A., & Marias, K. (2017). Integrated care solutions for the citizen: Personal health record functional models to support interoperability. *EJBI*, *13*(1), 41–56.

Katehakis, D. G., & Tsiknakis, M. (2006). *Electronic Health Record. Wiley Encyclopedia of Biomedical Engineering*. Hoboken, NJ: John Wiley & Sons, Inc.

Kerr, M. E. (1988). *Family evaluation: an approach based on Bowen theory*. New York: Norton.

Kessel, K. A., Vogel, M. M., Kessel, C., Bier, H., Biedermann, T., Friess, H., ... Combs, S. E. (2017). Mobile health in oncology: A patient survey about app-assisted cancer care. *JMIR mHealth and uHealth*, *5*(6), e81. doi:10.2196/mhealth.7689 PMID:28615159

Klasnja, P., Hartzler, A., Powell, C., Phan, G., & Pratt, W. (2010). Health weaver mobile: Designing a mobile tool for managing personal health information during cancer care. *AMIA ... Annual Symposium Proceedings - AMIA Symposium. AMIA Symposium*, *2010*, 392–396. PMID:21347007

Kondylakis, H., Bucur, A., Dong, F., Renzi, C., Manfrinati, A., Graf, N., . . . Kiefer, S. (2017a). iManage-Cancer: Developing a Platform for Empowering Patients and Strengthening Self-Management in Cancer Diseases. *Computer-Based Medical Systems (CBMS), IEEE 30th International Symposium*, 755-760.

Kondylakis, H., Koumakis, L., Hänold, S., Nwankwo, I., Forgó, N., Marias, K., & Graf, N. (2017b). Donor's support tool: Enabling informed secondary use of patient's biomaterial and personal data. *International Journal of Medical Informatics*, *97*, 282–292. doi:10.1016/j.ijmedinf.2016.10.019 PMID:27919386

Kondylakis, H., Koumakis, L., Tsiknakis, M., & Marias, K. (2018). Implementing a data management infrastructure for big healthcare data. *IEEE EMBS International Conference on Biomedical & Health Informatics (BHI)*, 361-364.

Kondylakis, H., Spanakis, E. G., Sfakianakis, S., Sakkalis, V., Tsiknakis, M., Marias, K., . . . Dong, F. (2015). Digital patient: Personalized and translational data management through the MyHealthAvatar EU project. *Engineering in Medicine and Biology Society (EMBC), 2015 37th Annual International Conference of the IEEE*, 1397-1400.

Kotronoulas, G., Kearney, N., Maguire, R., Harrow, A., Di Domenico, D., Croy, S., & MacGillivray, S. (2014). What is the value of the routine use of patient-reported outcome measures toward improvement of patient outcomes, processes of care, and health service outcomes in cancer care? A systematic review of controlled trials. *Journal of Clinical Oncology*, *32*(14), 1480–1501. doi:10.1200/JCO.2013.53.5948 PMID:24711559

Koumakis, L., Kondylakis, H., Katehakis, D. G., Iatraki, G., Argyropaidas, P., Hatzimina, M., & Marias, K. (2018). A content-aware analytics framework for open health data. Precision Medicine Powered by pHealth and Connected Health, 59–64.

Kuo, T. T., Kim, H. E., & Ohno-Machado, L. (2017). Blockchain distributed ledger technologies for biomedical and health care applications. *Journal of the American Medical Informatics Association*, *24*(6), 1211–1220. doi:10.1093/jamia/ocx068 PMID:29016974

Kushi, L. H., Doyle, C., McCullough, M., Rock, C. L., Demark-Wahnefried, W., Bandera, E. V., ... Gansler, T. (2012). American Cancer Society Guidelines on nutrition and physical activity for cancer prevention: Reducing the risk of cancer with healthy food choices and physical activity. *CA: a Cancer Journal for Clinicians*, *62*(1), 30–67. doi:10.3322/caac.20140 PMID:22237782

Kussaibi, H., Macary, F., Kennedy, M., Booker, D., Brodsky, V., Schrader, T., ... Daniel, C. (2010). HL7 CDA implementation guide for structured anatomic pathology reports methodology and tools. *Studies in Health Technology and Informatics*, *160*(Pt 1), 289–293. PMID:20841695

Kvåle, K., & Bondevik, M. (2008). What is important for patient centred care? A qualitative study about the perceptions of patients with cancer. *Scandinavian Journal of Caring Sciences*, *22*(4), 582–589. doi:10.1111/j.1471-6712.2007.00579.x PMID:19000089

Linn, L. A., & Koo, M. B. (2016). Blockchain for health data and its potential use in health it and health care related research. In *ONC/NIST Use of Blockchain for Healthcare and Research Workshop*. Gaithersburg, MD: ONC/NIST.

Maher, E. J. (2013). Managing the consequences of cancer treatment and the English National Cancer Survivorship Initiative. *Acta Oncologica, 52*(2), 225–232. doi:10.3109/0284186X.2012.746467 PMID:23237053

Mandel, J. C., Kreda, D. A., Mandl, K. D., Kohane, I. S., & Ramoni, R. B. (2016). SMART on FHIR: A standards-based, interoperable apps platform for electronic health records. *Journal of the American Medical Informatics Association, 23*(5), 899–908. doi:10.1093/jamia/ocv189 PMID:26911829

Martínez-Pérez, B., De La Torre-Díez, I., & López-Coronado, M. (2015). Privacy and security in mobile health apps: A review and recommendations. *Journal of Medical Systems, 39*(1), 181. doi:10.100710916-014-0181-3 PMID:25486895

McCorkle, R., Ercolano, E., Lazenby, M., Schulman-Green, D., Schilling, L. S., Lorig, K., & Wagner, E. H. (2011). Self-management: Enabling and empowering patients living with cancer as a chronic illness. *CA: a Cancer Journal for Clinicians, 61*(1), 50–62. doi:10.3322/caac.20093 PMID:21205833

McGuire, S. (2016). World Cancer Report 2014. Geneva, Switzerland: World Health Organization.

Mobasheri, M. H., Johnston, M., King, D., Leff, D., Thiruchelvam, P., & Darzi, A. (2014). Smartphone breast applications - What's the evidence? *The Breast, 23*(5), 4–10. doi:10.1016/j.breast.2014.07.006 PMID:25153432

Nasi, G., Cucciniello, M., & Guerrazzi, C. (2015). The role of mobile technologies in health care processes: The case of cancer supportive care. *Journal of Medical Internet Research, 17*(2), e26. doi:10.2196/jmir.3757 PMID:25679446

National Center for Chronic Disease Prevention and Health Promotion, Division of Cancer Prevention and Control. (2014). *Implementation Guide for Ambulatory Healthcare Provider Reporting to Central Cancer Registries, HL7 Clinical Document Architecture (CDA), Release 1.1.* IHE International. Retrieved from https://www.cdc.gov/phin/resources/guides/documents/implementation_guide_for_ambulatory_healthcare_provider_reporting_to_central_cancer_registries_march_2014.pdf

OAuth 2.0 (2018). *An open protocol to allow secure authorization in a simple and standard method from web, mobile and desktop applications.* Retrieved from https://oauth.net/

Pai, A. L., Patiño-Fernández, A. M., McSherry, M., Beele, D., Alderfer, M. A., Reilly, A. T., ... Kazak, A. E. (2007). The Psychosocial Assessment Tool (PAT2. 0): Psychometric properties of a screener for psychosocial distress in families of children newly diagnosed with cancer. *Journal of Pediatric Psychology, 33*(1), 50–62. doi:10.1093/jpepsy/jsm053 PMID:17609228

Parkin, D. M., Boyd, L., & Walker, L. C. (2011). 16. The fraction of cancer attributable to lifestyle and environmental factors in the UK in 2010. *British Journal of Cancer, 105*(S2), S77–S81. doi:10.1038/bjc.2011.489 PMID:22158327

Personal Connected Health Alliance. (2018). *Homepage.* Retrieved from http://www.pchalliance.org/

Regenstrief Institute. (2018). LOINC: *The universal standard for identifying health measurements, observations, and documents.* Retrieved from https://loinc.org/

Rincon, E., Monteiro-Guerra, F., Rivera-Romero, O., Dorronzoro-Zubiete, E., Sanchez-Bocanegra, C. L., & Gabarron, E. (2017). Mobile Phone Apps for Quality of Life and Well-Being Assessment in Breast and Prostate Cancer Patients: Systematic Review. *JMIR mHealth and uHealth*, *5*(12), e187. doi:10.2196/mhealth.8741 PMID:29203459

Roehrs, A., Da Costa, C. A., Da Rosa Righi, R., & De Oliveira, K. S. F. (2017). Personal health records: A systematic literature review. *Journal of Medical Internet Research*, *19*(1), e13. doi:10.2196/jmir.5876 PMID:28062391

Ruland, C. M., Andersen, T., Jeneson, A., Moore, S., Grimsbø, G. H., Børøsund, E., & Ellison, M. C. (2013). Effects of an internet support system to assist cancer patients in reducing symptom distress: A randomized controlled trial. *Cancer Nursing*, *36*(1), 6–17. doi:10.1097/NCC.0b013e31824d90d4 PMID:22495503

Schepers, S. A., Sint Nicolaas, S. M., Maurice-Stam, H., Haverman, L., Verhaak, C. M., & Grootenhuis, M. A. (2018). Parental distress 6 months after a pediatric cancer diagnosis in relation to family psychosocial risk at diagnosis. *Cancer*, *124*(2), 381–390. doi:10.1002/cncr.31023 PMID:28902391

Sheikh, A., Cresswell, K., Wright, A., & Bates, D. (2017). *Key Advances in Clinical Informatics: Transforming Health Care through Health Information Technology*. Academic Press.

SMART®. (2018). *An App Platform for Healthcare*. Retrieved from https://smarthealthit.org/

SNOMED International. (2018). *SNOMED CT: The Global Language of Healthcare*. Retrieved from https://www.snomed.org/snomed-ct

Stoyanov, S. R., Hides, L., Kavanagh, D. J., Zelenko, O., Tjondronegoro, D., & Mani, M. (2015). Mobile app rating scale: A new tool for assessing the quality of health mobile apps. *JMIR mHealth and uHealth*, *3*(1), e27. doi:10.2196/mhealth.3422 PMID:25760773

Valderas, J. M., Kotzeva, A., Espallargues, M., Guyatt, G., Ferrans, C. E., Halyard, M. Y., ... Alonso, J. (2008). The impact of measuring patient-reported outcomes in clinical practice: A systematic review of the literature. *Quality of Life Research: An International Journal of Quality of Life Aspects of Treatment, Care and Rehabilitation*, *17*(2), 179–193. doi:10.100711136-007-9295-0 PMID:18175207

Wang, J., Wang, Y., Wei, C., Yao, N., Yuan, A., Shan, Y., & Yuan, C. (2014). Smartphone interventions for long-term health management of chronic diseases: An integrative review. *Telemedicine Journal and e-Health*, *20*(6), 570–583. doi:10.1089/tmj.2013.0243 PMID:24787747

Warner, J. L., Rioth, M. J., Mandl, K. D., Mandel, J. C., Kreda, D. A., Kohane, I. S., ... Yao, H. (2016). SMART precision cancer medicine: A FHIR-based app to provide genomic information at the point of care. *Journal of the American Medical Informatics Association*, *23*(4), 701–710. doi:10.1093/jamia/ocw015 PMID:27018265

Wiljer, D., Leonard, K. J., Urowitz, S., Apatu, E., Massey, C., Quartey, N. K., & Catton, P. (2010). The anxious wait: Assessing the impact of patient accessible EHRs for breast cancer patients. *BMC Medical Informatics and Decision Making*, *10*(1), 46. doi:10.1186/1472-6947-10-46 PMID:20809950

World Health Oganization. (2018c). *Noncommunicable diseases and mental health.* Retrieved from http://www.who.int/nmh/ncd-tools/objectives-definition/en/

World Health Organization. (2011). *mHealth: new horizons for health through mobile technologies: based on the findings of the second global survey on eHealth* (Global Observatory for eHealth Series, Volume 3). WHO Press. Retrieved from http://www.who.int/goe/publications/goe_mhealth_web.pdf

World Health Organization. (2018a). *Cancer.* Retrieved from http://www.who.int/news-room/fact-sheets/detail/cancer

World Health Organization. (2018b). *International Classification of Diseases (ICD).* Retrieved from http://www.who.int/classifications/icd/en/

Yaqoob, I., Ahmed, E., Hashem, I. A. T., Ahmed, A. I. A., Gani, A., Imran, M., & Guizani, M. (2017). Internet of Things architecture: Recent advances, taxonomy, requirements, and open challenges. *IEEE Wireless Communications, 24*(3), 10–16. doi:10.1109/MWC.2017.1600421

ADDITIONAL READING

Böhme, C., von Osthoff, M. B., Frey, K., & Hübner, J. (2018). Qualitative evaluation of mobile cancer apps with particular attention to the target group, content, and advertising. *Journal of Cancer Research and Clinical Oncology, 144*(1), 173–181. doi:10.100700432-017-2533-0 PMID:29052039

COCIR. IHE-Europe, & The Personal Health Connected Alliance (2017). *We are all in this together: advancing eHealth interoperability.* Retrieved from http://www.cocir.org/fileadmin/Publications_2017/17022_COC_Interoperability_web.pdf

Corrigan, J. M. (2005). *Crossing the quality chasm. Building a better delivery system.* National Academies Press.

Holland, J. C. (Ed.). (2010). *Psycho-oncology.* Oxford University Press. doi:10.1093/med/9780195367430.001.0001

Information Resources Management Association (USA). (2016). *Web–based services: concepts, methodologies, tools, and applications* (Vols. 1–4). Information Science Reference (an Imprint of IGI Global).

Information Resources Management Association USA (in print). Chronic Illness and Long-Term Care: Breakthroughs in Research and Practice (2 Volumes). IGI Global.

Nasi, G., Cucciniello, M., & Guerrazzi, C. (2015). The Performance of mHealth in cancer supportive care: A research agenda. *Journal of Medical Internet Research, 17*(2), e9. doi:10.2196/jmir.3764 PMID:25720295

KEY TERMS AND DEFINITIONS

App: An application, especially as downloaded by a user to a mobile device.

Cancer: The uncontrolled growth and spread of cells. It can affect almost any part of the body. The growths often invade surrounding tissue and can metastasize to distant sites. Many cancers can be prevented by avoiding exposure to common risk factors, such as tobacco smoke. In addition, a significant proportion of cancers can be cured, by surgery, radiotherapy or chemotherapy, especially if they are detected early.

Electronic Health (eHealth): The use of information and communication technologies for health.

Electronic Health Record (EHR): The electronic health record (EHR) is a longitudinal electronic record of patient health information generated by one or more encounters in any care delivery setting. Included in this information are patient demographics, progress notes, problems, medications, vital signs, past medical history, immunizations, laboratory data and radiology reports. The EHR automates and streamlines the clinician's workflow. The EHR has the ability to generate a complete record of a clinical patient encounter—as well as supporting other care-related activities directly or indirectly via interface—including evidence-based decision support, quality management, and outcomes reporting.

Electronic Medical Record (EMR): An electronic record of health-related information on an individual that can be created, gathered, managed, and consulted by authorized clinicians and staff within one health care organization.

Health: Health is a state of complete physical, mental and social well-being and not merely the absence of disease or infirmity.

Interoperability: The ability of organizations to interact towards mutually beneficial goals, involving the sharing of information and knowledge between these organizations, through the business processes they support, by means of the exchange of data between their ICT systems.

Mobile Health (mHealth): The use of mobile and wireless devices to improve health outcomes, healthcare services and health research.

Personal Health Record (PHR): An electronic, lifelong resource of health information needed by individuals to make health decisions. Individuals own and manage the information in the PHR, which comes from healthcare providers and the individual. The PHR is maintained in a secure and private environment, with the individual determining rights of access. The PHR does not replace the legal record of any provider.

Quality of Life: An individual's perception of their position in life in the context of the culture and value systems in which they live and in relation to their goals, expectations, standards and concerns. It is a broad ranging concept affected in a complex way by the person's physical health, psychological state, personal beliefs, social relationships and their relationship to salient features of their environment.

Chapter 4
Management of Obese Pediatric Patients in the Digital Era

Elpis Vlachopapadopoulou
Children's Hospital "P. & A. Kyriakou", Greece

Eleni I. Georga
University of Ioannina, Greece

Dimitrios I. Fotiadis
University of Ioannina, Greece

ABSTRACT

In this chapter, state of the art in mHealth solutions for monitoring and treatment of children suffering from obesity is presented and discussed. mHealth solutions are used for self-management, remote monitoring, and counseling of several chronic conditions including diabetes mellitus, heart failure, Parkinson's disease, etc. Concerning childhood obesity, those solutions can combine targeted games and motivational approaches towards both physical activity and diet, which could help in addressing this serious and global health issue in the direction of minimizing co-morbidities and eventually preventing serious, life-threatening events. Management of obese children requires behavior change. Multi-component intervention programs via a mobile platform can play a significant role in weight control during childhood and adolescence. In continuation of the chapter, the authors report on the newest advances in the field of digital health interventions addressing childhood obesity.

INTRODUCTION

During 1990s, in association with the extensive use of the Internet, a variety of applications have been developed using e-technology. The introduction of e-Health promised to improve health care delivery and health care access through increased availability of information and enhanced communication. Although the word used is "health", it refers to healthcare. There are several definitions for e-Health. Most of the definitions use technology: (i) as a tool to enable a process or improve function, and (ii) as effective means to enhance human activities (Oh, Rizo, Enkin, & Jadad, 2005). The most commonly used definition is

DOI: 10.4018/978-1-5225-8021-8.ch004

Copyright © 2019, IGI Global. Copying or distributing in print or electronic forms without written permission of IGI Global is prohibited.

that of (Eysenbach, 2001). mHealth is an abbreviation for mobile health, a term coined for the practice of medicine and public Health interventions, using mobile devices. mHealth broadly encompasses the use of mobile telecommunications and multimedia technologies, within or along with conventional health care delivery systems. mHealth, today, is closely related to smartphones, which can provide connectivity to various devices and provide a means for receiving the feedback from the healthcare professional.

A definition formulated during the 2010 mHealth Summit for the Foundation of the National Institute of Health defines mHealth as "the delivery of health care services via mobile communication devices". We could differentiate mHealth and eHealth by elaborating on their fundamental functions, as eHealth supports health systems while mHealth provides healthcare access. mHealth offers an unparalleled opportunity to reach individuals and implement changes. With mHealth applications, the individual is at the center and the most important link: the technology responds to an individual's needs. Everything starts with the need of an individual, either a healthcare worker or a patient, in our case the patient, and the mobile technology application is viewed as the potential lever of the solution. Effective technologies are those that will undergo extensive modifications based on users' needs. Patient groups that can benefit include, but are not limited, to patients with asthma, diabetes, obesity, heart failure, neurogenerative diseases, multiple sclerosis, malignancies and bipolar disorders. In this chapter, we will review and elaborate on the published experience regarding interventions using mobile technology targeting childhood obesity, as well as, on the future potential, benefits and limitations of this emerging technology.

Childhood obesity is considered by the WHO as a new epidemic and has been characterized as the number one health problem worldwide (Ng et al., 2014). The American Academy of Pediatrics guidelines target the reduction of total and abdominal obesity through increased physical activity and healthy nutrition (Pediatrics, 2011). Although, recent research has demonstrated the efficacy of these lifestyle changes on weight loss and weight maintenance as well as on the prevention of comorbidities, promotion and maintenance of such changes continues to be a challenge (Teixeira et al., 2015).

It appears that there is a significant and growing opportunity for eHealth obesity intervention designers to leverage the widespread public adoption of rapidly converging information and communication technologies—most notably the World Wide Web, wireless PDAs and cellular telephones (Tufano & Karras, 2005). Communication technologies such as smartphones offer a potentially powerful approach to support and maintain behavior changes, through delivering of convenient individually tailored, in line with the guidelines, behavioral interventions (Allen, Stephens, Dennison Himmelfarb, Stewart, & Hauck, 2013). There is research evidence suggesting that mobile phones provide a powerful tool for interventions seeking to improve and maintain health outcomes (Allen et al., 2013; Cole-Lewis & Kershaw, 2010; Krishna, Boren, & Balas, 2009). This is supported by a multitude of applications ranging from graphical outputs, diaries, games, motivational platforms, etc. and of course connectivity to social media. More importantly, the child in this framework, is placed at the center of the mHealth solution, but at the same time it is connected with other players who are involved in his/her healthcare activities, such as caregivers, mainly family, pediatrician, another medical doctor, the psychologist, the nutritionist, the hospital, the school, etc. By those means, there is hope and expectation that the positive effect can be maximal.

This article is a continuation of our previous chapter on mHealth solutions to pediatric obesity management (Vlachopapadopoulou & Fotiadis, 2016). Herein, the literature overview has been enhanced by analyzing and discussing the recent developments in the field. Emphasis is placed on mHealth interventions adopting a solid theoretical model of behavior change and combining electronic recording of diet, physical activity monitoring via wearable devices, personalized feedback, educational support and positive reinforcement.

BACKGROUND

The number of smartphone users worldwide will grow to 2.87 billion in 2020, according to new figures from Statista—after nearly getting there in 2014. In 2018, there will be around 2.53 billion smartphone users across the globe; just over 36 percent of the world's population is projected to use a smartphone by 2018. Mobile applications (apps) can help people manage their health and wellness, promote healthy living, and gain access to useful information when and where they need it. These tools are being adopted almost as quickly as they can be developed. Statista reports mention that "the digital health market is expected to reach 206 billion U.S. dollars by 2020, driven particularly by the mobile and wireless health market". Thus, it would appear that smartphones would be the preferred hardware platform for mHealth obesity interventions for reasons of both enabling effective intervention design features and for promoting rapid public adoption and acceptance (Tufano & Karras, 2005). The trend is to merge mobile phones with tablets.

FDA encourages the development of mobile medical apps that improve healthcare and provide consumers and healthcare professionals with valuable health information. The FDA also has a public health responsibility to oversee the safety and effectiveness of medical devices – including mobile medical apps. The FDA intends to exercise enforcement discretion for mobile medical apps that help patients/users self-manage their disease or condition without providing specific treatment suggestions; provide patients with simple tools to organize and track their health information; provide easy access to information related to health conditions or treatments; help patients document, show or communicate potential medical conditions to health care providers; automate simple tasks for health care providers.

Childhood obesity is considered by WHO as a new epidemic, and it has been characterized as the number one health problem worldwide. It has been on the rise for the past decades, specifically, the prevalence of combined overweight and obesity rose by 47.1% for children between 1980 and 2013 (Ng et al., 2014). Researchers have associated the increased body mass index (BMI) in childhood with comorbidities during childhood and adolescence, but also with comorbidities in adult life. Childhood obesity is associated with increased blood pressure, hyperlipidemia and insulin resistance, triad that constitutes the metabolic syndrome (Litwin, 2014), type 2 diabetes, sleep apnea, increased likelihood of asthma, increased risk for orthopedic problems, psychological problems and social maladjustment. A correlation of childhood obesity with the premature development of diabetes and cardiovascular disease is well established (Litwin, 2014). Of special concern is the recently established association of childhood obesity with increased cancer risk during adulthood. The prevalence of several cancers is increased including thyroid cancer, colon, endometrial, and breast cancer. Contrary with previous findings, promising recent data provide supportive evidence that weight loss and attainment of normal weight during childhood or adolescence decreases the risk of malignancy later on in life. However, there are longitudinal studies that suggest that morbidity and mortality from complications of diabetes and cardiovascular disease is increased independently of the adult BMI (Kelsey, Zaepfel, Bjornstad, & Nadeau, 2014).

mHEALTH SOLUTIONS FOR PATIENTS WITH OBESITY

The need for interventions, in order to achieve primary prevention (preventing normal weight children from developing obesity) as well as secondary prevention (treating obese children and adolescents in order to revert to a normal BMI) to minimize health consequences, is obvious. Due to cost and resource limitations, effective obesity interventions can be challenging to deliver to the adolescent population in need of care. The low cost and availability of mobile phones make mHealth an important player in encouraging change and sustaining healthy behaviors (Dijkstra & De Vries, 1999; Kreuter & Wray, 2003).

One serious limitation of the traditional approach to childhood obesity is the difficulty parents have to adhere to the healthy lifestyle habits as suggested by the physicians and the difficulty to keep the medical appointments, due to work or school obligations. Additionally that parents and children recognize a burden in self-monitoring practices. Self-monitoring of energy expenditure, caloric intake and weight are hallmarks of long-term weight control (R. R. Wing & J. O. Hill, 2001; Rena R. Wing & James O. Hill, 2001). Despite the evidence that self-monitoring is very important for weight control the majority of adults and children find it quite difficult to adhere to a specific program. Previous studies have reported that in the first month of a weight control intervention for morbidly overweight children, 44% self-monitored at least 3.5 days per week (Germann, Kirschenbaum, & Rich, 2007; Kirschenbaum, Germann, & Rich, 2005); however, only 25% continued at six months (Germann et al., 2007). Compliance can be improved if a diary system can be used. Electronic communication systems also provide electronic diaries. Electronic diaries may increase adherence via immediate feedback as well as time recording (Bartlett, Lukk, Butz, Lampros-Klein, & Rand, 2002; Stone, Shiffman, Schwartz, Broderick, & Hufford, 2003).

There are reports documenting, that the use of a personal digital assistant (PDA), significantly increased the rate of adherence from 11% to 94% (Stone et al., 2003). Children use electronic devices regularly; 45% of US teenagers ages 12–17 own a mobile phone, and 33% use the short message service regularly (SMS; text messaging) (Shapiro et al., 2008). Researchers and physicians should look for protocols that will involve more modern ways of communication. Cost-effectiveness as compared to traditional therapy, telephone, email, web-based intervention or SMS should also be examined.

Globally, an estimated 43 million preschool children (under age 5) were overweight or obese in 2010, a 60 percent increase since 1990. The problem affects both countries rich and poor. Of the world's 43 million overweight and obese preschoolers, 35 million live in developing countries. By 2020, if the current epidemic continues unabated, 9 percent of all preschoolers will be overweight or obese—nearly 60 million children (de Onis, Blössner, & Borghi, 2010). Over 200 million school-age children are overweight, making this generation the first one predicted to have a shorter lifespan than their parents, as stated by the World Obesity Federation (2014). The necessity of implicating secondary prevention programs accessible to the large population of patients can be met by the development of web-based programs. To implicate such programs, the field of digital therapeutics has emerged. Furthermore, the vast majority of children are tentatively candidates for developing obesity in an older age and therefore in need of having accessible information regarding healthy nutrition, physical activity and other daily habits proven to be important in maintaining a normal weight. Digital therapeutics is evidence-based behavioral treatments delivered online that can increase accessibility and effectiveness of healthcare. Those approaches offer a new opportunity for healthcare delivery, which can enrich the range of applications in mHealth.

To date, several systematic reviews have found that Web-based interventions may be a moderately effective way to facilitate lifestyle change and weight loss. Many people do not read books, they might not explore the internet, but 90% of the people in most developed countries have a mobile phone, usually smartphone, which they carry all the time with them. These mobile phones have a camera and microphone, they can send and receive text, they can provide information about location, they make applications always available, and they are handy and chargeable anywhere and anytime. Mobile technology offers access; access offers knowledge and mHealth applications to empower individuals to take an active role in their health and promote their well-being. Thus, there is a substantial need for credible, trustworthy, understandable, concise but simple health information that is relevant, culturally sensitive and easy to apply. mHealth expands the definition of personalized medicine while maintaining and enhancing the integrity of the individual, delivering to the right person, the right information, at the right place, at the right time. Mobile means anytime and anywhere, at the discretion of the individual. Health issues and queries do not only arise when we are in front of a computer screen, but they can also arise anytime, anywhere. Via mobile technology, it is feasible to adapt face to face obesity interventions to a mobile platform and deliver effective remote care (Krishna et al., 2009; E. B. Tate et al., 2013).

Given the chronic health conditions associated with obesity, physicians, and other health providers are faced with the challenge to implement programs for both immediate and long-term weight loss. Predictive models have been published for adults that can predict weight change based on the daily energy imbalance. Based on historical controls they have estimated that an excess intake of 30kcal per day can lead to a weight gain of 1.8-2.0 lbs per year (Hill, Wyatt, Reed, & Peters, 2003). Another model used the method of doubly labeled water to measure total energy expenditure and introduces equation to estimate the difference in energy flux between two different weights (Swinburn et al., 2009). Hall and Jordan developed a spreadsheet-based model of the change in steady-state body weight that included the effect of both total energy intake together with physical activity changes and metabolic adaptation (Hall & Jordan, 2008). The application of predictive models for children is more complex as the energy needed for growth and the changing energy expenditure of the growing organism need to be considered. At present, there are no validated predictive models for childhood obesity. Predictive models can be implicated in intervention strategies, and they can increase the acceptance and accuracy of weight loss intervention plans, implicating nutrition, physical activity, and behavior changes.

There are several behavioral interventions that have demonstrated encouraging short-term results, but they do not have consistent results as far as the long-term maintenance of weight loss (D. F. Tate, Wing, & Winett, 2001). Thus, research for better models that can easily be delivered and sustained over time, is needed. To that end, mobile health development intervention could greatly benefit from the application of the health behavior theory (Khaylis, Yiaslas, Bergstrom, & Gore-Felton, 2010).

Smartphones can be easily connected to sensors that measure physiological parameters. Several protocols are available and continuous or no measurements can be collected. Features of those signals can be extracted, and those, or the raw signals can be uploaded in the cloud for storage and processing. Mainly the processing is related to the fusion of signals that characterize activity, lifestyle, physiological measurements, etc. Recently, those data have been enriched with the collection of environmental data, e.g. temperature, humidity, etc. which are also fused. The idea is to create decision support systems that can provide monitoring of the patient and support his/her treatment and wellbeing. As technology progresses, several players participate in this monitoring procedure and provide and exchange data. For example, caregivers can play a role in patient monitoring, and they can receive data even from patients otherwise unable to do so, concerning their vital signs, health status, activity, and medications. So parents, medical and school personnel become active and interactive players for the care of children with obesity and related disorders. The smartphone becomes a tool for data collection, data pre-processing and sometimes data processing and decision making. The old fashion telemedicine approach provides those data to the medical doctor, who is responsible for taking decisions regarding the patient. Those decisions can be transferred to the mobile, and the patient can receive an SMS or an alert on his/her smartphone. In that regard, we say that the loop is closed. In some cases, and this soon will become a reality, readings of the sensors and decisions made by the system can be fed to an actuator, e.g. a pump, in the case of diabetes an insulin pump and the system is again closed, meaning that the artificial pancreas is operational.

Internet of Things can be used to provide additional measurements which are related to blood pressure, weight, fat, and other, which can be combined in the same framework with other environmental and lifestyle measurements, which might come from sensors which can be placed in a refrigerator, in the ground, inside the house, etc. This results in a wider environment, which acts in the direction of collecting continuous measurements, which easily can be transferred to the cloud for storage, processing and decision making. The general framework of developing such an approach within the healthcare ecosystem for obese children is given in Figure 1.

Figure 1 mHealth solutions within the healthcare ecosystem for obese children. In that framework, the participation of other healthcare ecosystem stakeholders becomes more evident and active. Parents, teachers, relatives and, in general, formal and informal caregivers become more informed and aware of the status of the patient and can participate in an active process, which is patient-centric, highly personalized, but at the same time holistic since the medical doctor, the patient, the caregiver, the nurse and other actors can communicate and keep active in the ecosystem. The mHealth systems now are driven by the concept of self-management. Self-management can be defined as the decisions and behaviors that patients with chronic illness engage that affect their health. Self- management support is the care.

Moreover, encouragement provided to people with chronic conditions and their families to help them understand their central role in managing their illness, make informed decisions about care and engage in healthy behaviors. The question is how this can be achieved through a mHealth system. Figure 2 presents the evolution of self-management devices from 2004 to today in terms of connectivity, measurements and functionalities (Georga, Protopappas, Bellos, & Fotiadis, 2014). The first row presents the functionalities, the second the measurements and the third the connectivity technology. Lately, to those platforms apart from the use of sensors, several biosensors have been included. A biosensor is an analytical device incorporating a biological or biologically derived sensing element either intimately associated with or integrated within a physicochemical transducer. The usual aim is to produce an electronic digital signal that is proportional to the concentration of a chemical or set of chemicals (A. Turner, Karube, & Wilson, 1987). At present, those sensors can become small. Key enabling technologies, such as microfluidics, nanotechnology, and flexible electronics can be utilized to provide us with miniature sensors, which can analyze blood, saliva or other biological fluids and communicate the result to the smartphone (Figure 2)

Figure 1. mHealth solutions within the healthcare ecosystem for obese children

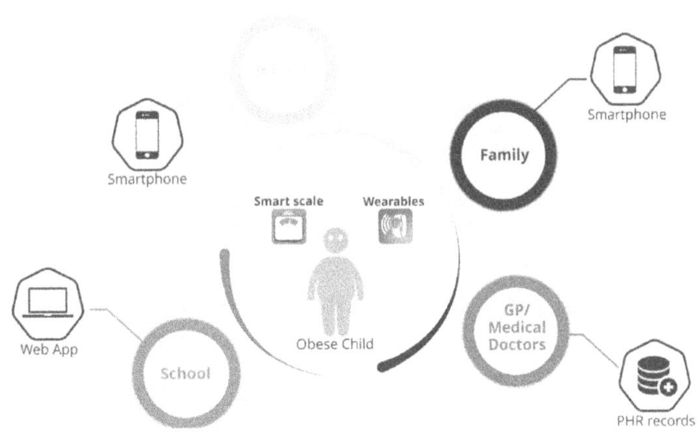

Figure 2. The evolution of self-management devices from 2004 to today in terms of connectivity, measurements and functionalities (Georga et al., 2014)

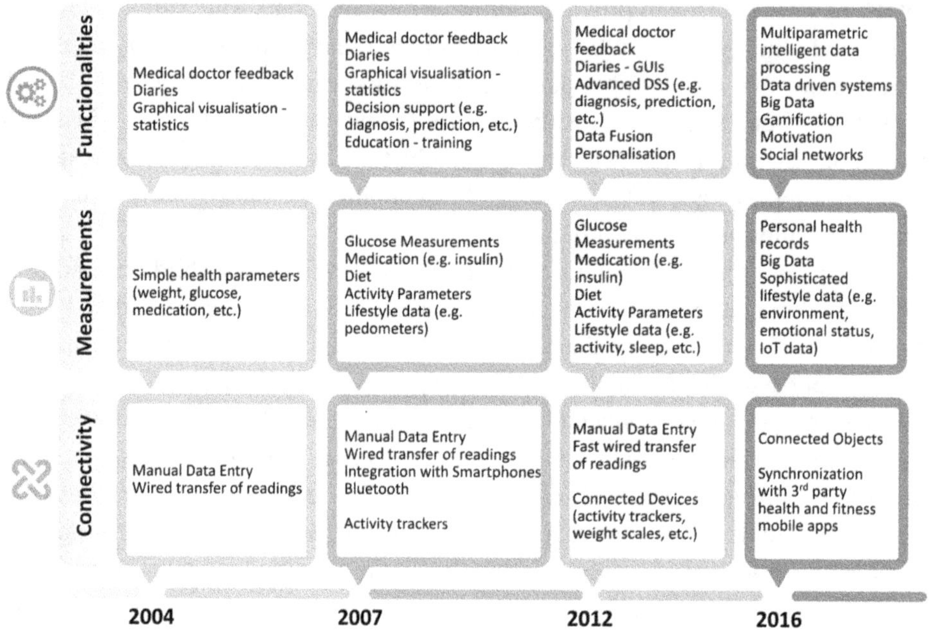

Previous Experience

Behavioral weight loss interventions consist of diet, exercise and behavior therapy. Behavioral modification strategies usually include the following: self-monitoring, goal-setting, shaping, reinforcement and stimulus control (Wadden & Butryn, 2003). The use of the web or mobile technology to support these strategies can augment the results. To date, several systematic reviews have found that Web-based interventions may be a moderately effective way to facilitate lifestyle change and weight loss (Neve, Morgan, Jones, & Collins, 2010; Norman et al., 2007).

Khaylis et al. have reviewed 21 studies and concluded that five elements are the key components in technology-based behavior interventions to be successful in weight loss (Khaylis et al., 2010). These features are self-monitoring; counselor feedback and communication; social support; structured program; and individually tailored program (Khaylis et al., 2010). The authors comment that a technology-based model of behavior change for weight management using the above mentioned five key components is advantageous over traditional methods in several aspects. The internet is a cost-effective way to deliver relevant information and stepwise instructions to individuals of different backgrounds, age range, and location. Using their mobile phone or digital music players, participants can have interactive communication with the physician, dietitian or counselor via online diaries and self-reports. They can also have access to lessons and healthy lifestyle information. A factor that is highly appreciated by the participants is that this approach is time-saving and can be incorporated into busy lifestyles, thus reducing resistance to engage in a weight reduction program. One of the most important reasons for drop outs of long-term programs in outpatient clinics is time restraint. On the other hand, portable devices such as handheld PDAs or pedometers, give the opportunity for continuous monitoring that has been shown to increase weight loss when compared with traditional methods. Of utmost importance is that technology-based interventions can provide individuals with a sense of control that is essential for developing and implementing short- and long-term behavioral change (Khaylis et al., 2010).

The program "Prevent" was created to apply the principles of Diabetes Prevention Program (DPP) into a digital form and make it available to millions of people. The effectiveness of "Prevent" when used by adults with obesity and pre-diabetes in lowering BMI and hemoglobin A1c was assessed. Participants were enrolled in the "Prevent" program that they were able to access via any Internet-enabled desktop or mobile device (prevent by Omada Health) (Salber, 2014). "Prevent" is an Internet-based translation of the DPP lifestyle intervention, which includes small group support, personalized health coaching, a weekly DPP-based curriculum, and digital tracking tools. Participants were demographically matched into groups of 10-15 participants and placed into a private online social network resembling Facebook where they could discuss goal progress and provide social support to one another. At any convenient time or place using Internet-enabled devices, they could asynchronously complete weekly DPP-based health education lessons, privately message and call a health coach for individual counselling, track weight loss, and physical activity using a wireless weight scale and pedometer, and monitor their engagement and weight loss progress. The participants were enrolled for one year, and they were followed for two years. The program was proven to be successful in weight reduction and amelioration of HbA1c even one year after the program discontinuation (S. Cameron Sepah, Jiang, & Peters, 2014; S Cameron Sepah, Jiang, & Peters, 2015).

Shapiro et al. used SMS texting to assure compliance with a program and adherence to self- monitoring. Children and parents participated in a total of three group education sessions (one session weekly for three weeks) to encourage increasing physical activity and decreasing screen time, and sugar-sweetened beverage consumption (Shapiro et al., 2008). All randomized children received a brief psychoeducational intervention and then were randomized into three groups either monitored target behaviors via SMS with feedback, via paper diaries or participated in a no monitoring control group for eight weeks. Children who were randomized to the SMS group were given one phone each to share for the duration of the study. They were instructed not to use the phone for anything except study-related SMS. They were instructed to send two SMSs per day (one for parent and one for child), daily for the full eight weeks of the study, and for each SMS sent, they would each receive an immediate, automated SMS feedback message from the program hosted on a secure server. The feedback message was automated to provide instant responses to the participants regardless of the time of day. This group of children had significantly higher adherence to self-monitoring than children who kept a paper diary, 43% vs. 19%. The children appear to prefer the assignment using mobile technology (Shapiro et al., 2008). The authors concluded that according to the cognitive, social learning theory, perhaps the support and positive reinforcement led to adherence and acceptability of the self-monitoring program (Shapiro et al., 2008). Moreover, SMS is more reliable regarding the date and time that is recorded automatically as opposed to paper diaries that are possible to be backfilled (Stone et al., 2003).

Bauer et al. (Bauer, de Niet, Timman, & Kordy, 2010) generated text messages based on weekly input from the overweight children in the study, but these messages were reviewed and modified by staff before sending. Diet, weight, and exercise data were provided via self-report for all interventions except the one by Hurling et al. (Hurling et al., 2007) which used accelerometer data wirelessly transmitted via Bluetooth to the mobile phone. Output from these interventions was predominately text although tabular and graphic comparisons to targets/goals were provided by some interventions (Beasley, Riley, Davis, & Singh, 2008; Burke et al., 2011; Haapala, Barengo, Biggs, Surakka, & Manninen, 2009). The intervention used a mobile phone program that adjusted music tempo to encourage an appropriate walking pace (Liu et al., 2008). Riley WT et al. criticized these studies for the fact that although they have based the protocol on a theoretical basis, they did not evaluate the changes in the targeted factors (W. T. Riley, Cesar, Martin, & Rivera, 2014; William T. Riley & Rivera, 2014). On the other hand, a positive outcome can be foreseen if there is a dynamical system model with algorithms that are used in real time and adapt the timing and the dose of the intervention (W. T. Riley et al., 2014; William T. Riley & Rivera, 2014).

The effectiveness of mHealth interventions as regards the prevention and treatment of pediatric as well as adult obesity has been largely reviewed, showing heterogeneous BMI or weight reduction outcomes which are, however, accompanied by a clearly increased adherence to treatment and improved eating and physical activity patterns (Chaplais, Naughton, Thivel, Courteix, & Greene, 2015; Stephens & Allen, 2013; T. Turner & Spruijt-Metz, 2015; Wang, Xue, Huang, Huang, & Zhang, 2017). Table 1 presents the main characteristics (i.e., population, study design, intervention period, mHealth intervention, and outcomes) of the most recent mHealth randomized control or quasi-experiment interventional studies targeting at the management or prevention of pediatric obesity. Their effectiveness was demonstrated through either the between-group or the within-group comparative assessment of a number of quantitative (e.g. weight, BMI, consumption of specific food categories, screen time) and qualitative outcomes (e.g. self-esteem, control over food), including usability and user acceptability metrics of the underlying mHealth system. Each study outcomes are closely connected to the study sample, the intervention period, and the employed mobile technologies.

In addiction model-based treatment intervention was delivered through a smartphone app supporting: (i) the daily self-monitoring of weight using a connected wireless body weight scale, and (ii) the graduated withdrawal of specific food categories as well as reduction of food portion sizes (Pretlow, Stock, Allison, & Roeger, 2015). Being combined with weekly 15-min phone meetings with a health professional, frequent text messages, four 2- to 4-hour in-person group meetings and peer support, it yielded significantly improved BMI indices, and it improved the overall self-esteem and problematic eating behaviors (i.e. emotional eating).

The SmartMoms smartphone-delivered intervention, which aimed at reducing primarily parent-provided sugar-sweetened beverage and juice consumption in preschool-aged children, and, secondarily, the maternal weight, encompassed: (i) self-monitoring of maternal weight and diet, and monitoring of the child's servings of sugar-sweetened beverage and juice intake through a paper diary or a smartphone app, (ii) lessons on behavioral strategies primarily to reduce caloric beverages and foods, which were accessed via a mobile website, (iii) tailored feedback sent through email, (iv) monthly progress reports on goal achievement, (v) text messages (tips, motivational messages and goal progress assessment), and (vi) child reinforcement charts (Nezami, Lytle, & Tate, 2016; Nezami, Ward, Lytle, Ennett, & Tate, 2017). This multi-component interventional strategy resulted in a statistically significant reduction in child's sugar-sweetened beverage and juice intake as compared with the control group[1.2 (-2.8, 5.1) vs 9.9 (5.8, 14.0) fl. oz. / day, $p < 0.01$], and, additionally, the maternal weight was significantly reduced [-2.7 (95% CI: -4.8, -0.7) vs. 1.1 (95% CI:-1.1, 3.2) ($p < 0.01$)]; however the child BMI z-score change did not reflect the effectiveness of the intervention. Similarly, a mobile app intervention, grounded in behavioral weight control principles and encompassing goal self-monitoring and reinforcement feedback, improved (though not significantly) fruits/vegetables consumption, sugar-sweetened beverages consumption and screen time both between- and within- group, which behavior was also reflected to improved BMIs (Nollen et al., 2013).

The comprehensive monitoring of physical activity through the Empatica E4 wristband and the electronic recording of food-intake through an app, enabled the provisioning of weekly feedback on the adequacy of the diet and the physical activity and the achievement of goals; all participants were given

Table 1. mHealth interventions to pediatric obesity treatment

Study	Population	Study Design	Intervention Period	mHealth Intervention	Outcomes
(Schiel, Kaps, & Bieber, 2012)	**Intervention Group** **(*n*=124)** Age (years): 13.5 ± 2.8 BMI (kg/m²): 31.3 ± 5.2	QE	36.5±13.0 days	A structured treatment and teaching programme (STTP) for weight reduction consisted of 28 therapeutic sessions with a duration of 45 min each. Physical activity monitoring via an in-house activity sensor, and physical activity self-recording using standardized questionnaires. Food intake recording via an in-house mobile app	**Primary Outcomes** Weight reduction (kg) 7.1±3.0 kg $(p < 0.01)$ BMI reduction (kg/m2) From 31.3±5.2 to 28.7±4.9 $(p < 0.01)$
(Sharifi et al., 2013)	**Intervention Group** **(*n* = 27)** Child Characteristics Age (years): 8.7±1.9 Parent Characteristics Age (years): 41.1±6.3	QE	3 weeks	Mobile phone text-messaging; parents received 3 text messages a week	**Qualitative Results** Parents were generally enthusiastic about receiving text messages (preferably via email and through links to a website) to support healthy behaviors for their children. Parents anticipated high responsiveness to messaging endorsed by their child's doctor as long as content remains relevant.
(Nollen et al., 2014)	**Intervention Group** **(*n* = 26)** Child Characteristics Female Age (years): 11.3±1.5 BMI (kg/m²): 22.5±4.8 **Control Group** $(n = 25)$ Child Characteristics Female Age (years): 11.3±1.7 BMI (kg/m²): 25.0±6.3	RCT	12 weeks	A mobile app intervention targeting fruits/vegetables consumption (Weeks 1–4), sugar-sweetened beverages consumption (Weeks 5–8), and screen time (Weeks 9–12), grounded in behavioral weight control principles (Nollen et al., 2013). - Goal-setting, planning, and self-monitoring of goal progress. - Feedback and reinforcement on goal attainment through a song-based reward system.	**Primary Outcomes** *Between Group (intervention vs. the control group)* Fruits and vegetables, daily servings 3.35±1.81 vs. 2.32±1.73 $(p = 0.13)$ Sugar-sweetened beverages, daily servings 0.87±0.93 vs. 1.05±0.85 $(p = 0.25)$ Screen time, hours per day 3.72±2.44 vs. 3.77±1.99 $(p = 0.76)$ BMI 22.55±4.56 vs. 24.50±5.93 $(p = 0.91)$ *Within Group (change with respect to baseline)* Fruits and vegetables, daily servings * 0.88±2.36 $(p = 0.08)$ vs. -0.12±2.16 $(p = 0.79)$ Sugar-sweetened beverages, daily servings * -0.33±0.93 $(p = 0.09)$ vs. 0.02±1.14 $(p = 0.94)$ Screen time, hours per day* 0.32±2.32 $(p = 0.53)$ vs. 0.12±2.05 $(p = 0.80)$ BMI* -0.21±2.20 $(p = 0.66)$ vs. -0.27±1.17 $(p = 0.33)$ *intervention vs. the control group

continued on following page

Table 1. Continued

Study	Population	Study Design	Interven-tion Period	mHealth Intervention	Outcomes
(Smith et al., 2014)	**Intervention Group** **(n =181)** Child Characteristics Male Age (years): 12.7±0.5 BMI (kg/m^2): 20.5±4.1 **Control Group)** Child Characteristics Male Age (years): 12.7±0.5 BMI (kg/m^2): 20.5±4.1	RCT	8 months	**ATLAS (Active Teen Leaders Avoiding Screen-Time); a multicomponent, school-based obesity prevention intervention among adolescent boys attending school in low-income areas.** - Teacher professional development including two 6 h workshops and one fitness instructor session. - 4 parent newsletters - 3 researcher-led 20-min seminars were provided to students - 20 enhanced 90-min school sport sessions - Six 20-min lunchtime physical activity-mentoring sessions - Smartphone app and Web site for physical activity monitoring, recording of fitness challenge results, tailored motivational messaging, peer assessment of RT skills, and goal setting for physical activity and screen-time (15 weeks)	**Primary Outcomes** BMI change (kg/m2) * 0.60±0.9 vs.0.61±0.08 $(p = 0.84)$ Waist circumference change (cm) * 0.0±0.33 vs.-0.5±0.31 $(p = 0.16)$ Body fat change (%)* 1.3±0.35 vs. 1.3±0.33 $(p = 0.99)$ **Secondary Outcomes** Overall activity change (mean counts per minute) * -23±18.08 vs -3±14.69 $(p = 0.41)$ Screen-time change (min) * 3±7.25 vs. 33±7.0 $(p = 0.03)$ SSB intake change (glass/day) * -0.8±0.19 vs. -0.1±0.18 $(p = 0.01)$ *intervention vs. the control group
(Pretlow et al., 2015)	**Intervention Group** **(n=43)** Age (years): 16.0±0.43 % over BMI: 77.4±4.6	QE	20 weeks	**An addiction model-based treatment intervention being delivered through a smartphone app which supports:** - Daily weight self-monitoring using a wireless body weight scale connected to the smartphone app. - Staged withdrawal of specific foods, snacking/grazing, and excessive amounts of foods. - Weekly 15-min phone meetings with a health professional, frequent text messages, and four 2- to 4-hour in person group meetings. - Peer support	**Primary Outcomes** % over BMI (with respect to baseline) Males: 82.6 vs. 95.9 $(p < 0.01)$ Females: 67.1 vs. 70.9 $(p < 0.01)$ **Secondary Outcomes** Improved control over food $(p < 0.01)$ Improved self-esteem $(p < 0.01)$ Improved control of emotional eating $(p < 0.01)$
(Hull et al., 2017)	**Intervention Group** **(n = 63)** *Black Children* $(n = 33)$ Child Characteristics * Age: 2 years: 18 (54) 3 years: 14 (42) 4 years: 1 (3) Gender: Male: 17 (52) Female: 16 (49) Maternal Characteristics* Age: 18-24 years: 5 (17) 25-34 years: 14 (47) 35-44 years: 11 (37) *Hispanic Children* (n = 30) Child Characteristics* Age: 2 years: 13 (45) 3 years: 10 (35) 4 years: 6 (21) Gender: Male: 17 (57) Female: 13 (43) Maternal Characteristics* Age: 18-24 years: 1 (3) 25-34 years: 18 (60) 35-44 years: 11 (37) *n(%)	Observational study- Betta Testing (Usage, Usability, Perceived Barriers)	3 months	**The Children Eating Well (CHEW) smartphone app developed as a supporting tool for the Special Supplemental Nutrition Program for Women, Infants, and Children (WIC) in the United States.** *The WIC Program* - Approved food packages are assigned to each WIC participant in the family, which list the specific types, brands, sizes, and quantities of products that can be purchased. - A cash value voucher (CVV) provides a flat dollar amount per WIC participant that can be spent on fruits or vegetables, currently $8 for children and $10 for mothers. *CHEW App Components* - WIC Shopping Tools, including a Barcode Scanner feature and Calculator Tools concerning the use of the CVVs. - Nutrition Education, focused on healthy snacks and beverages, including a Yummy Snack Gallery and Healthy Snacking Tips.	**Primary Outcomes** **Usage** Frequency of CHEW app sessions based on log files 12.57±14.98 Duration of CHEW app sessions (min) based on log files 4.67±4.29 Self-reported Usage* Used any feature at least once 57 (90.5) Used WIC Shopping Tools at least once 51 (81.0) Used Yummy Snack Gallery at least once 43 (68.3) Viewed Healthy Snacking Tips at least once 47 (74.6) *n(%) **Usability (5-point Likert scales ranging from 1=strongly disagree to 5=strongly agree, with higher values indicating greater usability).** *WIC Shopping Tools* $(n = 51)$ Easy of Use: 3.98±1.12 Helpfulness: 4.40±0.90 Usefulness: 4.29±1.15 *Yummy Snack Gallery* $(n = 43)$ Easy of Use: 4.81±0.50 Helpfulness: 4.95±0.21 Usefulness: 4.77±0.43 *Healthy Snacking Tips* $(n = 47)$ Helpfulness: 4.68±0.59 Usefulness: 4.40±0.83

continued on following page

Table 1. Continued

Study	Population	Study Design	Intervention Period	mHealth Intervention	Outcomes
(Nezami et al., 2017)	**Intervention Group** ($n = 27$) Child Characteristics Age (months): 56.4±10.5 BMI z-score: 0.30±1.02 Maternal Characteristics Age (years): 36.6±5.7 BMI (kg/m²): 33.1±4.8 **Control Group** ($n = 24$) Child Characteristics Age (months): 51.3±9.2 BMI z-score: 0.49±0.90 Maternal Characteristics Age (years): 36.2±4.3 BMI (kg/m2): 32.0±5.9	RCT	6 months	**The SmartMoms smartphone-delivered intervention (Nezami et al., 2016)** - One 75-min in-person group session at the beginning of the study. - Self-monitoring of weight and diet, and the child's servings of sugar sweetened beverage and juice intake through a paper diary or a smartphone app. - 18 lessons on behavioral strategies primarily to reduce caloric beverages and foods; they were accessed via a mobile website and were updated weekly for the first 12 weeks and biweekly for weeks 13-24. - Tailored feedback through email. Feedback was sent weekly for the first 12 weeks, and biweekly for weeks 13-24. - Monthly progress reports on goal achievement. - 3-4 text messages a week sent at random intervals (tips, motivational messages and goal progress assessment). - Child reinforcement charts	**Primary Outcome** Child's sugar sweetened beverage and juice intake (fl. oz./day)* 1.2 (-2.8, 5.1) vs. 9.9 (5.8, 14.0) $(p < 0.01)$ **Secondary Outcomes** Maternal percent weight change* -2.7 (-4.8, -0.7) vs. 1.1 (-1.1, 3.2) $(p < 0.01)$ Child BMI z-score * 0.40 (-0.05, 0.84) vs. 0.43 (-0.01, 0.87) $(p = 0.33)$ Maternal beverages (fl. oz. /day) * 5.6 (-1.2, 12.5) vs. 19.0 (11.9, 26.1) $(p < 0.01)$ *Values are model adjusted means and 95% confidence intervals.
(Yang et al., 2017)	**Intervention Group** **($n = 558$)** Child Characteristics Age (years): 10-12 **Control Group** **($n = 288$)** Child Characteristics Age (years): 10-12	Non RCT	6 months	**Childhood obesity prevention intervention in a school setting using a mobile system, HAPPY ME; a smartphone app coupled with a wearable activity tracker. Tailoring of nutrition information messages and educational content is performed according to the Transtheoretical Model (Lee et al., 2017).** *HAPPY ME for Children* - Self-monitoring of dietary habits, screen time, sleep duration (measured in hours), and physical activity. - Tailored feedback and encouraging messages. - Gamification *HAPPY ME for Parents* - Monitoring of their child's dietary habits and physical activity. - Educational materials about obesity, healthy eating habits, and nutrition. - Tailored messages once a week concerning the child's performance and offering guidance on how to create a healthier home environment. *HAPPY ME for Teachers* - Website with teacher-friendly educational material about nutrition and physical activity, test results of physical fitness measures among participants, and monitoring capabilities regarding application data on participating students from their classes. - Teachers in charge of classes with participating students can encourage participants using a bulletin or sending messages via the website, which can then be shown in an individual's smartphone application.	**Primary Outcomes** Behavioral changes, including healthy eating and increased physical activity. **Secondary Outcomes** Changes in anthropometric parameters (body weight, height, BMI z-score and waist circumference), and BMI percentiles. Changes in psychological variables, such as self-body perception and sleep hours.

continued on following page

Table 1. Continued

Study	Population	Study Design	Intervention Period	mHealth Intervention	Outcomes
(Mameli et al., 2018)	**Intervention Group** (n = 16) Child Characteristics Age (years): 12.6±1.7 BMI (kg/m²): 29.6±3.3 **Control Group** $(n = 14)$ Child Characteristics Age (years): 12.4±2.2 BMI (kg/m²): 28.6±2.6	RCT	3 months	**Intervention Group** - Physical activity monitoring through the Empatica E4 wristband. - Food intake recording via an app (METEDA, Italy). - Weekly feedback on the basis of the adequacy of the diet and the physical activity sent via SMS. A positive feedback was sent each time a goal was achieved. - All participants were given a Mediterranean diet, and were instructed to practice 1 h day^{-1} of moderate to vigorous physical activity and minimize sedentary time by reducing screen time (<2 h day-1).	**Primary Outcome** Between-group difference (intervention vs. the control group) in weight change -0.06 kg (95% CI: 3.29 to 3.14) $(p = 0.96)$ **Secondary Outcome** Between-group difference (intervention vs. the control group) in BMI change 0.01 kg/m² (95 CI: 0.15 to 0.18) $(p = 0.87)$ **Ancillary Outcome** The change in weight was not associated with the number of days of use of the app and the wristband.

Data are mean±standard deviation

a Mediterranean diet, and were instructed to practice 1 h day^{-1} of moderate to vigorous physical activity and minimize sedentary time by reducing screen time (<2 h day^{-1}) (Mameli et al., 2018). A -0.06 (95% CI: 3.29 to 3.14) kg between-group (intervention vs control) mean difference in weight loss at three months, as well as a 0.01 (95% CI: 0.15 to 0.18) between-group, mean difference in BMI z-score could not substantiate statistically significant outcomes. On the other hand, the combination of physical activity monitoring and electronic food-intake recording with a structured treatment and teaching program for weight reduction significantly reduced both the weight and BMI in overweight children and adolescents as compared with the baseline [weight reduction: 7.1±3.0 kg $(p < 0.01)$, BMI reduction: from 31.3±5.2 to 28.7±4.9 $(p < 0.01)$].

Yang et al. presented a childhood obesity prevention intervention relying on the transtheoretical model (Lee et al., 2017; Yang et al., 2017). In particular, the HAPPY ME mobile system couples a smartphone app with a wearable activity tracker and provides a multitude of features to participating children, parents and teachers, ranging from self-monitoring of a child's dietary habits, screen time, sleep duration (measured in hours), and physical activity to tailored nutrition information messages and educational content. The primary outcomes of this study are behavioral changes, including healthy eating and increased physical activity, whereas changes in anthropometric parameters (body weight, height, BMI z-score and waist circumference), and BMI percentiles, as well as changes in a psychological variable (self-body perception and sleep hours).

A smartphone intervention protocol for adolescent obesity was recently published. The program is ongoing with the primary aim to assess the impact of a smartphone application compared with usual care on body mass index SDS over 12 months in adolescents (age range from 12-17 years) who are obese. Secondary outcome measures are waist circumference, insulin sensitivity, quality of life, physical activity and psychosocial health (O'Malley et al., 2014). It is an investigator blinded protocol of one-year duration. The obese adolescents, after the initial evaluation by a multidisciplinary team, are randomized into two groups; one receiving standard care and the other following the experimental smartphone intervention protocol. The smartphone application incorporates evidence-based behavioral change tools such as self-monitoring, goal setting, and peer support. Evidence-based tips are sent to the user in the form of a text tip, a video tip or an image tip. The tips aim to increase the knowledge of the participant concerning healthy eating, physical activity, physical fitness, and sleep. The user is encouraged to engage in daily goal setting to increase the physical activity level and sleep, increase water intake, reduce intake of sugar and fat and to increase intake of fiber, fruits and vegetables. Also, the users are encouraged to monitor their progress by reviewing their goals daily and by entering their height and weight measurements. The findings are expected to guide further development of a telemedicine system for the management of clinical obesity in adolescence (O'Malley et al., 2014). Preliminary results of a pilot study of the above intervention project reveal that the majority of the adolescents were satisfied with the ease of use the benefit of the weight tracking and reward systems and the appealing look and feel of the app (O'Malley et al., 2014).

The use of social media and especially Facebook was integrated with a pilot study targeting college students. The study examined the feasibility, acceptability, and initial efficacy of a technology-based 8-week weight loss intervention among college students. Students were randomly assigned to one of the three arms: Facebook, Facebook Plus text messaging and personalized feedback. Waiting List control with assessments at four weeks and eight weeks post-treatment. At eight weeks, the Facebook Plus group had significantly greater weight loss than the Facebook alone and control group, indicating the potential use of social media in weight control interventions, particularly when targeting large groups of adolescents and young adults (Napolitano, Hayes, Bennett, Ives, & Foster, 2013).

The term Ecological Momentary Interventions [EMI] was used for treatments that are provided to people during their everyday lives (i.e., in real time) and in natural settings (i.e., real world). King and colleagues (King et al., 2008) developed a palmtop computer-delivered intervention aimed at increasing middle- and older-aged adults' physical activity using a palmtop computer-based EMI. The researchers demonstrated that a relatively short-term, low-intensity palmtop computer-based EMI could increase middle and older-aged adults physical activity. More, it provides an example of an automated, palmtop-computer based EMI that requires limited clinician time during the intervention (E. & M., 2010; Heron & Smyth, 2010; King et al., 2008).

The first RTC using smartphone technology aiming to increase daily physical activity was published in 2013. The smart move intervention program included obese patients older than 16 years of age who owned a smartphone and were randomly assigned to the intervention or controlled group. The intervention group was instructed in the usability features of the smartphone application and encouraged to achieve 10,000 steps per day as an exercise goal and was given an exercise promotion leaflet. The control group was encouraged to walk an additional 30 minutes per day along with their normal activity (the equivalent of 10,000 steps) as an exercise goal and was given an exercise promotion leaflet. The primary outcome was the mean difference in daily step count between baseline and follow-up (Glynn et al., 2013).

Future Implications for Weight Management

Several systematic reviews have found that web-based interventions are moderately effective in promoting weight loss. A personalized approach and intervention, with two-way feedback, sets a much more effective plan of action. Current technology offers the ability to measure and track several biological and environmental factors. At present, there are devices that can record weight, calories, sleep time, physical fitness, heart rate, sports performance. Shortly, we expect them to be able to measure and record nutrients, microbiome, sweat and tear production, medication concentrations in the blood, comprehensive stresses of the spine and many other variables. Some of these functions are already incorporated into smartphones while other measurements come from sensors that transmit data through USB or wireless connections. The sensors needed to capture these data have become miniscule, durable and highly effective. Currently, the data are personalized, and they can be exported in raw numbers or the form of graphs. Cloud sourcing and remote data accumulation and manipulation are already feasible and applicable. There are several health devices, usually sensors that connect to the body and they are used to acquire the recordings needed. In more details, we already have devices that can track calorie intake, activity and sleep round the clock using multiple sensors, others that can track weight, body fat, and BMI, or measure steps, distance and calories burned.

Furthermore, other devices can monitor sleep or track distance covered pace and calories. The use of GPS-enabled data recording and modulation enhances such a fitness watch. Blood pressure, heart rate, and pulse rate can be monitored and tracked, as well. iHealth Smart gluck monitoring system measures and records blood glucose levels, as this is measured and recorded using a portable testing kit. Similar sensors and apparatuses to collect similar biological data measurements are being developed at an enhanced pace.

Furthermore, of special interest and with fast development are the smart clothes. The world of electronics and textiles is collaborating, and they are creating smart clothes and e-textiles. These new materials are promising to detect an amazing number of physiological parameters, including thermal, mechanical, chemical, electrical, optical and magnetic signals. The availability of such diverse and relevant measurements and parameters highly enhances our ability to establish algorithms and models for health status analysis, prompt and effective intervention, with the ability of real-time data feedback and the ability to further fine-tune our actions.

Once the sensors detect the signal, it is collected, processed, stored and transmitted appropriately. There are several other developments, as the industry is currently researching extensively, to manufacture small, state-of-the-art health tools and useful gadgets. The main theory behind all that excitement is that by measuring and tracking your everyday activities, you can help improve your quality of life and health. Specifically, all of the above mentioned traceable parameters and factors are of great interest and significance for weight management and weight loss interventions.

All the information captured can be easily transferred to a smartphone and can be associated with location, date, time and other information contained on the phone such as calendar events, phone calls or mails. Thus, individuals and their physician can develop a good understanding of the real factors influencing their health and health-related behaviors. Based on that, a reaction plan can be available to lead decisions and actions, mainly regarding food choices and nutrition but also sleep and stress management techniques. In order to promote self-management, personalized predictive models can be combined with captured data (clinical, biological, lifestyle, diet) and empower the patient to participate in the management of his or her health, with application in lifestyle changes and disease monitoring. This will improve patient compliance, adherence to the intervention plan and possibly improve the quality of life and prevent later advert events.

Today's technology offers various ways to encourage children to adopt a certain type of behavior. Mobile technology is one of them since several alerts can be provided based on the understanding of unhealthy behavior. Also, messages can encourage the child to change the unhealthy behavior. In that respect, serious games provide with a means to entertain children, and in that way it is guaranteed that the children will use it, and, on the other hand, to provide with a means to change their behavior. The game must have a balance between "fun – ness" and "serious – ness" elements which can entertain and at the same time impose rules on their behavior (Thompson, 2014). For diabetes and self-management tools, several video games are distributed commercially to cover all ages (Lieberman, 2012). They are experimental and interactive, permitting the player to immerse in worlds offering challenges and progress feedback (Lieberman, 2012). In that sense, a game enhances learning about his/her health and stimulates behavioral change. To enhance access to those games, the cloud has been employed to provide content, recommendation, and evaluation and in that sense with guidance to change behavior (Hassan et al., 2012). A game can be used to fight obesity in children if energy expenditure can be increased, education on nutrition is provided, and healthy eating physical activity is promoted (Selmanovic, 2010).

A serious game can be combined with a mHealth solution. Smartphones can be utilized to deliver to children the high quality and attractive in that sense interfaces. From the point of view of frequent use, this is a real dangerous situation since the child can be addicted to the use of such a game. This somehow can be restricted, if mechanisms for delivering the game permit access only for certain time periods. The game must be carefully designed to include characters, which are familiar and trustable to the child. The game must be viewed as a two edges utility. on one edge the child can be placed, on the other the caregiver, especially the parents. Both sides must be motivated in healthy behavior: The child to avoid any unhealthy behaviors, and the parents to be motivated in a healthy diet, activity, etc. The child in everyday life eats whatever is offered by his/her parents. He/she exercises if the parents exercise. In general, he/she mimics the parent behavior. In that sense, both participate in an active and self-management "game", which entertains, trains and motivates. The game design must be performed by experts, who have a better understanding of the life of an obese child. Providing strict rules does not help, does not really motivate. The game must entertain and at the same time gain the child and convince on healthy attitudes. The solution must be straightforward and not complicated, the healthy eating messages must be presented in an easy to understand way, and above all the provided solution to be attractive and feasible.

Serious games might also involve the school community, but the advice and training provided must be followed by the school personnel itself. Working with a virtual environment and living in a real world, those two actions must be compatible. If the motivation for a healthy lifestyle and weight decrease cannot be followed in the school environment, e.g. if the school canteen does not have, or it is not oriented to the suggestion given by the game, this is not going to work. The same happens with the family and the home. The child must be motivated, but this must be reflected the surrounding world, and the solutions must be there, other ways such games or motivation approaches do not work.

Future developments and implications include the following:

1. Text messaging is an easy and cheap way to obtain greater adherence to treatment and monitoring. It is also well- accepted by parents and children.
2. A theory-driven model of mobile intervention development promises improvement of these interventions.
3. Applications with the end or another involved user in mind that are age appropriate and easy to use will be of greater success.
4. The more interactive the interface is, the more efficacious and approved by the users it will prove to be. The ability to have advice on day to day changing internal and external circumstances can increase compliance and have the much needed sustainable results

5. Use of social support networks may augment the impact. Adolescents are already engaged in social media so they can move to another platform that of weight management and belong to a closed group. They retrieve information, set goals and have peer support. They can also download and upload materials. An application can request data from the user's profile (e.g., his "likes" and interests). The moderators post the task of the week. The members of the group can access the app themselves and be presented with a list of completed and uncompleted tasks. The participants can send material to the moderator through the mail or Facebook message.
6. Serious games can be engaged and implemented in order to provide an interaction between the children and their teachers and/or parents. The games offer the opportunity to "play" (really engage) with their chronic condition, to receive advice and alerts and in case they succeed to receive points to reach a certain goal. Those serious games have been transferred to a smartphone/ tablet platform and are part of any behavioral monitoring or motivation platform. The development of those games is guided by behavioral science principles, and it is a real lead for future developments (Thompson et al., 2010).

DISCUSSION

The options that technology can offer us are unlimited. However, the evaluation of their clinical effectiveness, as well as the users' satisfaction, is very important to improve outcomes and establish effective and sustained progress. At present few developers report whether their apps have been in line with best practice guidelines (E. B. Tate et al., 2013). It is important to have the needs of end users in mind. Kushniruk et al. published cognitive approaches for evaluation of information systems, and users interface (Kushniruk, Patel, & Cimino, 1997). Usability of a computer system can be defined as the capacity of the system to allow users to carry out their tasks safely, effectively, efficiently and enjoyably. Results indicated that subjects tended to rate the system in a very positive way on the questionnaire, despite the fact that video recording of their interaction with the system showed that they had encountered considerable problems in using the system, ranging from inability to navigate through the information contained in the program, to comments indicating that the program's content was out of date (Kushniruk et al., 1997). The practice of evaluating the usability of the electronic application in a small cohort, as O' Malley et al. did, is a valuable, important and necessary tool before applying the application in larger patient groups (O'Malley et al., 2014). Another study explored the usability of the self-management program for youth with juvenile idiopathic arthritis and their parents to refine the health portal proto- type (the usability of the self-management program for youth with juvenile idiopathic arthritis and their parents to refine the health portal prototype (Stinson et al., 2010). Adolescents and parents provided similar as well as differing suggestions on how the website user interface could be improved in terms of improving its usability. Many participants responded that the interactive features made them feel supported and "not alone" in their illness (Stinson et al., 2010). Adolescents and parents provided similar as well as differing suggestions on how the website user interface could be improved in terms of improving its usability. Many participants responded that the interactive features made them feel supported and "not alone" in their illness (Stinson et al., 2010). This creates a very positive attitude for the whole process and enhances effective interventions. This creates a very positive attitude for the whole process and enhances effective interventions.

Additionally, one very important issue is that the content and timing of the intervention can be tailored to patients. By integrating the assessment and intervention capacities of the mobile technology, applications can be developed that are sensitive to the participants' internal states (e.g., mood, cravings, physiological responses) and external cues and contexts (e.g., social interaction, location) (Heron & Smyth, 2010). This feature is of particular importance when dealing with adolescents, but of course, it is welcomed for any population group.

Strengths

mHealth-based child obesity interventions can capitalize on flexibility, speed, and power participant burden offered by mobile technology. The following can be considered:

- The prediction for wide use of smartphones as well as the availability of inexpensive smartphones are opening new opportunities for health applications and particularly for obesity prevention program reaching larger number of patients including lower socioeconomic status children, adolescents and their families.
- The use of mobile phone apps may be a motivational tool for sustainable weight control
- Individualized intervention can be an aspect of success for the intervention
- Sensors and IoT devices offer great flexibility in the collection of data related to weight and other behavioral/ lifestyle patterns.
- Cloud services can be used as a platform for data gathering, analysis, and decision support.
- mHealth advances may provide a new channel through which large audiences of obese young people can be reached and engaged.
- mHealth solutions improve the participation of the patient in the care process
- Use of predictive models augments preventive management
- The major actors in this healthcare process can be easily integrated through the use of mobile applications.
- Serious games can be developed based on the principles of behavioral science.
- Such an approach offers flexibility and is enjoyable for the young people.

Limitations

Still, there are many limitations, which must be faced in self-management systems, which limit the use of such systems and do not permit the wide spread of those approaches:

- Mobile health technologies are rapidly progressing, and they can support health behavior interventions that can be delivered in a personalized manner. A possible drawback is that if the concept behind the intervention is not based on behavior theory, then the content and the timing of the intervention may not be as effective.
- Researchers and practitioners should consider the theoretical basis of health interventions.
- Data protection is a major concern.
- The time that the child or adolescent spends in sedentary behavior and the screen time have to be accounted.

- Increased social isolation, addiction to gaming, or electromagnetic radiation exposure with high cell phone use should be monitored.
- There is a need for interdisciplinary collaboration and the development of appropriate assessment tools.
- The relatively slower speed of the scientific research versus the high development speed of the mobile technology industry.

CONCLUSION

Communication technologies such as mobile phones may serve as an effective medium to deliver affordable health promotion and disease prevention care to an array of people, due to their ubiquity and penetration into people's everyday lives. However, emerging and promising technologies must be matched with such content that can successfully motivate people to change and sustain healthy behaviors. mHealth systems offer opportunities for surveillance and research in childhood obesity as well as development, delivery and dissemination of treatment and prevention programs. Adherence seems improved for those following webbased programs. Online monitoring programs lead to decreased severity of the disease. These interventions provide patients with a sense of accountability. Interventions using mHealth technology can target not only the children but their mothers as well, in order to change child dietary habits and improve maternal weight.

Usability testing is a critical step in the development of Internet interventions and solicits end-user feedback in order to learn what really works, what does not work, and where gaps in information or functionality exist, using iterative cycles to refine the prototype (Currie, 2005; Wichansky, 2000). These factors may impact on the frequency of use, understanding, and the likelihood that a user will implement the recommendations (Currie, 2005; Wichansky, 2000). Usability testing can also help determine the appropriateness of the website interface and content (Gustafson & Wyatt, 2004), especially when it is designed for different audiences (e.g., youth and parents) and delivered in different languages.

REFERENCES

Allen, J. K., Stephens, J., Dennison Himmelfarb, C. R., Stewart, K. J., & Hauck, S. (2013). Randomized Controlled Pilot Study Testing Use of Smartphone Technology for Obesity Treatment. *Journal of Obesity*, *7*. doi:10.1155/2013/151597 PMID:24392223

Bartlett, S. J., Lukk, P., Butz, A., Lampros-Klein, F., & Rand, C. S. (2002). Enhancing medication adherence among inner-city children with asthma: Results from pilot studies. *The Journal of Asthma*, *39*(1), 47–54. doi:10.1081/JAS-120000806 PMID:11883739

Bauer, S., de Niet, J., Timman, R., & Kordy, H. (2010). Enhancement of care through self-monitoring and tailored feedback via text messaging and their use in the treatment of childhood overweight. *Patient Education and Counseling*, *79*(3), 315–319. doi:10.1016/j.pec.2010.03.014 PMID:20418046

Beasley, J. M., Riley, W. T., Davis, A., & Singh, J. (2008). Evaluation of a PDA-based dietary assessment and intervention program: A randomized controlled trial. *Journal of the American College of Nutrition, 27*(2), 280–286. doi:10.1080/07315724.2008.10719701 PMID:18689560

Burke, L. E., Conroy, M. B., Sereika, S. M., Elci, O. U., Styn, M. A., Acharya, S. D., ... Glanz, K. (2011). The effect of electronic self-monitoring on weight loss and dietary intake: A randomized behavioral weight loss trial. *Obesity (Silver Spring, Md.), 19*(2), 338–344. doi:10.1038/oby.2010.208 PMID:20847736

Chaplais, E., Naughton, G., Thivel, D., Courteix, D., & Greene, D. (2015). Smartphone Interventions for Weight Treatment and Behavioral Change in Pediatric Obesity: A Systematic Review. *Telemedicine Journal and e-Health, 21*(10), 822–830. doi:10.1089/tmj.2014.0197 PMID:26290954

Cole-Lewis, H., & Kershaw, T. (2010). Text Messaging as a Tool for Behavior Change in Disease Prevention and Management. *Epidemiologic Reviews, 32*(1), 56–69. doi:10.1093/epirev/mxq004 PMID:20354039

Currie, L. M. (2005). Evaluation frameworks for nursing informatics. *International Journal of Medical Informatics, 74*(11), 908–916. doi:10.1016/j.ijmedinf.2005.07.007 PMID:16099711

de Onis, M., Blössner, M., & Borghi, E. (2010). Global prevalence and trends of overweight and obesity among preschool children. *The American Journal of Clinical Nutrition, 92*(5), 1257–1264. doi:10.3945/ajcn.2010.29786 PMID:20861173

Dijkstra, A., & De Vries, H. (1999). The development of computer-generated tailored interventions. *Patient Education and Counseling, 36*(2), 193–203. doi:10.1016/S0738-3991(98)00135-9 PMID:10223023

E., H. K., & M., S. J. (2010). Ecological momentary interventions: Incorporating mobile technology into psychosocial and health behaviour treatments. *British Journal of Health Psychology, 15*(1), 1-39. doi:10.1348/135910709X466063

Eysenbach, G. (2001). What is e-health? *Journal of Medical Internet Research, 3*(2), e20. doi:10.2196/jmir.3.2.e20 PMID:11720962

Georga, E. I., Protopappas, V. C., Bellos, C. V., & Fotiadis, D. I. (2014). Wearable systems and mobile applications for diabetes disease management. *Health and Technology, 4*(2), 101–112. doi:10.100712553-014-0082-y

Germann, J. N., Kirschenbaum, D. S., & Rich, B. H. (2007). Child and Parental Self-Monitoring as Determinants of Success in the Treatment of Morbid Obesity in Low-Income Minority Children. *Journal of Pediatric Psychology, 32*(1), 111–121. doi:10.1093/jpepsy/jsl007 PMID:16775083

Glynn, L. G., Hayes, P. S., Casey, M., Glynn, F., Alvarez-Iglesias, A., Newell, J., ... Murphy, A. W. (2013). SMART MOVE - a smartphone-based intervention to promote physical activity in primary care: Study protocol for a randomized controlled trial. *Trials, 14*(1), 157. doi:10.1186/1745-6215-14-157 PMID:23714362

Gustafson, D. H., & Wyatt, J. C. (2004). Evaluation of ehealth systems and services. *BMJ (Clinical Research Ed.), 328*(7449), 1150. doi:10.1136/bmj.328.7449.1150 PMID:15142895

Haapala, I., Barengo, N. C., Biggs, S., Surakka, L., & Manninen, P. (2009). Weight loss by mobile phone: A 1-year effectiveness study. *Public Health Nutrition*, *12*(12), 2382–2391. doi:10.1017/S1368980009005230 PMID:19323865

Hall, K. D., & Jordan, P. N. (2008). Modeling weight-loss maintenance to help prevent body weight regain. *The American Journal of Clinical Nutrition*, *88*(6), 1495–1503. doi:10.3945/ajcn.2008.26333 PMID:19064508

Hassan, M. M., Hossain, M. S., Alamri, A., Hossain, M. A., Al-Qurishi, M., Aldukhayyil, Y., & Ahmed, D. T. (2012). *A cloud-based serious games framework for obesity*. Paper presented at the Proceedings of the 1st ACM multimedia international workshop on Cloud-based multimedia applications and services for e-health, Nara, Japan.

Heron, K. E., & Smyth, J. M. (2010). Ecological momentary interventions: Incorporating mobile technology into psychosocial and health behaviour treatments. *British Journal of Health Psychology*, *15*(Pt 1), 1–39. doi:10.1348/135910709X466063 PMID:19646331

Hill, J. O., Wyatt, H. R., Reed, G. W., & Peters, J. C. (2003). Obesity and the Environment: Where Do We Go from Here? *Science*, *299*(5608), 853–855. doi:10.1126cience.1079857 PMID:12574618

Hull, P., Emerson, S. J., Quirk, E. M., Canedo, R. J., Jones, L. J., Vylegzhanina, V., ... Husaini, A. B. (2017). A Smartphone App for Families With Preschool-Aged Children in a Public Nutrition Program: Prototype Development and Beta-Testing. *JMIR mHealth and uHealth*, *5*(8), e102. doi:10.2196/mhealth.7477 PMID:28768611

Hurling, R., Catt, M., De Boni, M., Fairley, B. W., Hurst, T., Murray, P., ... Sodhi, J. S. (2007). Using Internet and Mobile Phone Technology to Deliver an Automated Physical Activity Program: Randomized Controlled Trial. *Journal of Medical Internet Research*, *9*(2), e7. doi:10.2196/jmir.9.2.e7 PMID:17478409

Kelsey, M. M., Zaepfel, A., Bjornstad, P., & Nadeau, K. J. (2014). Age-Related Consequences of Childhood Obesity. *Gerontology*, *60*(3), 222–228. doi:10.1159/000356023 PMID:24434909

Khaylis, A., Yiaslas, T., Bergstrom, J., & Gore-Felton, C. (2010). A Review of Efficacious Technology-Based Weight-Loss Interventions: Five Key Components. *Telemedicine Journal and e-Health*, *16*(9), 931–938. doi:10.1089/tmj.2010.0065 PMID:21091286

King, A. C., Ahn, D. K., Oliveira, B. M., Atienza, A. A., Castro, C. M., & Gardner, C. D. (2008). Promoting Physical Activity Through Hand-Held Computer Technology. *American Journal of Preventive Medicine*, *34*(2), 138–142. doi:10.1016/j.amepre.2007.09.025 PMID:18201644

Kirschenbaum, D. S., Germann, J. N., & Rich, B. H. (2005). Treatment of morbid obesity in low-income adolescents: Effects of parental self-monitoring. *Obesity Research*, *13*(9), 1527–1529. doi:10.1038/oby.2005.187 PMID:16222054

Kreuter, M. W., & Wray, R. J. (2003). Tailored and Targeted Health Communication: Strategies for Enhancing Information Relevance. *American Journal of Health Behavior*, *27*(1), S227–S232. doi:10.5993/AJHB.27.1.s3.6 PMID:14672383

Krishna, S., Boren, S. A., & Balas, E. A. (2009). Healthcare via cell phones: A systematic review. *Telemedicine Journal and e-Health, 15*(3), 231–240. doi:10.1089/tmj.2008.0099 PMID:19382860

Kushniruk, A. W., Patel, V. L., & Cimino, J. J. (1997). Usability testing in medical informatics: cognitive approaches to evaluation of information systems and user interfaces. *Proceedings of the AMIA Annual Fall Symposium*, 218-222.

Lee, J. E., Lee, D. E., Kim, K., Shim, J. E., Sung, E., Kang, J.-H., & Hwang, J.-Y. (2017). Development of tailored nutrition information messages based on the transtheoretical model for smartphone application of an obesity prevention and management program for elementary-school students. *Nutrition Research and Practice, 11*(3), 247–256. doi:10.4162/nrp.2017.11.3.247 PMID:28584582

Lieberman, D. A. (2012). Video Games for Diabetes Self-Management: Examples and Design Strategies. *Journal of Diabetes Science and Technology, 6*(4), 802–806. doi:10.1177/193229681200600410 PMID:22920805

Litwin, S. E. (2014). Childhood Obesity and Adulthood Cardiovascular Disease*: Quantifying the Lifetime Cumulative Burden of Cardiovascular Risk Factors. *Journal of the American College of Cardiology, 64*(15), 1588–1590. doi:10.1016/j.jacc.2014.07.962 PMID:25301462

Liu, W.-T., Wang, C.-H., Lin, H.-C., Lin, S.-M., Lee, K.-Y., Lo, Y.-L., ... Kuo, H.-P. (2008). Efficacy of a cell phone-based exercise programme for COPD. *The European Respiratory Journal, 32*(3), 651–659. doi:10.1183/09031936.00104407 PMID:18508824

Mameli, C., Brunetti, D., Colombo, V., Bedogni, G., Schneider, L., Penagini, F., ... Zuccotti, G. V. (2018). Combined use of a wristband and a smartphone to reduce body weight in obese children: Randomized controlled trial. *Pediatric Obesity, 13*(2), 81–87. doi:10.1111/ijpo.12201 PMID:27900849

Napolitano, M. A., Hayes, S., Bennett, G. G., Ives, A. K., & Foster, G. D. (2013). Using Facebook and text messaging to deliver a weight loss program to college students. *Obesity (Silver Spring, Md.), 21*(1), 25–31. doi:10.1002/oby.20232 PMID:23505165

Neve, M., Morgan, P. J., Jones, P. R., & Collins, C. E. (2010). Effectiveness of web-based interventions in achieving weight loss and weight loss maintenance in overweight and obese adults: A systematic review with meta-analysis. *Obesity Reviews, 11*(4), 306–321. doi:10.1111/j.1467-789X.2009.00646.x PMID:19754633

Nezami, B. T., Lytle, L. A., & Tate, D. F. (2016). A randomized trial to reduce sugar-sweetened beverage and juice intake in preschool-aged children: Description of the Smart Moms intervention trial. *BMC Public Health, 16*(1), 837. doi:10.118612889-016-3533-8 PMID:27542357

Nezami, B. T., Ward, D. S., Lytle, L. A., Ennett, S. T., & Tate, D. F. (2017). A mHealth randomized controlled trial to reduce sugar-sweetened beverage intake in preschool-aged children. *Pediatric Obesity*. doi:10.1111/ijpo.12258 PMID:29119719

Ng, M., Fleming, T., Robinson, M., Thomson, B., Graetz, N., Margono, C., ... Gakidou, E. (2014). Global, regional, and national prevalence of overweight and obesity in children and adults during 1980–2013: A systematic analysis for the Global Burden of Disease Study 2013. *Lancet, 384*(9945), 766–781. doi:10.1016/S0140-6736(14)60460-8 PMID:24880830

Nollen, N. L., Hutcheson, T., Carlson, S., Rapoff, M., Goggin, K., Mayfield, C., & Ellerbeck, E. (2013). Development and functionality of a handheld computer program to improve fruit and vegetable intake among low-income youth. *Health Education Research, 28*(2), 249–264. doi:10.1093/her/cys099 PMID:22949499

Nollen, N. L., Mayo, M. S., Carlson, S. E., Rapoff, M. A., Goggin, K. J., & Ellerbeck, E. F. (2014). Mobile Technology for Obesity Prevention: A Randomized Pilot Study in Racial- and Ethnic-Minority Girls. *American Journal of Preventive Medicine, 46*(4), 404–408. doi:10.1016/j.amepre.2013.12.011 PMID:24650843

Norman, G. J., Zabinski, M. F., Adams, M. A., Rosenberg, D. E., Yaroch, A. L., & Atienza, A. A. (2007). A Review of eHealth Interventions for Physical Activity and Dietary Behavior Change. *American Journal of Preventive Medicine, 33*(4), 336–345.e316. doi:10.1016/j.amepre.2007.05.007 PMID:17888860

O'Malley, G., Clarke, M., Burls, A., Murphy, S., Murphy, N., & Perry, I. J. (2014). A smartphone intervention for adolescent obesity: Study protocol for a randomised controlled non-inferiority trial. *Trials, 15*(1), 43. doi:10.1186/1745-6215-15-43 PMID:24485327

Oh, H., Rizo, C., Enkin, M., Jadad, A., Powell, J., & Pagliari, C. (2005). What Is eHealth (3): A Systematic Review of Published Definitions. *Journal of Medical Internet Research, 7*(1), e1. doi:10.2196/jmir.7.1.e1 PMID:15829471

Pediatrics, A. A. (2011). Expert Panel on Integrated Guidelines for Cardiovascular Health and Risk Reduction in Children and Adolescents: Summary Report. *Pediatrics, 128*(Supplement 5), S213–S256. doi:10.1542/peds.2009-2107C PMID:22084329

Pretlow, R. A., Stock, C. M., Allison, S., & Roeger, L. (2015). Treatment of child/adolescent obesity using the addiction model: A smartphone app pilot study. *Childhood Obesity, 11*(3), 248–259. doi:10.1089/chi.2014.0124 PMID:25760813

Riley, W. T., Cesar, A. M., & Rivera, D. E. (2014). *The importance of behavior theory in control system modeling of physical activity sensor data.* Paper presented at the 2014 36th Annual International Conference of the IEEE Engineering in Medicine and Biology Society.

Riley, W. T., & Rivera, D. E. (2014). Methodologies for optimizing behavioral interventions: Introduction to special section. *Translational Behavioral Medicine, 4*(3), 234–237. doi:10.100713142-014-0281-0 PMID:25264463

Schiel, R., Kaps, A., & Bieber, G. (2012). Electronic health technology for the assessment of physical activity and eating habits in children and adolescents with overweight and obesity IDA. *Appetite, 58*(2), 432–437. doi:10.1016/j.appet.2011.11.021 PMID:22155072

Sepah, S. C., Jiang, L., & Peters, A. L. (2014). Translating the Diabetes Prevention Program into an Online Social Network:Validation against CDC Standards. *The Diabetes Educator, 40*(4), 435–443. doi:10.1177/0145721714531339 PMID:24723130

Sepah, S. C., Jiang, L., & Peters, A. L. (2015). Long-Term Outcomes of a Web-Based Diabetes Prevention Program: 2-Year Results of a Single-Arm Longitudinal Study. *Journal of Medical Internet Research, 17*(4), e92. doi:10.2196/jmir.4052 PMID:25863515

Shapiro, J. R., Bauer, S., Hamer, R. M., Kordy, H., Ward, D., & Bulik, C. M. (2008). Use of Text Messaging for Monitoring Sugar-sweetened Beverages, Physical Activity, and Screen Time in Children: A Pilot Study. *Journal of Nutrition Education and Behavior*, *40*(6), 385–391. doi:10.1016/j.jneb.2007.09.014 PMID:18984496

Sharifi, M., Dryden, E. M., Horan, C. M., Price, S., Marshall, R., Hacker, K., ... Taveras, E. M. (2013). Leveraging text messaging and mobile technology to support pediatric obesity-related behavior change: A qualitative study using parent focus groups and interviews. *Journal of Medical Internet Research*, *15*(12), e272. doi:10.2196/jmir.2780 PMID:24317406

Smith, J. J., Morgan, P. J., Plotnikoff, R. C., Dally, K. A., Salmon, J., Okely, A. D., ... Lubans, D. R. (2014). Smart-Phone Obesity Prevention Trial for Adolescent Boys in Low-Income Communities: The ATLAS RCT. *Pediatrics*, *134*(3), e723–e731. doi:10.1542/peds.2014-1012 PMID:25157000

Stephens, J., & Allen, J. (2013). Mobile phone interventions to increase physical activity and reduce weight: A systematic review. *The Journal of Cardiovascular Nursing*, *28*(4), 320–329. doi:10.1097/JCN.0b013e318250a3e7 PMID:22635061

Stinson, J., McGrath, P., Hodnett, E., Feldman, B., Duffy, C., Huber, A., ... White, M. (2010). Usability Testing of an Online Self-management Program for Adolescents With Juvenile Idiopathic Arthritis. *Journal of Medical Internet Research*, *12*(3), e30. doi:10.2196/jmir.1349 PMID:20675293

Stone, A. A., Shiffman, S., Schwartz, J. E., Broderick, J. E., & Hufford, M. R. (2003). Patient compliance with paper and electronic diaries. *Controlled Clinical Trials*, *24*(2), 182–199. doi:10.1016/S0197-2456(02)00320-3 PMID:12689739

Swinburn, B. A., Sacks, G., Lo, S. K., Westerterp, K. R., Rush, E. C., Rosenbaum, M., ... Ravussin, E. (2009). Estimating the changes in energy flux that characterize the rise in obesity prevalence. *The American Journal of Clinical Nutrition*, *89*(6), 1723–1728. doi:10.3945/ajcn.2008.27061 PMID:19369382

Tate, D. F., Wing, R. R., & Winett, R. A. (2001). Using internet technology to deliver a behavioral weight loss program. *Journal of the American Medical Association*, *285*(9), 1172–1177. doi:10.1001/jama.285.9.1172 PMID:11231746

Tate, E. B., Spruijt-Metz, D., O'Reilly, G., Jordan-Marsh, M., Gotsis, M., Pentz, M. A., & Dunton, G. F. (2013). mHealth approaches to child obesity prevention: Successes, unique challenges, and next directions. *Translational Behavioral Medicine*, *3*(4), 406–415. doi:10.100713142-013-0222-3 PMID:24294329

Teixeira, P. J., Carraça, E. V., Marques, M. M., Rutter, H., Oppert, J.-M., De Bourdeaudhuij, I., ... Brug, J. (2015). Successful behavior change in obesity interventions in adults: A systematic review of self-regulation mediators. *BMC Medicine*, *13*(1), 84. doi:10.118612916-015-0323-6 PMID:25907778

Thompson, D. (2014). What Serious Video Games Can Offer Child Obesity Prevention. *JMIR Serious Games*, *2*(2), e8. doi:10.2196/games.3480 PMID:25654589

Thompson, D., Baranowski, T., Buday, R., Baranowski, J., Thompson, V., Jago, R., & Griffith, M. J. (2010). Serious Video Games for Health: How Behavioral Science Guided the Development of a Serious Video Game. *Simulation & Gaming*, *41*(4), 587–606. doi:10.1177/1046878108328087 PMID:20711522

Tufano, J. T., & Karras, B. T. (2005). Mobile eHealth Interventions for Obesity: A Timely Opportunity to Leverage Convergence Trends. *Journal of Medical Internet Research, 7*(5), e58. doi:10.2196/jmir.7.5.e58 PMID:16403722

Turner, A., Karube, I., & Wilson, G. S. (Eds.). (1987). *Biosensors: Fundamentals and Applications* (1st ed.). Oxford, UK: Oxford University Press.

Turner, T., & Spruijt-Metz, D. (2015). *Prevention and treatment of pediatric obesity using mobile and wireless technologies: a systematic review*. Academic Press. doi:10.1111/ijpo.12002

Vlachopapadopoulou, E., & Fotiadis, D. (2016). The Contribution of mHealth in the Care of Obese Pediatric Patients. In M. Anastasius (Ed.), *M-Health Innovations for Patient-Centered Care* (pp. 126–146). Hershey, PA: IGI Global. doi:10.4018/978-1-4666-9861-1.ch007

Wadden, T. A., & Butryn, M. L. (2003). Behavioral treatment of obesity. *Endocrinology and Metabolism Clinics of North America, 32*(4), 981–1003. doi:10.1016/S0889-8529(03)00072-0 PMID:14711071

Wang, Y., Xue, H., Huang, Y., Huang, L., & Zhang, D. (2017). A Systematic Review of Application and Effectiveness of mHealth Interventions for Obesity and Diabetes Treatment and Self-Management. *Advances in Nutrition, 8*(3), 449–462. doi:10.3945/an.116.014100 PMID:28507010

Wichansky, A. M. (2000). Usability testing in 2000 and beyond. *Ergonomics, 43*(7), 998–1006. doi:10.1080/001401300409170 PMID:10929833

Wing, R. R., & Hill, J. O. (2001). Successful weight loss maintenance. *Annual Review of Nutrition, 21*(1), 323–341. doi:10.1146/annurev.nutr.21.1.323 PMID:11375440

Wing, R. R., & Hill, J. O. (2001). Successful weight loss maintenance. *Annual Review of Nutrition, 21*(1), 323–341. doi:10.1146/annurev.nutr.21.1.323 PMID:11375440

Yang, H., Kang, J.-H., Kim, O., Choi, M., Oh, M., Nam, J., & Sung, E. (2017). Interventions for Preventing Childhood Obesity with Smartphones and Wearable Device: A Protocol for a Non-Randomized Controlled Trial. *International Journal of Environmental Research and Public Health, 14*(2), 184. doi:10.3390/ijerph14020184 PMID:28208839

KEY TERMS AND DEFINITIONS

Behavior Interventions: Protocols targeting body mass index reduction, implementing behavior modification and/or diet change, and increased physical activity. The strategy as well as the personnel involved, the duration, and the means used vary.

Biosensors: A biosensor is a device, based on a biological sensing element, whose output signal is proportional to a concentration of a chemical or chemicals.

Childhood Obesity: Increased body weight associated with increased adiposity which is best reflected by an increased body mass index. Body mass index cut offs points differ according to age and sex. There is no universal agreement regarding the cut-offs.

Cloud: Cloud computing refers to a model which permits users to access servers and storage resources through the internet using a web browser or a client code.

Comorbidities: Childhood obesity is potentially associated with some complications that include insulin resistance, glucose intolerance, diabetes mellitus, fatty liver disease, dyslipidemia, hypertension, metabolic syndrome, sleep apnea, depression.

Internet of Things (IoT): Is a concept which describes a network of "things" (sensors, electronic devices, other hardware, etc.) and their capability to exchange data.

Lifestyle: The sets of daily habits that include meal frequency and composition, exercise frequency and duration, hours of sleep, hours of sedentary activities, hours of physical activity mainly walking.

Sensors: A sensor is a device which can detect input from its physical environment, in our case from the human body. The sensor output is an electronic signal which can be transmitted and displayed.

Smartphones: A smartphone is a small device that can be used as a cellphone and a personal computer having the advantage of mobility. The disadvantage of the small screen has been overcome by its high-resolution screen.

Chapter 5
Mobile Health (M-Health) for Tele-Wound Monitoring:
Role of M-Health in Wound Management

Chinmay Chakraborty
Birla Institute of Technology, India

ABSTRACT

This chapter describes the implementation of tele-wound monitoring (TWM) for a patient's chronic wound using a smartphone. The system proved to be quick and reliable for providing healthcare at the doorstep. The smartphone-enabled a tele-wound monitoring (TWM) framework, which is used for remote wound monitoring, has been highlighted. The TWM is effective for both rural as well as urban people; it provides good performance in terms of wound monitoring and diagnosis. The objective of this chapter is to design and develop a TWM system model that can acquire, process and monitor chronic wound-related problems by using a low-cost smartphone to increase the overall performance of the system. Specifically, the TWM system is developed for biomedical information like chronic wound processing to monitor important patient information inexpensively and accurately. The implementation is carried out using hypertext preprocessor (PHP) and MySql database and especially by Firebase cloud database, which is used for improving the efficiency.

INTRODUCTION

The Information and Communication Technology (ICT) plays a vital role in the healthcare domain to improve the overall performance of the system. Efficient communication is needed for adjusting care and preventing serious issues as interventions can be done faster. The ICT is used for storing and retrieval of the information and provides the patients with better services at a reduced cost. The advantages of ICTs are as follows: (a) faster accessibility to clinicians and other medical resources, (b) technology helps to improve the hospital administration for better care, (c) quick critical patient monitoring, and (d) all medical related information is available via the social media. Currently ICT faces a lot of challenges due to the following reasons: lack of medical data standards, (b) poor infrastructure, (e) environmental chal-

DOI: 10.4018/978-1-5225-8021-8.ch005

Copyright © 2019, IGI Global. Copying or distributing in print or electronic forms without written permission of IGI Global is prohibited.

lenges, (f) Poor government policy, (g) lack of consistent power supply, (g) poor internet connectivity, and (h) lack of skilled people to operate the system, (i) lack of awareness respectively in today's health care system. Bashshur et al. (2011) explained the importance of ICT for health domains consisting of (a) telemedicine, (b) telehealth, (c) e-Health and (d) m-Health.

Telemedicine

The smartphone has been recognized as a possible tool for a telemedicine system. (Chinmay et al., 2016). The smartphone used in telemedicine with an inbuilt high-resolution camera to capture digital images and computing and networking features which allow direct interaction. The acquired wound data using a smartphone app process is the central hub for better treatment. Appropriate returning messages will be routed to local providers through physical delivery to ensure information integrity. Telemedicine systems are becoming more demanding by providing advanced features of the smartphone and better computing services. Telemedicine systems also maintain stored patient's data in the database. Telemedicine (Wood et al., 2008) is an emerging field in advanced communication systems and medical informatics, able to deliver the healthcare data and to share medical expertise using wireless technologies in the span of tele-oncology, telepathology, teleradiology, emergency healthcare and teledermatology. The high featured smartphones (Xolo, Apple, Nokia, Samsung Galaxy Tab, Windows Phone, Blackberry, iOS, Jio, Canon, Adobe, Android) can be used for sensing, acquiring a variety of medical data collection and monitoring applications.

Telehealth

Telehealth acts as a bridge between a patient and a healthcare provider via an electronic medium to monitor medical services at distant sites. Telehealth systems examine patients who are in a critical condition with medical facilities anytime. It provides the patient's vital signs monitoring on a regular basis reducing time and cost. This system created its network-based telehealth wound management system to address the systematic issue in the provision of wound care. It improves the access to healthcare technology and reduces costs. Telehealth can be applied to chronic wounds monitoring over a long distance because it can transfer audio and visual patient information from remote to expert clinics with specialized wound knowledge and technical skill.

E-Health

The electronic health (e-Health) services are driven by computers and other medical devices in the global market. Smartphone usability has increased drastically in recent years. e-Health improves the access efficiency, quality of care, effectiveness, and connected medical organizations, practitioners, patients, medical personnel in an effort to enhance the patient health status.

M-Health

Mobile health (m-Health) technology is the most demanding and developing factor in healthcare today providing better and more efficient care. The m-Health is a part of e-Health used in the delivery of healthcare services or medical information with a smartphone. m-Health technology plays an important role in monitoring the remote wound diseases. There is limited access to modern technology for managing the chronic wounds. According to clinical experience, high-quality regular care, especially for patients, self-management is necessary for accelerating wound healing. International statistics providing the complete depiction of the disability, occurrence, and impairment of wounds are difficult to acquire. The wound affected region information is collected by m-health technology through the faster network connectivity for processing and analysis. More advanced smartphone-enabled m-Health technology supports the remote diagnosis, telemedicine, and web-browsing, access to web-based patient data, GPS navigation, post-visit patient surveillance, and better healthcare management. Meum (2012) implemented the electronic medication management system using new technology to reduce the incidence of serious errors. A smartphone application page enables patients to remotely send wound images for monitoring by clinicians. M-Health allows the patient to be continuously monitored, and includes mobile telemedicine, various healthcare units, electronic health records (EHR), remote patient monitoring, mobile patient monitoring, hospital information system, hospital management system, decision support systems, medical survey and awareness raising which can play a major role to enhance the healthcare services. This technology provides fast, secure, reliable, accurate, economical and time-saving, reduce hospital visits for regular health monitoring. M-Health allows new technologies in sensing, medical imaging and wireless data communications with much lower cost, enabling the development of new widespread remote medicine initiatives.

m-Health = Smartphone with application page + patient + remote healthcare service provider + cloud framework + clinician's feedback processing

The above-mentioned platforms have been providing continuous supports towards remote chronic wound status monitoring. Nowadays, the chronic wounds (CWs) signify an important health issue. The wound status monitoring is also a vital task in healthcare globally. Mostly, older adults (over 60 years) are more prone to suffering due to chronic wounds. The non-healing wounds can persist for years, causing pain to patients and placing them at risk for secondary infections and loss of a limb. All types of wounds may become chronic due to various conditions that stop or slow the wound healing process. These may include any of the following: (a) poor blood supply or ischemia, (b) infections, (c) immune suppression, (d) tissue swelling, (e) age, and (f) malignancy respectively. Patients are affected in many ways by various problems caused by the CWs such as pain, restricted mobility, economic burden and psychological stress which all lead to a reduced quality of life. The open wound is an injury, involves an internal or external break in body tissue. The five types of open wounds are abrasion (topmost layer of the skin is removed, painful), incision (smooth edges), laceration (irregular edges), puncture (deep, narrow wound) and avulsion (bleed heavily) respectively. In a closed wound, the skin surface is not broken so tissue damage and any bleeding occur below the surface.

Wound Types

More broadly, wounds are classified into two types acute and chronic wound. ***Acute wound*** – it is defined as the disruption in the integrity of skin and underlying tissue that progresses through the healing process in a timely and uneventful manner that results in sustained restoration of anatomic and functional integrity. ***Chronic wound*** – according to Mustoe et al. (2006), chronic wound healing process is slow and stagnated; it does not heal through an orderly and timely reparative process over a period of three months to restore anatomic and functional integrity. Moreo (2005), and Mustoe (2004) discussed that CWs are mainly classified into four categories: diabetic ulcer (DU), pressure ulcer (PU), venous ulcer (VU) and ischemic or arterial ulcer (IU) respectively.

Classification of Wounds

The chronic wound tissue can be classified into three major categories like granulation, slough, and necrosis. Granulation (G) tissue represents the growth of new tissue with a red color area that requires moist wound healing products, slough (S) tissue indicates infection with a yellow color area, requiring autolytic debridement and moist wound healing and necrotic (N) tissue represents the area of black dead tissue, which needs to be removed. Chinmay et al. (2016) discussed that the clinicians are used to the red-yellow-black (RYB) color coding scheme for classifying the different wound tissue and digital image commonly represented as red-green-blue (RGB) color. Figure 1 depicts the various tissue types with color variation.

Status of Chronic Wounds Treatment

In India, there is a scarcity of wound data on the prevalence of diabetes, atherosclerosis, tuberculosis, leprosy, and trauma, all of which lead to the development of CWs by one or other mechanism. There is also a lack of adequate health facilities and appropriate treatment in rural areas where 70% of the population lives, very few studies have been conducted to address the problem of CWs. The inappropriate treatment of acute traumatic wounds was the most widespread cause of the CW. In many poor counties, a lot of patients' cannot meet the expenses of many of the wound-related investigations. The different kinds of ulcers are debilitating and more painful, mainly reducing patient's quality of life. The wound assessment is a tedious assignment for clinicians as it requires periodic evaluation. The 5-7 million chronic or complex wounds occur each year in North America. An occurrence of patients with a wound was 3.55 per 1000 population in the United Kingdom. The popularity of wounds was surgical/trauma (48%), leg/foot (28%), and pressure ulcers (21%). In the United States, the healing cost of a single pressure ulcer can be as much as $50 billion, and CWs affect around 6.4 million patients annually. The United Nations - 2009 report showed that it affects more than 2 billion European populations and the

Figure 1. Three important tissue types - granulation, slough, and necrotic tissue

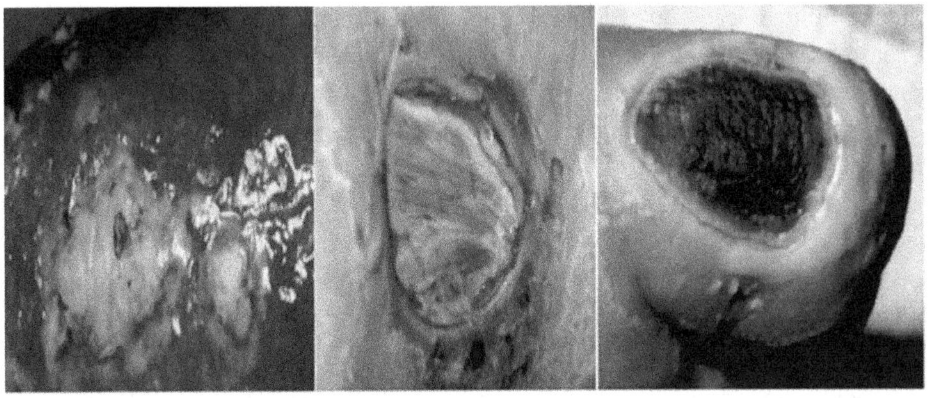

related cost of treatment is about 8 billion Euros per year. In 2012, there were 24 million people who faced CWs problems worldwide. Also, it is anticipated that worldwide 380 million people will suffer from this highly branded disease by the year 2025 (Inter., 2006). The treating foot ulcers cost is estimated at around $5 billion annually (Arthur, 2010). Although there is little variation in the treatment of the different CWs, appropriate management seeks to address the root cause of CWs, including ischemia, infection, and imbalance of proteases (Mustoe, 2004).

A typical treatment protocol is based on the combination of the following interventions:

1. Proper cleansing of the wound with sterile water to reduce the possibility of infection.
2. Debridement of dead necrotic tissue, foreign objects such as small stones, glass particles, and dirt that can delay healing and lead to infection.
3. Use of external compression bandages to reduce edema by encouraging a movement of lymphatic fluids and blood through the veins.
4. Use of wound dressings to absorb the wound exudate and maintain the moisture in the wound area to promote and speed healing.
5. Infection should be controlled by the application of topical or oral antibiotics.
6. If required wound should be treated surgically to promote wound healing.

Healing wounds have mostly red granulation tissue that shows proper blood circulation in the wound region and absence of any infection. Whereas yellow slough tissue is due to the presence of pus, fibrous material and other cellular components which accumulate as a result of infection in the wound. The black tissue is due to adherent necrotic tissue in the wound which should be removed to improve the wound healing. Information about the size of the wound area and percentage of each tissue in the wound area are important factors for determining the healing state of the wound and to evaluate and make necessary changes for the further treatment of the wound.

BACKGROUND

The preventive measures can be taken to bring low-cost screenings to the patients. The major limitations of chronic wound treatments are the lack of qualitative assessment, mostly dependent on color information, while more ambiguities are there in detecting the CW type. There is no information about the percentage of wound tissue, inaccurate estimation of area and its monitoring over time, which is highly expert-dependent, limited access to modern technology for managing chronic wounds and there is no standard database available in present days respectively. There is, however, a demand for a practical tool for automatic wound assessment, combining dimensional measurements and tissue classification in a single user-friendly system which is not only used in therapeutic follow-up in hospitals but could also be used for telemedicine purposes and clinical research, where repeatability and accuracy of wound assessment are critical. Automatic wound assessment tools integrated with the m-health facility will drastically reduce the health care cost as patient monitoring could be carried out from a distance, outside a hospital environment, in private homes properly equipped for telemedicine practice. The clinician needs an objective for wound characterization method to decide if the current treatment is adequate or requires adjustments. The accurate wound measurement is an important task in CWs treatments because changes in the wound size and proportions of different tissue types are indicators of the wound healing.

Professionals dealing with wounded patients need to make treatment decisions principally, but not solely based on their visual perception.

Traditionally only empirical traditional or manual methods are used by the healthcare professionals for spatial measurements such as rulers, sketches, transparency tracings and alginate moldings (Gethin, 2005). These methods give an only rough approximation of total wound area and no information about the proportion of different wound tissue types. Also, these methods are time-consuming, inaccurate and result in pain, infection, and allergy to the patient. These evaluations depend on the experience of the clinicians and are non-objective thus not eligible for validation of the wound healing process. Normal digital cameras and the smartphone could be used to acquire the wound image quickly and store it for further processing. The different methods required for analyzing the wound image such as preprocessing, segmentation, feature extraction, and classification are easily done by the automated diagnostic tool, although it is a difficult task for a human being (Albouy, 2005). Evaluation should be more accurate, reproducible and faster. Affordability of high-speed computers makes possible the implementation of sophisticated classification algorithms. The wound analysis should include measurement of the wound area and analysis of the color distribution within the wound affected portion. As manual methods of wound area calculation are invasive and inaccurate, the non-invasive digital planimetry method has the advantage of reducing the possibility of imparting infection as well as being faster and reproducible.

Challenges in Chronic Wound Monitoring Methods: Conventional vs. Recent Advances

There is limited access to modern technology for managing CWs. The current traditional clinical wound assessments depend on simple spatial measurements like ruler-based methods, tape measurement methods, transparency tracing, and alginate cast. Such types of subjective evaluations are inaccurate, inconsistent, inefficient and painful. The ambiguities and intra-observer variation affect wound classification. The manual errors include inconsistency of the data, loss of reliability and redundancy. The physical dangers to the data are aging of the paper documents, water, and bugs respectively. Several features contribute to making an automatic classification difficult. First, wound image acquisition requires technical skill, especially in the patient room where lighting is not controlled. At close range, the depth of field remains always limited in macro-mode; ambient light is insufficient and may easily result in fuzzy images. Moreover, the patient is rarely able to maintain a convenient posture for a snapshot. Figure 2 depicts the manual, error-prone patient monitoring systems.

The treatments of chronic wounds include monitoring of the color and size of the wound at regular intervals. Most of the people reported re-occurrences even after a long period of treatment. The critical task is to perform an accurate diagnosis and select a suitable treatment. The important parameter like color may provide relevant information about the tissue type and inflammation. The semi-automatic and or automatic process gives better results with respect to traditional methods. Mankar et al. (2013) have discussed 2D and 3D techniques for wound measurement. Two-dimensional techniques are influenced by lighting conditions, camera position, and angle of acquisition. 3D techniques could produce more metrics from the wound such as perimeter, depth, area, and volume. The new non-traditional techniques are required that increases accuracy in size measurements while reducing inter and intra-observer variability. They are low-cost, multispectral, hyperspectral, hi-tech medical imaging combined with a 3D surface and user-friendly. The computer-based diagnosis gives a good result concerning manual observation. The wound shape and size are the vital parameters in clinical and basic research for test

Figure 2. Manual, error-prone patient's monitoring system

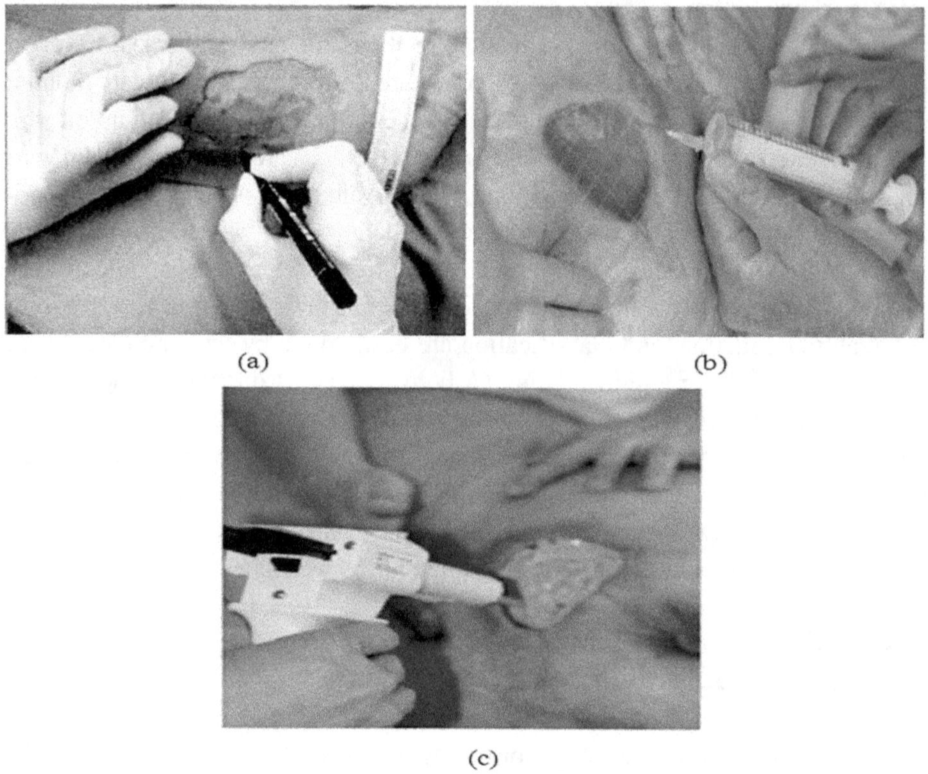

and effectiveness. The computerized wound documenting systems like digital VERG (Vista Medial Ltd., Winnipeg, Manitoba, Canada) and VISITRAK give the capability to measure the wound length and width automatically (Haghpanah, 2006). The VERG and VISITRAK software provide estimates of the length, width, area, and volume. DigiSkin software uses digital photography for picture processing that provides length, width, depth, area, and volume (Korber et al., 2006). Table 1 depicts the features of different devices for CW healing monitoring.

M-Health for Remote Wound Monitoring

M-Health is used for the delivery of public health and the sharing of medical information supported by smartphones. The aim is to provide expert based medical care service to any place that health care is needed. The shortage of good medical doctors, nurses, clinics or hospitals, and high expenditure incurred during medical treatment, increase the seriousness of the problem. Due to the unavailability of these factors m-health is needed to collect the vital patient's information remotely through computer-aided diagnosis and or high-resolution camera based smartphones. M-health aims to improves access to healthcare facilities for rural areas, gives clinicians better accessibility to tertiary consultation, gives clinicians access to conduct remote examinations, improve patient care, reduces health-care costs and patient transfers to secondary and tertiary care centers respectively. In the real-time mode, the clinician is present during the capture process through a video conferencing system, and streaming can be sent to TMH. The store-and-forward approach in a telemedicine system consists of a tele-medical Agent (TMA)

Table 1. Characteristics of various medical devices for CWs

Devices	*Main Features*	*Limitation*	*Cost*
Measurement of Area and Volume Instrument System (MAVIS) (Plassmann et al., 1998)	To measure area and volume of skin wounds, ulcers, and pressure sores Small and deep wounds can be measured with greater precision It is fast and comparably more precise than existing traditional techniques Frequently monitoring is possible with higher consistency	It cannot measure the depth of wound or ulcer Lacking interconnectivity between patients and clinics	Expensive
Stereophotogramm-etry (SPG) (Sprigle et al., 2006)	Multiple images are taken of the same wound with a slightly different angle Easy to perform Gives an accurate and repeatable result	Lacks accuracy Complex systems	Expensive
Wound measurement device (WMD) (Nemeth et al., 2010)	Depth measurement is possible Increased reliability as compared to conventional methods with high precision	Poor accuracy	Moderate
ARANZ Medical Silhouette (Silhousette, 2010)	High-quality wound image handling capability Robust, portable, easy to use and gives an accurate outcome	Poor accuracy	Expensive
Advanced Wound Assessment and Measurement System (AWAMS) (Casas et al., 2011)	Interface of a video camera with touch pad Calculate wound area and percentage of tissue types	----	Expensive
Medical Digital Photogrammetric System (MEDPHOS) (Malcolm, 2013)	Provide high speed and simple application Robustness and reliability Precision and accuracy	----	Low
DERMA device (Nila et al., 2013)	Measure the time evolution of CWs Provides uniform interface to manage data High precision	Complicated	Moderate
Verge Videometer (VeV) (Williams, 2009)	Determine wound measurement using an accurate perimeter-based algorithm	Lack of accuracy	Quite costly
Stereophotogrammetry (SPG) (Thawer et al., 2002)	Wound volume determination performed Reliable and precise computer-assisted technique	Inaccuracy	Low cost
Compression Therapy Device (Robson et al., 2006)	To reduce the swelling and aid in the healing of a CW Used for chronic venous insufficiency	Poor healing rate Complex	Moderate

capturing patient data independently (images, text files, patient symptoms in a text file, etc.) and then sending them over the Internet to a clinician who can asynchronously and non-interactively perform a diagnosis (Chakraborty et al., 2014). The m-Health provides TMA to monitor physiological changes, test results, images with proper clinical evidence. Here, the TWM framework under the m-health scenario has been highlighted for remote wound monitoring. This framework is very effective for rural peoples as well as urban areas; it gives better performance in terms of wound data monitoring and advanced diagnostics. The different sensors are associated with telemedicine systems for acquiring the medical images from the patient. Oduncu et al. (2004) discussed that the most acceptable automatic or semiautomatic wound analysis is color image processing. The wound image could be quickly acquired using ordinary cameras and or smartphones and storing for further processing. Accurate and faster-wound image analysis is possible with the help of a digital image processing technique rather than error-prone manual observation. The wound analysis includes estimation of the wound area and color distribution within the infected portion of the wound. The area of the wound is measured based on the total number of pixels in the region multiplied by a suitable scaling factor.

Wireless Body Sensor Networks (WBSN)

A wireless body sensor network plays an important role in data acquisition from the patient body via sensors. The WBSNs related issues and challenges were addressed which include emergency medical care, reliable transmission of vital patient's data, low cost and better quality of service, need for extremely low power operation, lightweight, avoidance of wearable/implantable sensors, maintenance of security and privacy, real-time connectivity to heterogeneous networks, low complexity, standardization, and interoperability. The Advanced Topometric sensor (ATOS-II) is a stereo-photographic system that measures a 3D map of the wound surface. Present and emerging developments in today's communications integrated with the developments in Microelectronics and embedded system technologies will have a drastic impact on future patient monitoring and health information delivery systems. The major challenges are bandwidth limitations, power consumption, and skin or tissue protection. The body sensor network is a set of several nodes distributed over the body to collect the physiological information. These networks are usually meant for the acquisition of data. The WBSN infrastructures are complex and need many functional support elements. Biosensors are attached to the human body for remote patient's health monitoring with extremely high mobility. The wireless body area network consists of three types of nodes like (a) *Implant-BAN* – used for internal communication between the inside of the body where sensors and actuators are connected to the BAN coordinator that serves as a data acquisition centre (DAC), (b) *External-BAN* - for external communication between sensor nodes surrounding the body and the outside world, no contact with human skin, (c) *Surface-BAN* – placed on the surface of the human skin (Reinzo et al., 2009). These data are collected by m-Health through the faster network connectivity, processing, and analysis. Chen et al. (2011) present the difference between the wireless sensor network and BAN in terms of mobility, data rate, latency, node density, power supply, network topology, node replacement, security level etc and also compare with the existing body sensor nodes (Omeni et al., 2007), (Sofia et al., 2011), (Deena et al., 2012). A number of ongoing projects like firmware based *CodeBlue* (Shnayder et al., 2005), *MobiHealth* (Konstantas et al., 2003), *AlarmNet* (Wood et al., 2008), Advanced care and alert portable telemedical monitor (*AMON*) (Anliker et al., 2004), *MagIC* (Rienzo, 2005), Medical remote monitoring of clothes (*MERMOTH*) (Weber et al., 2006), Microsystems platform for mobile services and applications (*MIMOSA*) (Jantunen, 2008), Wireless sensor node for a motion capture systems with accelerometers (*WiMoCA*) (Farella et al., 2008), *CareNet* (Jiang et al., 2008), Advanced Health and Disaster Aid Network (*AID-N*) (Gao et al., 2007), *SMART* (Curtis et al., 2008), *ASNET* (Sheltami et al., 2006), *MITHril* (Pentland, 2004), Wearable health monitoring systems (*WHMS*) (Mienkovic et al., 2006), *NASA-LifeGuard* (Montgomery et al., 2004), non-invasive *LifeShirt* (VivoMetrics, 2002), *iSIM* (iSIM, 2015), *HealthGear* (Oliver et al., 2006), Ubiquitous Monitoring (*Ubimon*) (Jason et al., 2004), *eWatch* (Maurer et al., 2006), *Vital jacket* (Cunha et al., 2010), *m-Health* (Jovanov, 2005), Personal Care Connect (Blount, 2007) and *HeartToGo* (Jin et al., 2009) have contributed to establish a practical solution for WBAN that is detailed in Table 2. Sana et al. (2009) highlight the efficient power solutions towards in-body and on-body sensor networks. According to the World Health Organization (WHO's) report, approximately 17.5 million people die due to heart attacks each year, more than 246 million people suffer from diabetes; it will be increasing up to 380 million by 2025 and almost 20 million people will die from cardiovascular disease in 2025 (World, 2010). So, these deaths can be prevented with the help of the WBSN based telemedicine system. A typical WBSN consists of several sensor nodes with a low power constraint, each acquiring a specific physiological parameter from the human body. These nodes act as a bridge between the patient and technology-enabled devices. We can easily diagnose the patient

Table 2. Detailed description of various projects

Projects	Main Features
CodeBlue	Provides higher priority based on scalable and robust patient's medical monitoring.
MobiHealth	Allows continuous health monitoring fastly and reliably.
AlarmNet	Uses for medical data analysis and long-term health monitoring
AMON	Provides continuous collection and evaluation of various medical vital signs.
MERMOTH	Used to monitor patient's vital signs comfortably using wearable interface and supports parallel data management service.
WiMoCA	Used to monitor the patient's movement with high flexibility.
CareNet	Monitors remote healthcare with a highly reliable and secure way.
AID-N	Performs data delivery efficiently and treats a large number of patient's.
SMART	Provides a viable method for monitoring patient's at-risk in the waiting areas of an emergency department.
ASNET	Provides dynamic data query to allow the clinicians to monitor patients at any place via the web or Smartphones.
MITHril	Provides healthcare with a highly flexible way and reduce medical costs.
LifeGuard	Monitors patient's vital signs.
LifeShirt	Monitors patient's health in real time.
HealthGear	Monitors visualize and analyze a patient's physiological data.
Ubimon)	Monitors patient's physiological states continuously.
eWatch	Used in elderly monitoring and context-aware notification.
(Blo'07)	Provides timely accessibility to the patient's health status remotely. Improves patient's quality care and life.
HeartToGo	Detects abnormality of cardiovascular disease.
MagIC	Detects ECG, respiratory activity and monitors patient data via wireless transmission scheme remotely.
Vital jacket	Monitors patient's vital signs
M-Health	Continuously monitors ambulatory settings, early detection of abnormalities and supervised rehabilitation.
iSIM	Supports sensing of location; position; obstacles; range finding; temperature; sound; and vision.
WHMS	Monitors patient's vital signs closely and provides optimal health status.
MIMOSA	Uses low-power, optimized for flexibility and smart sensor based architecture.

health status and early detection of abnormalities is also possible using sensor nodes. So the mortality rate can be minimized. An efficient WBSN requires portable, lightweight, low-power, miniature sensors, and autonomous sensor nodes that monitor the health-related applications.

TELE-WOUND MONITORING FOR REMOTE HEALTHCARE

Most of the population living in rural areas has been facing many problems due to the shortages of healthcare capacity in India. The affordable connectivity is required in rural areas where connectivity is dense. M-Health which integrated the TWM system has the potential to provide cost-effective treatment to the rural area. The proposed system suggests the following high-level requirements for the right solution: (1) ***Accessibility*** – to implement the methods to collect, process, analyze and monitor the patient's vital signs. (2) ***Scalability*** - to support efficient remote monitoring and computerized data analysis of large patient populations. (3) ***Reliability*** – to provide reliable communication between TMA and tele-medical hub (TMH). (4) ***Manageability*** - to manage all patient-centric control information. (5) ***Flexibility*** – to be open, flexible and extensible. (6) ***Security*** – to protect the data, when processing for getting best treatment over the networks. (7) ***Throughput*** – to provide high throughput in terms of data processed over heterogeneous networks. (8) ***Storage*** – to increase the large volume of patient's data storage. (9) ***Cost*** – to minimize the cost. The cost is associated with network bandwidth, use of computation, storage space, monitoring, accounting and billing, software services and content delivery. The cost can be increased using paid networks, but the TWM minimizes the cost by the minimal use of network involvement. (10) ***Optimization*** – to provide the network to the patient inexpensively. (11) **Visualization** – powerful visualization is required by the advanced processor for patients' data analysis. (12) **Easy up-gradation** – the TWM can be upgraded easily with the changes in the medical information from time to time. This TWM is the system used to collect patient's vital signs automatically via the internet from medical sensors to TMH for storage, processing, analyzing and distribution. This tool has four important features like (a) voice, and video, (b) the web-based electronic health records, and cloud services, (c) wireless broadband, and (d) advanced wound healing products. The accurate wound assessment in the TWM system is an essential skill required by all practitioners able to plan effectively, implement and evaluate patient's care. This system helps to develop a proper management plan for resolving the wound-related issues. Every CW might require at least three to six months, so a regular medication-related update is required. The TWM provides such patient medication. The TWM system maintained clinical documentation accurately and carefully for identifying vital signs of improvement or deterioration. The TWM followed the National Institutes of Health and Agency (NIHA) for Health Research and Quality guidelines for wound care and programmed them into its electronic health record system to standardize protocols for its TMA. The TWM system is needed for minimizing morbidity and possible mortality.

Smartphones enable the TWM healthcare platform to provide low-cost and high-quality medical services. TWM is applied for acquiring, transmitting, and monitoring wound status from rural to good clinics by wound app in smartphone technologies. It provides clinicians with the possibility to monitor emergency homebound patients using m-Health fastly, accurately, and precisely. The huge numbers of rural people in the world have been suffering from different types of wounds. However, due to the lack of trained clinicians, this adds up in suffering populations. The major improvement and development in mobile communication throughout the world reduce the problem up to some extent. The telemedicine-based wireless body area networks can be used for continuous remote patient monitoring (Chinmay et al., 2013) where a wound image is collected by a high-resolution camera based on a smartphone and using the image sensor.

Operation

The TWM system aims to take off the chronic wound patients at each level. It provides a clinician module, registers patients, emergency call services, sends a report. The smartphone can be used to capturing high-quality wound images and acquiring clinical information and send it to the TMH through a secure, web-based medium. Chronic wound images are automatically converted to the JPEG format by the camera and transferred to a compatible computer. Some limitations of wound image acquisition are low image resolution, color quality and constancy, pose uncertainty due to target movement, reflections due to skin nature and illumination constraints, shading and noise and variable environment illumination.

Figure 3. TWM system model for remote patient's monitoring

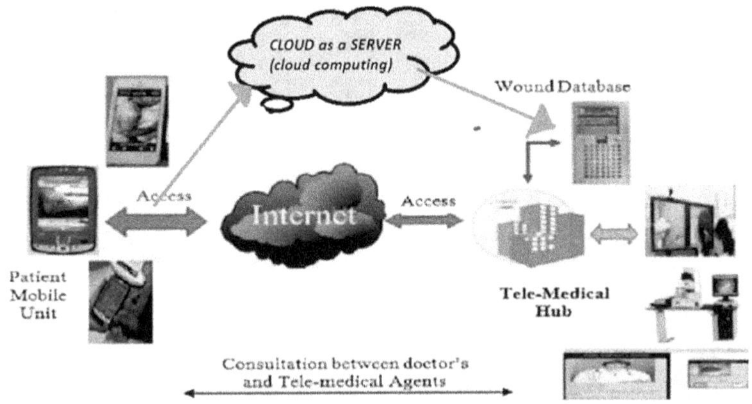

The noise can be eliminated using superior adaptive filtering methods (Chinmay et al., 2016). Therefore, images must be pre-processed to correct the variations in illumination. Automation of manual digital planimetry by replacing the task of manual delineation with a wound measurement technique will exclude dependency on clinician and reduce the probability of error due to the human factor. Results remain too dependent on image capture conditions, sample database building, region descriptor selection, tissue class learning protocol, etc., preventing reproducible results from being obtained within the complete color image processing chain. The cloud computing framework provides resources to patients or TMA on an on-demand basis through the web service interface. The TWM system can collect remote CW related information and send it via a communication platform to the TMH for better treatment (Figure 3).

The medical images are taken care of by the Image Recognition APIs and are progressively dependent on chronic wound images for screening, diagnosis, treatment planning, and routine check-ups. A smartphone integrated low cost and a greater quality based metadata creation process for wound image acquisition at the patient. It provides a smooth interaction between experts and patients remotely. The end-to-end routine diagnostic and maintaining patient history are also explained here. This chapter describes a prototype system that demonstrates and validates the approach. The implementation and simulation are carried out using Hypertext Preprocessor (PHP) and MySql database and especially by Firebase cloud database and also Wamp server, localhost database, Backendless and its API, OpenWeatherMap, Org API, artificial intelligence in Microsoft image cognitive APIs which are used for improving the efficiency. Each patient is assigned a unique PATIENT ID and password for authorization. Figure 4 shows that the screenshots of the TWM app using m-Health related to patients, doctors, medicine etc information.

FIREBASE CLOUD DATABASE

It is the main database used in the TWM app to store clinical data. Both the patient's and doctor's information is stored in this database. Data of patients includes their name, date-of-birth, patient identification number, address at the time of diagnosis, wound site, patient history, year of diagnosis, previous visit history, contact number, comments along with their wound images. Images require much memory and hence would accumulate in the server if used there. Therefore, Firebase cloud is used for this purpose

Figure 4. TWM application screenshots

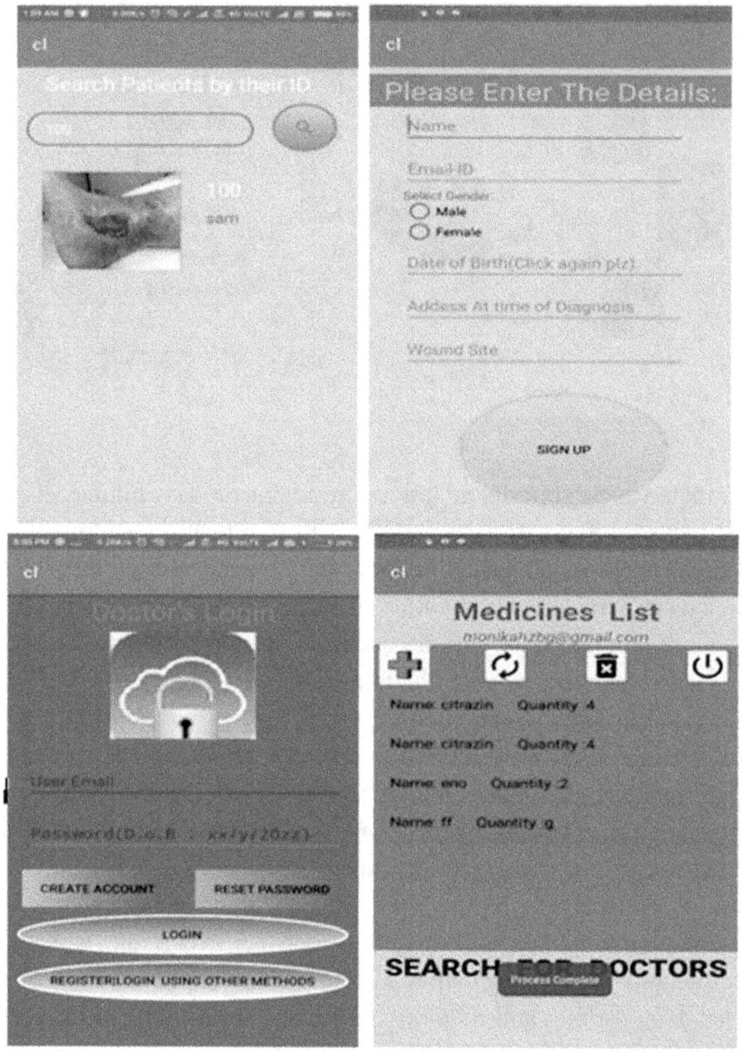

to store patient health records on a cloud server that is shown in Figure 5. This data can be accessed at any place, at any specified time. Firebase is a web application and a mobile tool that helps developers build high-quality apps. The storage space is 1 GB for uploading and 10 Gb for downloading data. The most powerful, simple and cost-effective tool like Firebase storage is applied to store wound images, video, patient-centric contents.

FUTURE RESEARCH DIRECTIONS

The captured wound images, with clinical information, are processed via the TWM app to server-end. The clinician gives feedback related to wound status to the patients. In the future, a better medical data protection algorithm is required for sending patient's information through the transmission medium.

Figure 5. Firebase database for wound data management

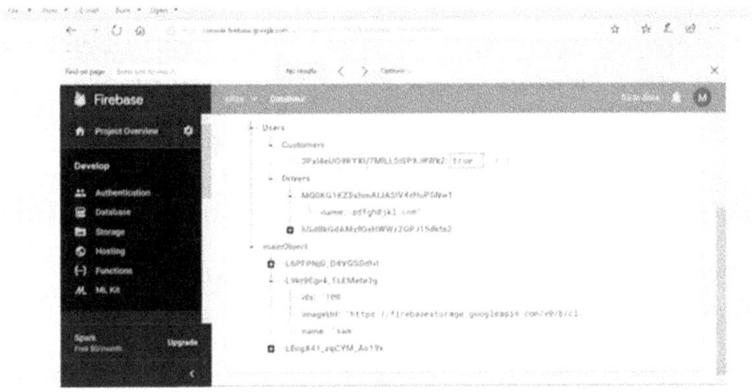

Availability of video conferencing and the TWM problems provide more flexibility and improvement in rural, remote care. In the future, tele-trauma case will be enhanced with patients uploading their images and videos of the wound for better treatment. The major challenge is to manage the large medical data that can be integrated with electronic health records (EHR) for big data analytics purposes. This novel approach can be used in data mining applications and remote health monitoring systems.

CONCLUSION

M-Health technology is becoming the solution for providing a fast and efficient diagnosis in the treatment of CWs, and several other diseases. The TWM has been a breakthrough in providing quick and effective service to the patients. They can also maintain an electronic-prescription for referral case. Hence, time and cost could be saved, and clinicians can work from anywhere using a smartphone. CWs represent not only a burden to individuals affected but also a burden to the medical health care system. Information about the percentage of wounded tissues is the determining factor for the healing state, allowing evaluation of the treatment efficiency and further treatment decisions. The TWM care provides the recording of clinical information, communication of clinical data, treatment planning, billing, quality assurance, standardization of care and medico-legal reasons. The m-health increases the accessibility, quality of patient's care and focuses on preventive medicine through early intervention, reduces the overall healthcare cost, provides better services, reduces the need for the transportation of patients from their house to specialized clinics, getting the best consultation by medical experts, makes specialty care more accessible to rural and medically underserved areas, improves communication between rural-to-urban providers, supports high patient and provider satisfaction.

REFERENCES

Albouy, B., Treuillet, S., Lucas, Y., Barre, H., & Pichaud, J. C. (2005). Depth and color analysis of wounds using digital camera. *ITBM-RBM*, *26*(4), 240–242. doi:10.1016/j.rbmret.2005.06.001

Anliker, U., Ward, J. A., Lukowicz, P., Tröster, G., Dolveck, F., Baer, M., ... Vuskovic, M. (2004). AMON: A wearable multi parameter medical monitoring and alert systems. *IEEE Transactions on Information Technology in Biomedicine*, *8*(4), 415–427. doi:10.1109/TITB.2004.837888 PMID:15615032

Arthur, G. (2010). *Wound care: Innovation and chronic care drives market growth.* Retrieved from http://www.trilogy-capital.com/sci/sci_woundcare.pdf

Bashshur, R., Shannon, G., Krupinski, E., & Grigsby, J. (2011). Policy: The taxonomy of telemedicine. *Telemedicine Journal and e-Health*, *17*(6), 484–494. doi:10.1089/tmj.2011.0103 PMID:21718114

Blount, M., Batra, V. M., Capella, A. N., Ebling, M. R., Jerome, W. F., Martin, S. M., ... Wright, S. P. (2007). Remote health-care monitoring using personal care connect. *IBM Systems Journal*, *46*(1), 95–115. doi:10.1147j.461.0095

Casas, L., Castaneda, B., & Treuillet, S. (2011). *Imaging technologies applied to chronic wounds: a survey*. ACM.

Chakraborty, C., Gupta, B., & Ghosh, S. K. (2014). Mobile metadata assisted community database of chronic wound. *International Journal of Wound Medicine, 6*, 34–42. doi:10.1016/j.wndm.2014.09.002

Chen, M., Gonzalez, S., Vasilakos, A., Cao, H., & Leung, V. (2011). *Body area networks: A survey*, Springer. *Mobile Networks and Applications*, *16*(2), 171–193. doi:10.100711036-010-0260-8

Chinmay, C., Bharat, G., & Soumya, K. G. (2013). *A review on telemedicine-based WBAN framework for patient monitoring*. Telemedicine and e-health, Marry Ann Liebert *Inc*.

Chinmay, C., & Gupta, B. (2016). Adaptive Filtering Technique for Chronic Wound Image analysis under Tele-Wound Network. *International Journal of Communication, Navigation, Sensing and Services, 1*, 57–76.

Chinmay, C., Gupta, B., & Ghosh, S. K. (2016), *Mobile Telemedicine Systems for Remote Patient's Chronic Wound Monitoring*. IGI.

Cunha, J. P. S., Cunha, B., Xavier, W., Ferreira, N., & Meireles, L. (2010). *Vital-Jacket®: A wearable wireless vital signs monitor for patients' mobility in cardiology and sports*. IEETA/Dep. Electron. Telecommunication & Information, *4th International Conference on Pervasive Computing Technologies for Healthcare (PervasiveHealth)*.

Curtis, D., Shih, E., Bailey, J., Stair, T., & Greenes, R.A. (2008). Physiological signal monitoring in the waiting areas of an emergency room. *International Procedings of BodyNets,* 1-8.

Deena, M., & Muhammad, A. (2012). A survey of challenges and applications of wireless body area network (WBAN) and role of a virtual doctor server in existing architecture. *IEEE 3rd International Conference on Intelligent Systems Modelling and Simulation*, 214-219.

Farella, E., Pieracci, A., Benini, L., Rocchi, L., & Acquaviva, A. (2008). Interfacing human and computer with wireless body area sensor networks: The WiMoCA solution. *Multimedia Tools and Applications, 38*(3), 337–363. doi:10.100711042-007-0189-5

Gao, T., Massey, T., Selvo, L., Crawford, D., Chen, B., Lorincz, K., ... Welsh, M. (2007). The advanced health and disaster AID network: A light-weight wireless medical system for triage. *IEEE Transactions on Biomedical Circuits and Systems, 1*(3), 203–216. doi:10.1109/TBCAS.2007.910901 PMID:23852414

Gethin, G., & Cowman, S. (2005). Wound measurement comparing the use of acetate tracings and Visitrak digital planimetry. *Journal of Clinical Nursing, 15*(4), 422–427. doi:10.1111/j.1365-2702.2006.01364.x PMID:16553755

Gottrup, F., Holstein, P., Jorgensen, B., Lohmann, M., & Karlsmar, T. (2001). A new concept of a multidisciplinary wound healing center and a national expert function of wound healing. *Archives of Surgery, 136*(7), 765–772. doi:10.1001/archsurg.136.7.765 PMID:11448387

Haghpanah, S., Bogie, K., Wang, X., Banks, P. G., & Ho, C. H. (2006). Reliability of electronic versus manual wound measurement techniques. *Archives of Physical Medicine and Rehabilitation, 87*(10), 1396–1402. doi:10.1016/j.apmr.2006.06.014 PMID:17023252

Han, J., & Kamber, M. (Eds.). (2006). *Data mining: Concepts and techniques*. Morgan Kaufmann.

International Diabetes Federation. (2006). *Diabetes Atlas* (3rd ed.). Brussels: Author.

iSIM Project. (2015). Retrieved from http://www.cs.uoregon.edu/research/mds/iSIM/

Jantunen, I., Laine, H., Huuskonen, P., Trossen, D., & Ermolov, V. (2008). Smart sensor architecture for mobile-terminal-centric ambient intelligence. *Sensors and Actuators, 142*(1), 352–360. doi:10.1016/j.sna.2007.04.014

Jason, W. P., Benny, P. L. L., Oliver, W., Morris, S., Nick, P., Ara, D., Chris, T., & Guang, Z.Y. (2004). Ubiquitous monitoring environment for wearable and implantable sensors (UbiMon). *UbiComp'04, The 6th International Conference on Ubiquitous Computing, Poster Proc.*, 1-2.

Jiang, S., Cao, Y., Iyengar, S., Kuryloski, P., Jafari, R., Xue, Y., ... Wicker, S. (2008). CareNet: an integrated wireless sensor networking environment for remote healthcare. *International Conference on Body Area Networks, 9*, 1-3.

Jin, Z., Oresko, J., Huang, S., & Cheng, A. C. (2009). HeartToGo: a personalized medicine technology for cardiovascular disease prevention and detection. *Proceedings of IEEE/NIH LiSSA*, 80-83.

Jovanov, E. (2005). Wireless technology and system integration in body area networks for m-health applications. *Proceedings of the IEEE Engineering in Medicine and Biology, 27th Annual International Conference, 7*, 7158-7160.

Konstantas, D., & Herzog, R. (2003). Continuous monitoring of vital constants for mobile users: the MobiHealth approach. *25th Annual International Conference of the IEEE EMBS*, 3728-3731.

Korber, A., Rietkoo, T. J., Grabbe, S., & Dissemond, J. (2006). Three-dimensional documentation of wound healing: First results of a new objective method for measurement. *Journal of the German Society of Dermatology*, *4*(10), 848–854. PMID:17010174

Malcolm, S. (2013). *Smartphone apps, permissions and privacy concerns and next steps.* TEKDESK: A division of the community opportunity and innovation network. Retrieved from http://rebootpeterborough.ca/wp-content/uploads/2013/04/Smartphone-Apps-Permissions-and-Privacy-Report.pdf, 1-93.

Mankar, N. B., & Nagdeve, U. T. (2013). *Comparison of different imaging techniques used for chronic wounds.* IJRET. *International Journal of Research in Engineering and Technology*, *2*(7), 68–70. doi:10.15623/ijret.2013.0207009

Maurer, U., Rowe, A., Smailagic, A., & Siewiorek, P. (2006). eWatch: a wearable sensor and notification platform. *Proceedings of International Workshop on BSN, Wearable and Implanted Body Sensor Networks*, 144-145.

Milenkovic,, A., Otto, C., & Jovanov. (2006). Wireless sensor networks for personal health monitoring: Issues and an implementation. *Current Communication*, *29*, 13–14.

Montgomery, K., Mundt, C., Tellier, A., Udoh, V., Berker, R., Giovangrandi, L., … Kovacs, G. (2004). Lifeguard – a personal physiological monitor for extreme environments. *IEEE International Conference of EMBS*.

Moreo, K. (2005). Understanding and overcoming the challenges of effective case management for patients with chronic wounds. *The Case Manager*, *16*(2), 62–67. doi:10.1016/j.casemgr.2005.01.014 PMID:15818347

Mustoe, T. (2004). Understanding chronic wounds: A unifying hypothesis on their pathogenesis and implications for therapy. *American Journal of Surgery*, *187*(5), 65–70. doi:10.1016/S0002-9610(03)00306-4 PMID:15147994

Mustoe, T. A., O'Shaughnessy, K., & Kloeters, O. (2006). Chronic wound pathogenesis and current treatment strategies: A unifying hypothesis. *Plastic and Reconstructive Surgery*, *117*, 35–41. doi:10.1097/01.prs.0000225431.63010.1b PMID:16799373

Mustoe, T. A., O'Shaughnessy, K., & Kloeters, O. (2006). Chronic wound pathogenic and current treatment strategies: A unifying hypothesis. *Plastic and Reconstructive Surgery*, *117*, 35–41. doi:10.1097/01.prs.0000225431.63010.1b PMID:16799373

Muto, N. (2012). *Basic smartphone workshop*. Retrieved from http://www.saultcareercentre.ca/wp-content/uploads/2012/09/PREVIEW-SMARTPHONE.pdf, *1-5*.

Nemeth, M., Sprigle, S., & Gajjala, A. (2010). Clinical usability of a wound measurement device. *36th Annual American Spinal Injury Conference*, 1-17.

Nila, B. (2013). *Comparison of different imaging techniques used for chronic wounds. International Journal of Research in Engineering and Technology*, *2*(7), 68–70. doi:10.15623/ijret.2013.0207009

Oliver, N., & Flores, F. (2006). HealthGear: a real-time wearable system for monitoring and analyzing physiological signals. *International Workshop on Wearable and Implanted Body Sensor Networks*, 3-5.

Omeni, O. C., Eljamaly, & Burdett, A.J. (2007). Energy efficient medium access protocol for wireless medical body area sensor networks. *Proceedings of the 4th IEEE EMBS*, 19-22.

Pentland, S. (2004). *Healthwear: medical technology becomes wearable*. Academic Press.

Plassmann, P., & Jones, T. D. (1998). MAVIS: A non-invasive instrument to measure area and volume of wounds. *Medical Engineering & Physics*, *20*(5), 332–338. doi:10.1016/S1350-4533(98)00034-4 PMID:9773686

Rienzo, M., Rizzo, F., Parati, G., Brambilla, F. M., & Castiglioni, P. (2005). MagIC system: A new textile-based wearable device for biological signal monitoring applicability in daily life and clinical setting. *Proceedings of the 27th Annual International IEEE EMBS Conference*, 7167–7169.

Robson, M. C., Cooper, D. M., Aslam, R., Gould, L. J., Harding, K. G., Margolis, D. J., ... Bryant, L. W. (2006). Guidelines for the treatment of venous ulcers. *Wound Repair and Regeneration*, *14*(6), 649–662. doi:10.1111/j.1524-475X.2006.00174.x PMID:17199831

Sheltami, T., Mahmoud, A., & Abu, A. (2006). Warning and monitoring medical system using sensor networks. *18th National Computer Conference*, 63-68.

Shnayder, V., Chen, B., Lorincz, K., Jones, T., & Welsh, M. (2005). Sensor networks for medical care, *3rd International Conference on Embedded Networked Sensor Systems*. 10.1145/1098918.1098979

Silhousette, T. M. (2010). *Advanced wound assessment and management system*. Retrieved from http://www.aranzmedical.com

Snyder, R. J. (2005). Treatment of non-healing ulcers with allografts. *Clinics in Dermatology*, *23*(4), 388–395. doi:10.1016/j.clindermatol.2004.07.020 PMID:16023934

Sofia, N., & Rabiah, A. (2011). Surveying the wireless body area network in the realm of wireless communication. *IEEE 7th International Conference on Information Assurance and Security*.

Sprigle, S., Nirmal, P., Aditya, J., & Thad, S. (2006). Handheld, non-contact wound measurement device. *Clinical Symposium on Advances in Skin & Wound care*, 379.

Thawer, H. A., Houghton, P. E., Woodbury, G., Keast, D., & Campbell, K. A. (2002). Comparison of computer-assisted and manual wound size measurement. *Ostomy/Wound Management*, *48*, 46–53. PMID:12378003

Cuzzell. (1988). The new RYB color code. *The American Journal of Nursing*, *88*(10), 1342–1346. PMID:3177488

VivoMetrics. (2002). Three More Studies Use LifeShirt System to Assess Treatment Protocols, Ambulatory Intelligence. *The Journal of Ambulatory Monitoring*, *1*(1).

Weber, J., & Porotte, F. (2006). Medical remote monitoring with clothes. *International Workshop on PHealth.*

Williams, C. (2009). The Verge Videometer wound measurement package. *British Journal of Nursing (Mark Allen Publishing)*, *9*(4), 237–239. doi:10.12968/bjon.2000.9.4.6383 PMID:11033643

Wood, A., Stankovic, J., Virone, G., Selavo, L., He, Z., Cao, Q., ... Stoleru, R. (2008). Context aware wireless sensor networks for assisted living and residential monitoring. *IEEE Network*, *22*(4), 26–33. doi:10.1109/MNET.2008.4579768

World Health Organizations. (2010). *Global status report on noncommunicable diseases.* WHO.

KEY TERMS AND DEFINITIONS

M-Health: It is used in smartphones and other mobile technology in healthcare services.

Remote Monitoring: It is applied to collect clinical information in advanced communication technology that is interconnected with remote devices.

Tele-Wound Monitoring: The main purpose is to collect the patient's wound image using a smartphone under the telemedicine system for remote monitoring.

Wound Database: A large volume of patient's wound images along with vital signs which can be stored at a particular place called wound database.

Wound Tissue: Wound tissue is a biological cellular structure which has been injured. The wound tissue can be classified into three major categories: granulation, slough, and necrotic.

Chapter 6
Mobile Health Applications in Prehospital Emergency Medicine

Bibiana Metelmann
Greifswald University, Germany

Camilla Metelmann
Greifswald University, Germany

ABSTRACT

Prehospital emergency medicine treats time-critical diseases at the emergency site to reduce preventable disabilities and deaths. mHealth can assist in prehospital emergency medicine in multiple ways. This chapter provides insights into emergency medicine and presents three different forms of mHealth in this field. One is a retrieval of medical data (e.g., with aid of smartphone applications). A second one uses unmanned aerial vehicles. And the third one establishes real time communication with medical experts. Examples are given to illustrate the variety of mHealth in prehospital emergency medicine.

INTRODUCTION

Prehospital emergency medicine is an integral part of all health care systems worldwide. The goal of prehospital emergency medicine is to treat time-critical diseases and conditions as early as at the emergency site and hereby reduce preventable disabilities and deaths. MHealth offers the opportunity to balance existing healthcare disparities by using mobile information and communication technologies. It has huge advantages in emergency medicine, where the transfer of knowledge in a short time is critical and potentially lifesaving (Amadi-Obi, Gilligan, Owens, & O'Donnell, 2014). Mhealth applications support treatment of emergencies at the place of occurrence, whether it is at a patient's home or the site of a road accident. Thus, there has been a rapid development in the field of mHealth in prehospital medicine in the last years. The purpose of this chapter is to display different approaches, how mHealth might be beneficial in prehospital emergency medicine.

After introducing the role of paramedics and emergency doctors in prehospital emergency medicine, the three key emergency cases of myocardial infarction, stroke, and trauma are described. These life-threatening diseases belong to the leading causes of death worldwide and have a high economic impact.

DOI: 10.4018/978-1-5225-8021-8.ch006

Copyright © 2019, IGI Global. Copying or distributing in print or electronic forms without written permission of IGI Global is prohibited.

MHealth offers a possibility to increase the quality of treatment starting at the emergency site to save lives potentially. There are three main ways of applying mHealth in prehospital emergency medicine. One is to retrieve data, e.g. by using smartphone applications. Multiple uses of applications will be presented. The second is the use of unmanned aerial vehicles to deliver medical goods.

Moreover, the third way to use mHealth is real-time communication with a medical expert. This communication could be the transmission of audio, vital signs, photos or video. Four projects using high-definition real-time video communication from the emergency site to a remote emergency doctor will be presented and discussed. Experiences in mHealth in the field of prehospital emergency medicine gained in the European Union FP7-funded project LiveCity (Grant Agreement No. 297291) will be described. Within the project, a video camera was developed and tested in a medical simulation center. Key findings of this study will be presented and issues and problems, which arose, will be analyzed and possible solutions discussed. Future research is expected to solve some remaining technical challenges, making mHealth in prehospital emergency medicine very promising.

BACKGROUND

Prehospital Emergency Medicine

Prehospital emergency medicine summarizes all efforts made by medical professionals to treat acute illnesses, life-threatening conditions and pain at the emergency site and to transport the patient – if needed – to a hospital. Prehospital emergency medicine varies between countries (Callese et al., 2015; Roudsari et al., 2007). Most developed countries have an advanced life support system, which can be divided into the Anglo-American model and the Franco-German model. In the Anglo-American model, the prehospital emergency medicine is provided by paramedics (Wandling, Nathens, Shapiro, & Haut, 2016). The Franco-German model is similar to the Anglo-American model but differs in life-threatening conditions (Al-Shaqsi, 2010). The Franco-German model dispatches paramedics and additively dispatches emergency physicians in life-threatening conditions (Dick, 2003).

Three Key Emergencies: Myocardial Infarction, Stroke, Trauma

Medical emergencies, which happen outside a hospital, contribute immensely to the global morbidity and mortality. The World Health Organization published a fact sheet about "the top 10 causes of death", where ischaemic heart disease and stroke are the two leading causes of death worldwide (WHO, 2014). Myocardial infarction, as the acute and life-threatening form of ischaemic heart disease, is one of the leading causes of hospitalization and mortality worldwide (Filgueiras Filho et al., 2018). The European Society of Cardiology emphasizes the importance of the prehospital phase because this is the most critical phase for the occurrence of cardiac arrest. Early treatment is proven to reduce morbidity and mortality (Steg et al., 2012). Stroke, which also is a common diagnosis in prehospital emergency medicine, depends on early treatment, too. The European Stroke Organisation recommends priority treatment to reduce morbidity and mortality (The European Stroke Organisation Executive & Committee, 2008). In case of stroke, a telemedical consultation from the emergency department increases patient outcome (Bernetti et al., 2018). The implementation of telemedicine in stroke treatment was recommended by the American Heart Association and American Stroke Association already in 2009 (Schwamm et al., 2009). MHealth for stroke in prehospital emergency medicine is also feasible and beneficial (Hubert, Müller-Barna, & Audebert, 2014). Trauma, as in road injuries, also ranks in "the top 10 causes of death" and attempts are made to reduce trauma-related deaths (Dagal, Greer, & McCunn, 2014). Most deaths caused by injury and other medical emergencies occur outside of hospitals (Nilsen, 2012). The burden of traffic-related traumas is likely to increase further with further motorization, and the World Health Organization recognized the importance of prehospital emergency medicine in their developed action plans (Moroz & Spiegel, 2014). The prognosis for 2030 predicts ischaemic heart disease, stroke and trauma to be within the top five leading causes of death worldwide (WHO, 2010). This chapter will illustrate how different approaches in mHealth might improve the emergency treatment of these three severe emergencies.

MHealth in Prehospital Emergency Medicine

As shown in the three examples, the early beginning of the right treatment is crucial to improving the outcome of the patient. There are several concepts to make expertise available at the emergency site within a minimum of time. One possible way is by using mHealth. MHealth offers the transfer of knowledge over geographical distances in real time.

In contrast to the traditional telemedicine, mHealth has a huge advantage: it is not restricted to stationary devices anymore. Thus, a connection to a moving partner is possible. MHealth, therefore, allows telemedicine in the prehospital emergency medicine.

MHealth in prehospital emergency medicine can be grouped into three categories based on the kind of transmitted data: The first one is the retrieval of data, e.g. at the emergency site. This can, for instance, be made with smartphone applications (apps). The second one is the delivery of goods via unmanned aerial vehicles. Moreover, the third is real-time communication with a medical expert. It allows the transfer of knowledge from a remote expert to the emergency site.

Retrieval of Data

There is a variety of smartphone apps, which regard several different aspects of emergency medicine (Boulos, Brewer, Karimkhani, Buller, & Dellavalle, 2014). In January 2014, there were about 300 smartphone apps with a focus on emergency medicine available in the Apple App Store (Lin, Rezaie, & Husain, 2014) and there are more than 20.000 apps in the field of medicine (Wiechmann, Kwan, Bokarius, & Toohey, 2016). Looking at the dynamics of the past, this number is expected to grow rapidly. There is a tendency towards smartphones compared to stationary computers, especially in rural areas and low- and middle-income countries. This makes the use of mHealth especially appealing in these areas (WorldBank, 2012). The world of emergency apps is evolving swiftly, and some authors state, that emergency apps are becoming increasingly essential to medical emergency personnel as well as medical laypersons (Bachmann, Jamison, Martin, Delgado, & Kman, 2015). Smartphone apps are either designed for non-medical professionals or medical professionals or both; latter being the rarest. Apps for non-professionals aim to assist daily life and help to detect alarming symptoms. Exemplarily an app to detect and monitor possible concussions after a sports accident was developed by an interdisciplinary team of a neurosurgeon, graphic artist and computer programmer (Curaudeau, Sharma, & Rovin, 2011). There are also apps, which help medical laypersons to perform therapeutic procedures, e.g. cardiopulmonary resuscitation. Sakai and colleagues developed an app, which guides medical laypersons in real-time in a step-by-step approach through resuscitation and showed the higher quality of chest compressions in participants using the app (Sakai et al., 2015).

Apps for medical professionals enable retrieval of knowledge in multiple domains: While some apps offer textbooks and lookup tables, others offer interactive flowcharts and step-by-step instructions. As an example of helping prehospital decision making, an app assisting with the allocation of trauma patients to the appropriate hospital was successfully tested against a paper version (Freshwater & Crouch). Consistently it could be shown that the use of tablet PCs at the emergency site to help allocate patients, could reduce transportation times and costs (Yamada, Inoue, & Sakamoto, 2015).Several apps assist in finding the right medication dosage. Calculating medical scores can be very challenging, because of complex equations and numbers. Thus, apps assisting in these tasks were developed. For instance, it could be shown that an app calculating adequate fluid management for burn victims was feasible and accurate (Barnes et al., 2014). Another group of apps keeps the user up-to-date on the latest research to ensure high-quality medicine. Many medical professionals value apps because they support work by providing information in a structured way. The traditional textbooks, handwritten notes, and papers can be replaced by smartphone apps, which are ubiquitously available and allow fast retrieval of data. However, one has to be aware, that not all apps have been officially approved by medical committees and not all information displayed in apps is consistent with medical guidelines and current research. The Medicine and Healthcare Products Regulatory Agency of the United Kingdom published in August 2014 a "Guidance on what a software application medical device is and how to comply with the legal requirements"(MHRA, 2014).

Uncrewed Aerial Vehicles (Drones)

Over the last years, the technology of unmanned aerial vehicles (UAV) improved, and they became more easily available. This led to many reflections, how these drones might be helpful also in medicine (Bhatt, Pourmand, & Sikka, 2018). It could be shown, that UAV can transport medical products (e.g. automated external defibrillators) or medicine (e.g. vaccines or blood products) safely and fast from one point to another (Thiels, Aho, Zietlow, & Jenkins, 2015). This can be used in prehospital emergency medicine to deliver equipment to the emergency site. Initial obstacles, e.g. in the field of blood transportation, have been overcome (Wen, Zhang, & Wong, 2016). Drone networks, which are based on mathematical models, can provide automated external defibrillators substantially faster to patients with cardiac arrest than traditional systems do and, thus, might increase the likelihood of survival (Boutilier et al., 2017). UAVs can also be helpful in case of drowning. With the aid of an UAV, the exact location of the drowning person can be found, and a floating device can be provided (Seguin, Blaquiere, Loundou, Michelet, & Markarian, 2018). UAVs were shown to allow faster detection of victims and may thus lead to a faster start of resuscitation (Claesson et al., 2017). First reflections are done on how UAV might be helpful to detect hazards in case of a car crash with multiple vehicles involved (Jain, Sibley, Stryhn, & Hubloue, 2018).

Real-Time Communication With Medical Expert

The third category of mHealth in prehospital emergency medicine enables the user to have real-time communication with a medical expert. This allows a dynamic interaction and remote guidance. The kind of transmitted data differs between audio, vital signs (e.g. heart rate, blood pressure, oxygen saturation), photos, and video. One paramount example for transmission of audio to the emergency site is telephone-advised cardiopulmonary resuscitation (CPR). If a first aider calls the European emergency number "112" and the emergency dispatcher detects a cardiac arrest, the emergency dispatcher will then start assisting the layperson by explaining resuscitation. A video conference call from a bystander to the emergency dispatcher was shown to be possible with off-the-shelf products and to increase the confidence of the bystander (Melbye, Hotvedt, & Bolle, 2014). Thus, in the latest European Resuscitation Council Guidelines from 2015, the importance of telephone-guidance was stressed once more (Perkins et al., 2015). An example of the transmission of vital signs from the emergency site to a remote expert is the wireless transmission of a 12-lead electrocardiogram (ECG). In cases of acute transmural myocardial infarction, a change in the ECG in terms of ST-elevation is detectable. As mentioned above, the treatment of this ST-elevation-myocardial infarction has to start as early as possible. If a pathological 12-lead-ECG is transmitted to a cardiologist in the hospital, he can start preparing the therapy. Thus, many studies showed a benefit of wireless transmission of 12-lead ECGs (Kerem et al., 2014), so that it is recommended by the European Society of Cardiology (Steg et al., 2012). Although many ambulance cars are equipped with a digital camera, there is little research, how the transmission of photos can increase emergency treatment. In a trial by BERGRATH and colleagues paramedics mostly transmitted photos of medical records, physician's notes and medication lists (Bergrath, Rossaint, Lenssen, Fitzner, & Skorning, 2013). Even though the transmission of pictures is inferior to the transmission of videos to enable guidance by remote experts, there are still good reasons to take photos at the emergency site. For instance, in trauma patients, pictures of a traffic accident or wounds and injuries before emergency treatment can later help hospital doctors with further treatment and might be significant for forensic reasons. The video combines the two body senses hearing and seeing, which are essential for medical doctors to find the right diagnosis. While the patient's history and symptom description are assessed acoustically, visual impressions are of the same importance. High-definition video communication in realtime offers the highest amount of information-transfer currently available. It probably has the greatest potential for the application of mHealth in prehospital emergency medicine. Therefore, the following part of the chapter will focus on the use of video communication in prehospital emergency medicine.

VIDEO COMMUNICATION IN PREHOSPITAL EMERGENCY MEDICINE

Four Projects Using Real-Time Video Communication in Prehospital Emergency Medicine

Several different mHealth concepts of video communication in prehospital emergency medicine are currently under study or already implemented. They use the mHealth video technology to transmit the expertise of emergency doctors to support and guide paramedics at the emergency site (Czaplik et al., 2014). Exemplarily, pioneering projects from Germany, Belgium and USA will be outlined:

TemRas, based on the project Med-on-@ix (Aachen, Germany), developed a monitor, which automatically sends the vital signs of a patient in real time to an emergency doctor, who is stationed at the emergency dispatch centre.

Additionally, the ambulance car is equipped with a video camera at the ceiling of the ambulance car, which sends high-definition videos in real time to the emergency doctor. The remote emergency doctor can operate this camera. For instance, the emergency doctor can zoom to analyze small details. The technical feasibility of this system was enhanced further in the last years, and the concept was proven to be sufficient (Felzen et al., 2017). Thus, this concept, called "Telenotarzt" was successfully implemented as part of the emergency medical system in the city of Aachen in April 2014 (Buscher & Schilberg; Rortgen et al., 2013). Since then, the medical advantages were evaluated in several studies. It could be shown, that in cases of myocardial infarction, hypertensive crisis and pain management, the remote treatment by a tele emergency physician was equivalent or had an even higher guideline compliance than traditional treatment (Brokmann, Conrad, et al., 2016; Brokmann, Rossaint, et al., 2016; Brokmann et al., 2017).

In the project Land|Rettung in the county Vorpommern-Greifswald in northern Germany, the experiences of the city of Aachen are now adapted to a rural area (Brinkrolf, Scheer, Hasebrook, & Hahnenkamp, 2017). The project equipped six ambulance cars with the mHealth technologies, which treat patients in an agrarian area. Technical feasibility in areas with low internet connectivity is evaluated as well as medical advantages in a rural area. It is expected, that areas with long distances to hospitals benefit even further from real-time video support.

The FACT Study (Feasibility of AmbulanCe-based Telemedicine) in Brussels, Belgium, part of the PreSSUB Project, has a similar approach using real-time video connection between the ambulance car and a teleconsultant. In patients with suspected stroke, the teleconsultant examines the patient according to a standardized protocol, asking questions and evaluating for example movements of facial muscles. It could be demonstrated that remote stroke assessment in moving ambulances is possible and reliable(Van Hooff et al., 2013; Yperzeele et al., 2014). Additionally, cost-efficiency could be shown (Valenzuela Espinoza et al., 2017). The mHealth support was rated as beneficial by patients as well as paramedics and doctors, and a 24/7 service could be implemented (Valenzuela Espinoza, De Smedt, et al., 2016; Valenzuela Espinoza, Van Hooff, et al., 2016).

The Tucson ER-link Project (Tucson, USA) combined a video link from inside an ambulance car with additional videos taken by cameras attached to the outside of the ambulance car and the existing highway cameras. The advantages of this approach lie especially in trauma management when the emergency doctor can also look at the accident scene. The system was successfully implemented in ambulance cars in the city of Tucson and could reach approximately 95% of the city's inhabitants (Latifi, 2010; Latifi et al., 2007). Unfortunately, this project was terminated due to a shortage of funding.

One of the limitations of this Aachen-system and Brussels-system for telemedical consulting is that the video camera is fixed on the ceiling of the ambulance car (Thelen, Schneiders, Schilberg, & Jeschke, 2013; Yperzeele et al., 2014). That way, the first video connection between paramedics and the remote emergency doctor is not possible before the paramedics and the patient enter the ambulance car. For some emergency situations, this might be too late. In a patient with severe bleeding, shock or coma, the blood circulation of the patient has to be stabilized or the airway secured, e.g. by endotracheal intubation, before it is possible to start transportation (Arbabi et al., 2004; Kleber et al., 2012). It could be shown, that paramedics not always perform endotracheal intubation in situations, where it is strongly recommended because they are not practiced enough (Franschman et al., 2009). This stabilization and the airway management can be difficult, and in a meta-analysis, it has been shown that emergency doctors have a significantly higher success rate in emergency endotracheal intubation than paramedics (Lossius, Roislien, & Lockey, 2012). So, a video-based assistance by an emergency doctor for those tasks could be helpful. Thus, the Tucson ER-link Project already integrated video laryngoscopes into their prehospital telemedicine network (Sakles et al., 2011). Video laryngoscopes are intubation-devices, which transmit a real-time video showing the vocal chords on a screen.

Another lack of benefit when using a video camera system mounted on the ambulance car occurs at the other end of the emergency spectrum, where there are also situations, in which a video consultation before entering the ambulance car might be helpful. The decision, whether a patient has to be treated in a hospital or can be left at home, is a complex decision requiring consideration of a lot of additional surrounding facts, like the age of the patient, living situation, accessibility of family, friends and neighbours. It is especially difficult to decide on hospital admission in cases of allergies and anaphylaxis and altered level of consciousness (Cummins et al., 2013). Hence, it is a decision many paramedics want to be made by the emergency doctor. Emergency doctors are more confident than paramedics in deciding not to transport a patient to a hospital(Roberts, Blethyn, Foreman, & Bleetman, 2009). The moment a patient has been carried into the ambulance car just for video consultation, the emergency doctor and the paramedics will become reluctant to tell the patient, that he can be treated at home and can leave the ambulance car again. This could lead to a higher rate of patients admitted to the hospital, which in consequence increases the workload and costs in the health system(Patton & Thakore, 2013).

In all situations mentioned above, patients would benefit from a mobile camera that can build a video connection and can be brought directly to the emergency site. That way, the emergency doctor can get earlier visual information about the patient. In a pilot feasibility study, WU and co-workers tested a video camera attached to the stretcher, with which the patient can be transported in a lying position from the emergency site and the ambulance car to the hospital. They concluded that prehospital stroke evaluation using this camera was feasible and reliable(Wu et al., 2014).To further enhance the chance to obtain essential information, it might be important to see the surroundings of the emergency site and thus get a better picture of what might be the reason for the emergency. This requires a mobile camera, which is directed by the paramedics.

Nonetheless, it is essential that the camera should not restrict the work of the paramedic while keeping both hands free to work. Such a kind of mobile video camera is google glass, which is tested in numerous projects in different scientific areas. Among others, PORTER and co-workers tested the use of google glass for a dermatology examination in the emergency department at the Rhode Island Hospital in Providence, USA and HRONG and colleagues tested a modified version of google glass in the emergency department at Beth Israel Deaconess Medical Center in Boston, USA (Friedman, 2014; Rojahn, 2014). Google glass is also tested in the field of disaster management to assist in triage (Broach et al., 2018).

Because of the wide distribution of mobile phones with the ability to do video calls, the idea often arose, that telemedicine could be realized with commercial off-the-shelf products. Moreover, especially in emergency medicine, the idea seems appealing, that the patient or the first-aider calling the emergency dispatcher uses a mobile phone video call and thus increases the amount of information the emergency dispatcher gets. For example, dispatcher-assisted cardiopulmonary resuscitation with video-conference via mobile phones could be shown to be superior to audio-connection (Johnsen & Bolle, 2008; Yang et al., 2008). However, off-the-shelf products are not designed for this purpose and often technical issues regarding for instance light, and audio-quality limit the success of such projects (Bolle, Johnsen, & Gilbert, 2011; Melbye et al., 2014). Furthermore, the internet connection needs to “transport” a high amount of data within a short time in a stable and high quality, which limits the successful implementation of some telemedicine projects with off-the-shelf products (Mosier, Joseph, & Sakles, 2013).

Additionally, the telemedicine connection has to meet the high standards regarding the security of vulnerable patient data. Concerns about failures in data security are one of the main obstacles in telemedicine (Klack, Ziefle, Wilkowska, & Kluge, 2013). Therefore, individual devices with specially designed software and hardware for the specific purposes have to be developed. The camera, developed in the LiveCity project, was built to meet those challenges.

Experiences Gained During the LiveCity Project

LiveCity Project

Among the main goals of the European Union are the reduction of disparities and the sustainable gain of equal opportunities across borders and over geographical distances. The LiveCity Project ("Live Video-to-Video Supporting Interactive City Infrastructure") examined the technical and structural basis of live communication between individuals or groups of individuals in distant places by using high-definition (HD) video communication in realtime (I Chochliouros; I. Chochliouros, Stephanakis, Spiliopoulou, Sfakianakis, & Ladid, 2012). Such a concept is expected to positively contribute to the quality of life of citizens or communities within the European Union in various situations (I. Chochliouros et al., 2012; Weerakkody, El-Haddadeh, Chochliouros, & Morris, 2012). One approach is to use mHealth in the pre-hospital emergency medicine by connecting paramedics at the emergency site with a remote emergency doctor through a video camera. For this purpose, a HD real-time video camera, called LiveCity camera, was developed within this project (Goncalves, Cordeiro, Batista, & Monteiro, 2012; Palma et al., 2013). This camera enables paramedics to demonstrate the emergency situation and vital signs of the patient to the emergency doctor, and the emergency doctor can assess the emergency situation and advice the paramedics at the emergency site (B. Metelmann, C. Metelmann, D. Morris, et al., 2014).

LiveCity Camera

The LiveCity camera consists of (i) the video camera itself, worn with a headband above the right ear; (ii) a headphone with a mouthpiece to enable audio connection in both ways; and (iii) the micro-PC, which builds the internet connection. The position of the camera above the right ear was chosen to transmit the same perspective the paramedic has. Since the emergency doctor sees the emergency "through the eyes" of the paramedic, he can access all relevant information needed to evaluate the situation and can then guide manual activities. The transmitted video is dynamic and follows the head movements of the paramedics. Another advantage of this camera position is that the paramedic still has both hands free to work, which is of great importance in emergency medicine. Since the work of paramedics requires much bending and kneeling, the micro PC is placed in a small backpack. The transmitted video is received by the remote emergency doctor at a laptop provided with the special software. This software allows the emergency doctor to adapt the transmitted video according to the particular needs, e.g. regarding light, contrast and sound level (Metelmann, Metelmann, M.Wendt, K.Meissner, & Heyden, 2014). While the emphasis was put on reducing the time-lag to allow sufficient communication and guidance, high legal standards regarding data security were met.

Who Should Operate the Video Camera?

All four projects mentioned above, which establish a video communication from the emergency site to a remote expert, share the idea, that the communication device is brought to the emergency site by the approaching paramedics.

The prerequisite for mHealth is that two individuals or groups of individuals are connected with each other using communication technology. Often, this connection is built beforehand during a face-to-face-meeting when both partners apportion the communication devices. When using mHealth in prehospital emergency medicine, there is no possibility to meet beforehand and establish a connection. If an emergency patient is not already part of a telemedicine project, the connection has to be newly created, and the devices to build the connection have to be brought to the patient. In the LiveCity Project this communication device, the LiveCity camera, was brought to the emergency site by the approaching paramedics(C. Metelmann, B. Metelmann, D. Morris, et al., 2014). There are several advantages and some disadvantages if a paramedic operates the mHealth device and not the emergency patient. Because the paramedic is instructed into the operation of the camera and practiced in using it, the telemedicine connection can be established fast. However, the connection can only be established after the paramedics arrived at the emergency site. Patients and relatives are in an exceptional situation. For different reasons, their thoughts and actions are focused and reduced to the essential. Because of pain, anxiety and different levels of consciousness, the operation of a new device might be difficult or not possible. Therefore, it is of great value, when the paramedics establish the telemedicine connection, even if it is an additional burden for the paramedics. Another advantage is that the paramedics can integrate the maintenance of the device into their daily routine and, therefore, keep a high level of quality. Independent from the socioeconomic status of the emergency patient, this mHealth connection is accessible for all citizens. The patient does not need to have any prior knowledge in the use of computers or similar equipment. This is especially important for elderly people, who form one of the main groups of emergency patients. Because the device can be used for several emergency patients, this concept also has the economic advantage of cost reduction (B. Metelmann, C. Metelmann, K. Meissner, et al., 2014).

Examining the LiveCity Camera in Simulated Emergency Scenarios

In the LiveCity Project, the benefit of paramedics consulting an emergency doctor by use of the LiveCity camera was investigated in terms of professional workflow and outcome. To prevent potential harm to individuals, the initial phase of the study was performed in the fully equipped medical simulation center of the Department of Anesthesiology and Intensive Care Medicine at Greifswald University Medicine. A medical simulation center creates dynamic, realistic routine or emergency scenarios with computer-operated mannequins (Gaba, 2007). Simulation centers are commonly used for education and research in medicine worldwide and offer the possibility to learn and examine procedures without putting patients at risk (Levine, DeMaria, Schwartz, & Sim, 2013).

Ten typical emergency scenarios from five different categories were standardized and structured for a randomized two-armed protocol. Three of the chosen categories were myocardial infarction, stroke, and trauma. They were selected to represent life-threatening diseases, which require fast treatment. Because these emergencies often occur, lead to a high number of disability, inability to work and death, an improvement in treatment could have a notable economic impact (Wolfe, 2000). Apart from these emergency categories, two additional groups of emergencies were chosen, one being rare diseases and the other complications during pregnancy. Rare diseases do not have such an economic impact, but they are often a challenge in diagnostics and treatment. Thus, a transfer of knowledge through mHealth might improve the outcome of the individual patient.

Similarly, complications during pregnancy challenge the paramedic because special knowledge about changes in physiology and safe use of medication during pregnancy is required. Hence, the five different emergency scenarios aimed to represent the broad spectrum of emergencies, which occur in prehospital emergency medicine. For each emergency category, two cases with a similar level of difficulty in terms of diagnosis and treatment were created. This allowed a cross-over design: Paramedics encountered similar scenarios (i) without support by an emergency doctor and (ii) with support by a remote emergency doctor using the LiveCity camera. To assess the outcome in technical, practical and psychological aspects, paramedics and doctors were interviewed by the use of structured questionnaires.

Key Findings of the Simulated Emergency Scenarios

More than 100 emergency scenarios were simulated, and five key findings will be presented in the following.

In line with the theoretical reflections made above, the vast majority of paramedics perceived the video guidance by the remote emergency doctor as helpful. Both, emergency doctors and paramedics agreed, at least partly, that the video connection with the LiveCity video camera improved the quality of patient care. At the same time, emergency doctors predominantly stated, that a sole transmission of vital signs without audio or video connection would not have been sufficient. Indeed, even a combined transmission of vital signs and audio would not have been sufficient for most emergency doctors. Though, many emergency doctors could imagine working as a doctor, consulting paramedics through a video connection. Similarly, after having encountered the simulated emergency scenarios without and with a video consultation by an emergency doctor, nearly all paramedics concluded, that they could imagine working with such a video camera.

Issues, Controversies, Problems in the LiveCity Project

Although some technical hiccups occurred during the work with the LiveCity camera, there was a positive perception of the camera. The technical problems arose mostly due to interruptions of the data flow through the mobile network. This was intensified by the multiple demands on the data transmission, e.g. high definition video, real-time transmission and high requests for data security.

Discussion of Potential Solutions and Recommendations

One possible solution to prevent technical hiccups and breakdowns could be a decreased amount of data transmission. This approach is difficult to realize. As mentioned above, data security regulations must be met at all times. Although complex encryption mechanisms increase the amount of data transmission, they are fundamental. Users' trust in mHealth systems is essential, and data security has to be ensured permanently (Calleja-Castillo & Gonzalez-Calderon, 2018). Another approach would be to permit greater time latency. Yet, that would challenge a meaningful communication and could even make guidance by video communication impossible. To compare the LiveCity camera with off-the-shelf products, remote video guidance via the GoPro camera Hero 3® was also done. However, communication was severely hindered by a long time lag, and additionally, a handheld receiver had to be used to allow audio-communication in both ways. That made the Hero 3-camera, which wasn't originally designed for such purposes, unusable for video communication in prehospital emergency medicine. Another strategy to decrease the amount of data transmission is the reduction of video quality. But, this could make it impossible for the emergency doctor to detect important details. Moreover, a downgrade to mere photo and audio transmission instead of video transmission would make physical examinations from remote very challenging. For instance, the physical examination to detect a stroke includes the observation of facial movements. Thus, a reduction in video quality would strongly inhibit the potential of video communication in prehospital emergency medicine. In summary, the approach to decrease the amount of data transmission to prevent technical problems is currently not a feasible solution. Instead, the answer to this problem will be a further development of mobile networks.

FUTURE RESEARCH DIRECTIONS

With the fast evolving technology and immense successes in computer science, mHealth is bound to change and improve constantly. Looking at the progress made in the last decades, it is safe to predict, that mHealth devices will get smaller, more compact and even more user-friendly. At the same time, the mobile networks will optimize, and next generations of mobile telecommunication technologies will ensure that transmission of video will be more stable, of higher quality and faster. Thus, there is great promise in the use of video communication from the emergency site to a remote expert.

It will be very interesting to see, how the future achievements in mHealth will contribute to prehospital emergency medicine and as a result potentially safe lives.

CONCLUSION

Prehospital emergency medicine strives to treat (potentially) life-threatening conditions as early as possible. For instance, the three emergencies myocardial infarction, stroke, and trauma are frequent and require immediate therapy and could benefit from mHealth. MHealth offers the opportunity to transfer knowledge to the emergency site with high flexibility in real time. One example is the retrieval of medical knowledge, for instance with the help of smartphone applications. There is a multitude of smartphone apps for a variety of emergency conditions for both medical laypersons and medical professionals. Lately, mHealth in the field of unmanned aerial vehicles has developed rapidly, and several application fields are currently evaluated. MHealth also enables real-time communication with a remote medical expert by the transmission of audio, vital signs, photos, and/or video. High definition video communication in real time offers the highest amount of mHealth communication currently available in prehospital emergency medicine. Research projects in Germany and Belgium proved technical feasibility and medical benefits, e.g. in cases of stroke, myocardial infarction and pain management. In the LiveCity Project, a camera was developed and tested with realistic scenarios in a medical simulation center in a cross-over design. Paramedics were supported in diagnostics and treatment of emergencies by remote emergency doctors through the LiveCity camera. After having encountered the simulated scenarios, emergency doctors and paramedics rated the video connection as helpful, an improvement of the quality of patient care and could imagine working with such a video consultation. The impact of high-quality real-time video communication on prehospital emergency medicine is appreciated by potential users. MHealth has huge potential for the application in prehospital emergency medicine.

REFERENCES

Al-Shaqsi, S. (2010). Models of International Emergency Medical Service (EMS) Systems. *Oman Medical Journal, 25*(4), 320–323. doi:10.5001/omj.2010.92 PMID:22043368

Amadi-Obi, A., Gilligan, P., Owens, N., & O'Donnell, C. (2014). Telemedicine in pre-hospital care: A review of telemedicine applications in the pre-hospital environment. *International Journal of Emergency Medicine, 7*(1), 29. doi:10.118612245-014-0029-0 PMID:25635190

Arbabi, S., Jurkovich, G. J., Wahl, W. L., Franklin, G. A., Hemmila, M. R., Taheri, P. A., & Maier, R. V. (2004). A comparison of prehospital and hospital data in trauma patients. *The Journal of Trauma, 56*(5), 1029–1032. doi:10.1097/01.TA.0000123036.20919.4B PMID:15179242

Bachmann, D. J., Jamison, N. K., Martin, A., Delgado, J., & Kman, N. E. (2015). Emergency Preparedness and Disaster Response: There's An App for That. *Prehospital and Disaster Medicine, 30*(5), 486–490. doi:10.1017/S1049023X15005099 PMID:26369629

Barnes, J., Duffy, A., Hamnett, N., McPhail, J., Seaton, C., Shokrollahi, K., ... Pritchard Jones, R. (2014). The Mersey Burns App: Evolving a model of validation. *Emergency Medicine Journal.* doi:10.1136/emermed-2013-203416 PMID:25371408

Bergrath, S., Rossaint, R., Lenssen, N., Fitzner, C., & Skorning, M. (2013). Prehospital digital photography and automated image transmission in an emergency medical service - an ancillary retrospective analysis of a prospective controlled trial. *Scandinavian Journal of Trauma, Resuscitation and Emergency Medicine, 21*(1), 3. doi:10.1186/1757-7241-21-3 PMID:23324531

Bernetti, L., Nuzzaco, G., Muscia, F., Gamboni, A., Zedde, M., Eusebi, P., ... Corea, F. (2018). Stroke networks and telemedicine: An Italian national survey. *Neurology International, 10*(1), 7599. doi:10.4081/ni.2018.7599 PMID:29844893

Bhatt, K., Pourmand, A., & Sikka, N. (2018). Targeted Applications of Unmanned Aerial Vehicles (Drones) in Telemedicine. *Telemedicine Journal and e-Health*, tmj.2017.0289. doi:10.1089/tmj.2017.0289 PMID:29489441

Bolle, S. R., Johnsen, E., & Gilbert, M. (2011). Video calls for dispatcher-assisted cardiopulmonary resuscitation can improve the confidence of lay rescuers--surveys after simulated cardiac arrest. *Journal of Telemedicine and Telecare, 17*(2), 88–92. doi:10.1258/jtt.2010.100605 PMID:21139017

Boulos, M. N., Brewer, A. C., Karimkhani, C., Buller, D. B., & Dellavalle, R. P. (2014). Mobile medical and health apps: State of the art, concerns, regulatory control and certification. *Online Journal of Public Health Informatics, 5*(3), 229. doi:10.5210/ojphi.v5i3.4814 PMID:24683442

Boutilier, J. J., Brooks, S. C., Janmohamed, A., Byers, A., Buick, J. E., Zhan, C., ... Chan, T. C. Y. (2017). Optimizing a Drone Network to Deliver Automated External Defibrillators. *Circulation, 135*(25), 2454–2465. doi:10.1161/CIRCULATIONAHA.116.026318 PMID:28254836

Brinkrolf, P., Scheer, D., Hasebrook, J., & Hahnenkamp, K. (2017). Land|Rettung: Zukunftsfeste notfallmedizinische Neuausrichtung eines Landkreises. In Amelung (Ed.), Innovationsfonds (pp. 140-145). MWV.

Broach, J., Hart, A., Griswold, M., Lai, J., Boyer, E. W., Skolnik, A. B., & Chai, P. R. (2018). Usability and Reliability of Smart Glasses for Secondary Triage During Mass Casualty Incidents. *Proc Annu Hawaii Int Conf Syst Sci*, 2018, 1416-1422.

Brokmann, J. C., Conrad, C., Rossaint, R., Bergrath, S., Beckers, S. K., Tamm, M., ... Hirsch, F. (2016). Treatment of Acute Coronary Syndrome by Telemedically Supported Paramedics Compared With Physician-Based Treatment: A Prospective, Interventional, Multicenter Trial. *Journal of Medical Internet Research, 18*(12), e314. doi:10.2196/jmir.6358 PMID:27908843

Brokmann, J. C., Rossaint, R., Hirsch, F., Beckers, S. K., Czaplik, M., Chowanetz, M., ... Bergrath, S. (2016). Analgesia by telemedically supported paramedics compared with physician-administered analgesia: A prospective, interventional, multicentre trial. *European Journal of Pain (London, England), 20*(7), 1176–1184. doi:10.1002/ejp.843 PMID:26914284

Brokmann, J. C., Rossaint, R., Muller, M., Fitzner, C., Villa, L., Beckers, S. K., & Bergrath, S. (2017). Blood pressure management and guideline adherence in hypertensive emergencies and urgencies: A comparison between telemedically supported and conventional out-of-hospital care. *Journal of Clinical Hypertension (Greenwich, Conn.), 19*(7), 704–712. doi:10.1111/jch.13026 PMID:28560799

Buscher, C., & Schilberg, D. (n.d.). *TemRas Telemedizinische Rettungsassistenzsystem*. Retrieved 04.06.2013, from http://www.temras.de/

Calleja-Castillo, J. M., & Gonzalez-Calderon, G. (2018). WhatsApp in Stroke Systems: Current Use and Regulatory Concerns. *Frontiers in Neurology, 9*, 388. doi:10.3389/fneur.2018.00388 PMID:29904369

Callese, T. E., Richards, C. T., Shaw, P., Schuetz, S. J., Paladino, L., Issa, N., & Swaroop, M. (2015). Trauma system development in low- and middle-income countries: A review. *The Journal of Surgical Research, 193*(1), 300–307. doi:10.1016/j.jss.2014.09.040 PMID:25450600

Chochliouros, I. (n.d.). *Live Video-to-Video Supporting Interactive City Infrastructure*. Retrieved 03.06.2013, from http://www.livecity-psp.eu/

Chochliouros, I., Stephanakis, I., Spiliopoulou, A., Sfakianakis, E., & Ladid, L. (2012). Developing Innovative Live Video-to-Video Communications for Smarter European Cities. In L. Iliadis, I. Maglogiannis, H. Papadopoulos, K. Karatzas, & S. Sioutas (Eds.), *Artificial Intelligence Applications and Innovations* (Vol. 382, pp. 279–289). Springer Berlin Heidelberg. doi:10.1007/978-3-642-33412-2_29

Claesson, A., Svensson, L., Nordberg, P., Ringh, M., Rosenqvist, M., Djarv, T., ... Hollenberg, J. (2017). Drones may be used to save lives in out of hospital cardiac arrest due to drowning. *Resuscitation, 114*, 152–156. doi:10.1016/j.resuscitation.2017.01.003 PMID:28110000

Cummins, N. M., Dixon, M., Garavan, C., Landymore, E., Mulligan, N., & O'Donnell, C. (2013). Can advanced paramedics in the field diagnose patients and predict hospital admission? *Emergency Medicine Journal, 30*(12), 1043–1047. doi:10.1136/emermed-2012-201899 PMID:23407377

Curaudeau, G. A., Sharma, N., & Rovin, R. A. (2011). Development of an iPhone application for sideline concussion testing. *Neurosurgical Focus, 31*(5), E4. doi:10.3171/2011.8.FOCUS11186 PMID:22044103

Czaplik, M., Bergrath, S., Rossaint, R., Thelen, S., Brodziak, T., Valentin, B., ... Brokmann, J. C. (2014). Employment of telemedicine in emergency medicine. Clinical requirement analysis, system development and first test results. *Methods of Information in Medicine*, *53*(2), 99–107. doi:10.3414/ME13-01-0022 PMID:24477815

Dagal, A., Greer, S. E., & McCunn, M. (2014). International disparities in trauma care. *Current Opinion in Anaesthesiology*, *27*(2), 233–239. doi:10.1097/ACO.0000000000000049 PMID:24514036

Dick, W. F. (2003). Anglo-American vs. Franco-German emergency medical services system. *Prehosp Disaster Med, 18*(1), 29-35.

Felzen, M., Brokmann, J. C., Beckers, S. K., Czaplik, M., Hirsch, F., Tamm, M., ... Bergrath, S. (2017). Improved technical performance of a multifunctional prehospital telemedicine system between the research phase and the routine use phase - an observational study. *Journal of Telemedicine and Telecare*, *23*(3), 402–409. doi:10.1177/1357633X16644115 PMID:27080747

Filho, F., Menezes, N., Filho, F., Soares, G., Solla, D. J. F., Argôlo, F. C., ... Lopes, R. D. (2018). Implementation of a Regional Network for ST-Segment–Elevation Myocardial Infarction (STEMI) Care and 30-Day Mortality in a Low- to Middle-Income City in Brazil: Findings From Salvador's STEMI Registry (RESISST). *Journal of the American Heart Association*, *7*(14). doi:10.1161/jaha.118.008624 PMID:29980522

Franschman, G., Peerdeman, S. M., Greuters, S., Vieveen, J., Brinkman, A. C. M., Christiaans, H. M. T., ... Boer, C. (2009). Prehospital endotracheal intubation in patients with severe traumatic brain injury: Guidelines versus reality. *Resuscitation*, *80*(10), 1147–1151. doi:10.1016/j.resuscitation.2009.06.029 PMID:19632024

Freshwater, E., & Crouch, R. (n.d.). Technology for trauma: testing the validity of a smartphone app for pre-hospital clinicians. *International Emergency Nursing, 23*(1), 32-37. doi:10.1016/j.ienj.2014.04.003

Friedman, J. (2014). Rhode Island Hospital launches country's first Google Glass study in emergency department. *R I Med J (2013), 97*(4), 47.

Gaba, D. M. (2007). The future vision of simulation in healthcare. *Simulation in Healthcare*, *2*(2), 126–135. doi:10.1097/01.SIH.0000258411.38212.32 PMID:19088617

Goncalves, J., Cordeiro, L., Batista, P., & Monteiro, E. (2012). LiveCity: A Secure Live Video-to-Video Interactive City Infrastructure. In L. Iliadis, I. Maglogiannis, H. Papadopoulos, K. Karatzas, & S. Sioutas (Eds.), *Artificial Intelligence Applications and Innovations* (Vol. 382, pp. 260–267). Springer Berlin Heidelberg. doi:10.1007/978-3-642-33412-2_27

Hubert, G., Müller-Barna, P., & Audebert, H. (2014). Recent advances in TeleStroke: A systematic review on applications in prehospital management and Stroke Unit treatment or TeleStroke networking in developing countries. *International Journal of Stroke*, *9*(8), 968–973. doi:10.1111/ijs.12394 PMID:25381687

Jain, T., Sibley, A., Stryhn, H., & Hubloue, I. (2018). Comparison of Unmanned Aerial Vehicle Technology Versus Standard Practice in Identification of Hazards at a Mass Casualty Incident Scenario by Primary Care Paramedic Students. *Disaster Medicine and Public Health Preparedness, 1-4*. doi:10.1017/dmp.2017.129 PMID:29382398

Johnsen, E., & Bolle, S. R. (2008). To see or not to see--better dispatcher-assisted CPR with video-calls? A qualitative study based on simulated trials. *Resuscitation*, *78*(3), 320–326. doi:10.1016/j.resuscitation.2008.04.024 PMID:18583015

Kerem, Y., Eastvold, J. S., Faragoi, D., Strasburger, D., Motzny, S. E., & Kulstad, E. B. (2014). The role of prehospital electrocardiograms in the recognition of ST-segment elevation myocardial infarctions and reperfusion times. *The Journal of Emergency Medicine*, *46*(2), 202–207. doi:10.1016/j.jemermed.2013.08.084 PMID:24268634

Klack, L., Ziefle, M., Wilkowska, W., & Kluge, J. (2013). Telemedical versus conventional heart patient monitoring: A survey study with German physicians. *International Journal of Technology Assessment in Health Care*, *29*(4), 378–383. doi:10.1017/S026646231300041X PMID:24290330

Kleber, C., Giesecke, M., Tsokos, M., Haas, N., Schaser, K., Stefan, P., & Buschmann, C. (2012). Overall Distribution of Trauma-related Deaths in Berlin 2010: Advancement or Stagnation of German Trauma Management? *World Journal of Surgery*, *36*(9), 2125–2130. doi:10.100700268-012-1650-9 PMID:22610265

Latifi, R. (2010). *Telemedicine for Trauma, Emergencies, and Disaster Management*. Norwood: Artech House.

Latifi, R., Weinstein, R. S., Porter, J. M., Ziemba, M., Judkins, D., Ridings, D., ... Leyva, F. (2007). Telemedicine and telepresence for trauma and emergency care management. *Scandinavian Journal of Surgery*, *96*(4), 281–289. doi:10.1177/145749690709600404 PMID:18265854

Levine, A. I., DeMaria, S., Schwartz, A. D., & Sim, A. J. (2013). *The Comprehensive Textbook of Healthcare Simulation*. Springer. doi:10.1007/978-1-4614-5993-4

Lin, M., Rezaie, S., & Husain, I. (2014). Top 10 mobile apps in Emergency Medicine. *Emergency Medicine Journal*, *31*(5), 432–433. doi:10.1136/emermed-2014-203607 PMID:24567149

Lossius, H. M., Roislien, J., & Lockey, D. J. (2012). Patient safety in pre-hospital emergency tracheal intubation: A comprehensive meta-analysis of the intubation success rates of EMS providers. *Critical Care (London, England)*, *16*(1), R24. doi:10.1186/cc11189 PMID:22325973

Melbye, S., Hotvedt, M., & Bolle, S. (2014). Mobile videoconferencing for enhanced emergency medical communication - a shot in the dark or a walk in the park? -- A simulation study. *Scandinavian Journal of Trauma, Resuscitation and Emergency Medicine*, *22*(1), 35. doi:10.1186/1757-7241-22-35 PMID:24887256

Metelmann, B., Metelmann, C., Meissner, K., Wendt, M., Goncalves, J., Gilligan, P., & von der Heyden, M. (2014). The Potential of Telemedicine. In L. Iliadis, I. Maglogiannis, H. Papadopoulos, S. Sioutas, & C. Makris (Eds.), *Artificial Intelligence Applications and Innovations* (Vol. 437, pp. 30–37). Springer Berlin Heidelberg.

Metelmann, B., Metelmann, C., Morris, D., Cordeiro, L., Chochliouros, I., von der Heyden, M., . . . Wendt, M. (2014). *Live Video Transmission to Improve Emergency Medicine* [Videoübertragung in Echtzeit zur Verbesserung der Notfallmedizin]. Paper presented at the VDE-Kongress 2014 - Smart Cities, Frankfurt am Main, Germany.

Metelmann, C., Metelmann, B., Morris, D., Cordeiro, L., Chochliouros, I., von der Heyden, M., . . . Wendt, M. (2014). *The Potential of Telemedicine for Patients at Home* [Potenziale der Telemedizin bei Patienten in der Häuslichkeit]. Paper presented at the VDE-Kongress 2014 - Smart Cities, Frankfurt am Main, Germany.

Metelmann, C., Metelmann, B., Wendt, M., Meissner, K., & von der Heyden, M. (2014). LiveCity: The Impact of Video Communication on Emergency Medicine. *International Journal of Electronic Government Research, 10*(3), 47–65. doi:10.4018/ijegr.2014070104

MHRA, Medicines and Healthcare Products Regulatory Agency. (2014). *Medical device stand-alone software including apps*. Retrieved from https://www.gov.uk/government/publications/medical-devices-software-applications-apps

Moroz, P. J., & Spiegel, D. A. (2014). The World Health Organization's action plan on the road traffic injury pandemic: Is there any action for orthopaedic trauma surgeons? *Journal of Orthopaedic Trauma, 28*(Suppl 1), S11–S14. doi:10.1097/BOT.0000000000000105 PMID:24857989

Mosier, J., Joseph, B., & Sakles, J. C. (2013). Telebation: Next-generation telemedicine in remote airway management using current wireless technologies. *Telemedicine Journal and e-Health, 19*(2), 95–98. doi:10.1089/tmj.2012.0093 PMID:23215736

Nilsen, J. E. (2012). *Improving quality of care in the Emergency Medical Communication Centres (EMCC)*. Paper presented at the Konferanse for medisinsk nødmeldetjeneste, Sola, Norway.

Palma, D., Goncalves, J., Cordeiro, L., Simoes, P., Monteiro, E., Magdalinos, P., & Chochliouros, I. (2013). Tutamen: An Integrated Personal Mobile and Adaptable Video Platform for Health and Protection. In H. Papadopoulos, A. Andreou, L. Iliadis, & I. Maglogiannis (Eds.), *Artificial Intelligence Applications and Innovations* (Vol. 412, pp. 442–451). Springer Berlin Heidelberg. doi:10.1007/978-3-642-41142-7_45

Patton, G. G., & Thakore, S. (2013). Reducing inappropriate emergency department attendances--a review of ambulance service attendances at a regional teaching hospital in Scotland. *Emergency Medicine Journal, 30*(6), 459–461. doi:10.1136/emermed-2012-201116 PMID:22802457

Perkins, G. D., Handley, A. J., Koster, R. W., Castren, M., Smyth, M. A., Olasveengen, T., ... Soar, J. (2015). European Resuscitation Council Guidelines for Resuscitation 2015: Section 2. Adult basic life support and automated external defibrillation. *Resuscitation, 95*, 81–99. doi:10.1016/j.resuscitation.2015.07.015 PMID:26477420

Roberts, K., Blethyn, K., Foreman, M., & Bleetman, A. (2009). Influence of air ambulance doctors on on-scene times, clinical interventions, decision-making and independent paramedic practice. *Emergency Medicine Journal, 26*(2), 128–134. doi:10.1136/emj.2008.059899 PMID:19164630

Rojahn, S. (2014). *Why Some Doctors Like Google Glass So Much*. MIT Technology Review.

Rortgen, D., Bergrath, S., Rossaint, R., Beckers, S. K., Fischermann, H., Na, I. S., ... Skorning, M. (2013). Comparison of physician staffed emergency teams with paramedic teams assisted by telemedicine--a randomized, controlled simulation study. *Resuscitation, 84*(1), 85–92. doi:10.1016/j.resuscitation.2012.06.012 PMID:22750663

Roudsari, B., Nathens, A., Cameron, P., Civil, I., Gruen, R., Koepsell, T., ... Rivara, F. (2007). International comparison of prehospital trauma care systems. *Injury*, *38*(9), 993–1000. doi:10.1016/j.injury.2007.03.028 PMID:17640641

Sakai, T., Kitamura, T., Nishiyama, C., Murakami, Y., Ando, M., Kawamura, T., ... Iwami, T. (2015). Cardiopulmonary resuscitation support application on a smartphone - randomized controlled trial. *Circulation Journal*, *79*(5), 1052–1057. doi:10.1253/circj.CJ-14-1258 PMID:25740350

Sakles, J. C., Mosier, J., Hadeed, G., Hudson, M., Valenzuela, T., & Latifi, R. (2011). Telemedicine and telepresence for prehospital and remote hospital tracheal intubation using a GlideScope videolaryngoscope: A model for tele-intubation. *Telemedicine Journal and e-Health*, *17*(3), 185–188. doi:10.1089/tmj.2010.0119 PMID:21443441

Schwamm, L. H., Holloway, R. G., Amarenco, P., Audebert, H. J., Bakas, T., Chumbler, N. R., ... Wechsler, L. R. (2009). A review of the evidence for the use of telemedicine within stroke systems of care: A scientific statement from the American Heart Association/American Stroke Association. *Stroke*, *40*(7), 2616–2634. doi:10.1161/STROKEAHA.109.192360 PMID:19423852

Seguin, C., Blaquiere, G., Loundou, A., Michelet, P., & Markarian, T. (2018). Unmanned aerial vehicles (drones) to prevent drowning. *Resuscitation*, *127*, 63–67. doi:10.1016/j.resuscitation.2018.04.005 PMID:29653153

Steg, P., James, S., Atar, D., Badano, L., Lundqvist, C., Borger, M., ... Wallentin, L. (2012). ESC Guidelines for the management of acute myocardial infarction in patients presenting with ST-segment elevation: The Task Force on the management of ST-segment elevation acute myocardial infarction of the European Society of Cardiology (ESC). *European Heart Journal*. doi:10.1093/eurheartj/ehs215

The European Stroke Organisation Executive. (2008). Guidelines for Management of Ischaemic Stroke and Transient Ischaemic Attack 2008. *Cerebrovascular Diseases (Basel, Switzerland)*, *25*(5), 457–507. doi:10.1159/000131083 PMID:18477843

Thelen, S., Schneiders, M., Schilberg, D., & Jeschke, S. (2013). *A Multifunctional Telemedicine System for Pre-hospital Emergency Medical Services*. Paper presented at the eTELEMED 2013, The Fifth International Conference on eHealth, Telemedicine, and Social Medicine.

Thiels, C. A., Aho, J. M., Zietlow, S. P., & Jenkins, D. H. (2015). Use of unmanned aerial vehicles for medical product transport. *Air Medical Journal*, *34*(2), 104–108. doi:10.1016/j.amj.2014.10.011 PMID:25733117

Valenzuela Espinoza, A., De Smedt, A., Guldolf, K., Vandervorst, F., Van Hooff, R. J., Fernandez Tellez, H., ... Brouns, R. (2016). Opinions and Beliefs About Telemedicine for Emergency Treatment During Ambulance Transportation and for Chronic Care at Home. *Interactive Journal of Medical Research*, *5*(1), e9. doi:10.2196/ijmr.5015 PMID:27029999

Valenzuela Espinoza, A., Devos, S., van Hooff, R. J., Fobelets, M., Dupont, A., Moens, M., ... Putman, K. (2017). Time Gain Needed for In-Ambulance Telemedicine: Cost-Utility Model. *JMIR mHealth and uHealth*, *5*(11), e175. doi:10.2196/mhealth.8288 PMID:29175808

Valenzuela Espinoza, A., Van Hooff, R. J., De Smedt, A., Moens, M., Yperzeele, L., Nieboer, K., ... Brouns, R. (2016). Development and Pilot Testing of 24/7 In-Ambulance Telemedicine for Acute Stroke: Prehospital Stroke Study at the Universitair Ziekenhuis Brussel-Project. *Cerebrovascular Diseases (Basel, Switzerland)*, *42*(1-2), 15–22. doi:10.1159/000444175 PMID:26950076

Van Hooff, R. J., Cambron, M., Van Dyck, R., De Smedt, A., Moens, M., Espinoza, A. V., ... Brouns, R. (2013). Prehospital unassisted assessment of stroke severity using telemedicine: A feasibility study. *Stroke*, *44*(10), 2907–2909. doi:10.1161/STROKEAHA.113.002079 PMID:23920013

Wandling, M. W., Nathens, A. B., Shapiro, M. B., & Haut, E. R. (2016). Police transport versus ground EMS: A trauma system-level evaluation of prehospital care policies and their effect on clinical outcomes. *The Journal of Trauma and Acute Care Surgery*, *81*(5), 931–935. doi:10.1097/TA.0000000000001228 PMID:27537514

Weerakkody, V., El-Haddadeh, R., Chochliouros, I., & Morris, D. (2012). Utilizing a High Definition Live Video Platform to Facilitate Public Service Delivery. In L. Iliadis, I. Maglogiannis, H. Papadopoulos, K. Karatzas, & S. Sioutas (Eds.), *Artificial Intelligence Applications and Innovations* (Vol. 382, pp. 290–299). Springer Berlin Heidelberg. doi:10.1007/978-3-642-33412-2_30

Wen, T., Zhang, Z., & Wong, K. K. (2016). Multi-Objective Algorithm for Blood Supply via Unmanned Aerial Vehicles to the Wounded in an Emergency Situation. *PLoS One*, *11*(5), e0155176. doi:10.1371/journal.pone.0155176 PMID:27163361

WHO. (2010). *Injuries and violence: the facts*. Geneva: WHO.

WHO. (2014). *The top 10 causes of death* (Vol. Fact sheet N°310, pp. 5). World Health Organization.

Wiechmann, W., Kwan, D., Bokarius, A., & Toohey, S. L. (2016). There's an App for That? Highlighting the Difficulty in Finding Clinically Relevant Smartphone Applications. *The Western Journal of Emergency Medicine*, *17*(2), 191–194. doi:10.5811/westjem.2015.12.28781 PMID:26973750

Wolfe, C. (2000). The impact of stroke. *British Medical Bulletin*, *56*(2), 275–286. doi:10.1258/0007142001903120 PMID:11092079

World Bank. (2012). 2012 Information and Communications for Development: Maximizing Mobile. Washington, DC: Author.

Wu, T. C., Nguyen, C., Ankrom, C., Yang, J., Persse, D., Vahidy, F., ... Savitz, S. I. (2014). Prehospital utility of rapid stroke evaluation using in-ambulance telemedicine: A pilot feasibility study. *Stroke*, *45*(8), 2342–2347. doi:10.1161/STROKEAHA.114.005193 PMID:24938842

Yamada, K. C., Inoue, S., & Sakamoto, Y. (2015). An effective support system of emergency medical services with tablet computers. *JMIR mHealth and uHealth*, *3*(1), e23. doi:10.2196/mhealth.3293 PMID:25803096

Yang, C. W., Wang, H. C., Chiang, W. C., Chang, W. T., Yen, Z. S., Chen, S. Y., ... Lin, F. Y. (2008). Impact of adding video communication to dispatch instructions on the quality of rescue breathing in simulated cardiac arrests--a randomized controlled study. *Resuscitation*, *78*(3), 327–332. doi:10.1016/j.resuscitation.2008.03.232 PMID:18583016

Yperzeele, L., Van Hooff, R. J., De Smedt, A., Valenzuela Espinoza, A., Van Dyck, R., Van de Casseye, R., ... Brouns, R. (2014). Feasibility of AmbulanCe-Based Telemedicine (FACT) Study: Safety, Feasibility and Reliability of Third Generation In-Ambulance Telemedicine. *PLoS One*, *9*(10), e110043. doi:10.1371/journal.pone.0110043 PMID:25343246

KEY TERMS AND DEFINITIONS

Emergency Doctor: A doctor with special training in emergency medicine. In the Anglo-American model, the emergency doctor treats the patients in the emergency department of a hospital. In the Franco-German model, emergency doctors start the treatment of patients with (potentially) life-threatening conditions already at the emergency site.

Medical Simulation Center: Creates dynamic, realistic routine or emergency scenarios with computer-operated mannequins to learn or examine procedures without putting patients at risk.

Myocardial Infarction: Acute blockage of a coronary artery, stopping the blood flow to the heart muscle. This leads to severe damage to the heart and can result in cardiac arrest and death.

Paramedic: Paramedics receive a one- to three-year education in handling emergency situations and are the basis of prehospital emergency systems worldwide.

Prehospital Emergency Medicine: All efforts made by medical professionals to treat acute illnesses, life-threatening conditions and pain at the emergency site and to transport the patient—if needed—to a hospital.

Stroke: Acute lack of oxygen in brain cells, caused by either bleeding or blockage of an artery. A stroke can lead to massive disability or even death.

Trauma: Accidents, for example traffic accidents, leading to injuries. Severe accidents can result in massive bleeding, organ failure, and death.

Chapter 7
Cytopathology and the Smartphone:
An Update

Abraham Pouliakis
National and Kapodistrian University of Athens, Greece

Effrosyni Karakitsou
University of Barcelona, Spain

Niki Margari
Independent Researcher, Greece

ABSTRACT

Since George Papanicolaou proposed the famous test pap about 60 years ago, and due to heavy impact on cervical cancer reduction, cytopathology became a popular discipline, and in some countries, a medical specialty. The microscope is still the primary device in cytopathology laboratories; however, modalities for molecular tests and networks hosting laboratory information systems and imaging systems produce enormous data. Nowadays, competing mobile devices are integrated with the environment, always connected and always on the user side. Therefore, it is expected that applications for the mobile device targeting cytopathology would flourish. There is potential for applications to various activities of the laboratory including and not limited to training, reporting of results, diagnosis and consultation, management of the laboratory, whole slide imaging and still image capture, quality control and assurance, and numerous channels for interactions between patient-doctor or among medical specialists. The mobile device can enhance the cytopathology laboratory and offer numerous benefits.

INTRODUCTION

The practice of medicine and public health supported by mobile devices is called Mobile Health, in short mHealth or m-health (Adibi, 2015). Mobile computing and modern communication devices, mainly smart phones and tablet computers, has rapidly grown and nowadays are still growing. mHealth applications

DOI: 10.4018/978-1-5225-8021-8.ch007

Copyright © 2019, IGI Global. Copying or distributing in print or electronic forms without written permission of IGI Global is prohibited.

have been used vastly to collect health-related data, delivery of healthcare information, monitoring in real time patient vital signs, and provisioning of healthcare services, to mention the main application streams.

mHealth has been applied in ambulatory medicine (K. Banitsas, Perakis, Koutsouris, Konis, & Tachakra, 2005; K. A. Banitsas, Perakis, Tachakra, & Koutsouris, 2006; Kiselev, Gridnev, Shvartz, Posnenkova, & Dovgalevsky, 2012; Pavlopoulos, Kyriacou, Berler, Dembeyiotis, & Koutsouris, 1998; Rosales Saurer, Mueller-Gorchs, & Kunze, 2009; Zerth, Besser, & Reichert, 2012), management of diabetes (Miyamoto, Dharmar, Fazio, Tang-Feldman, & Young, 2018; Modzelewski, Stockman, & Steenkamp, 2018; Ribu et al., 2013; Spat et al., 2013; Torbjornsen, Smastuen, Jenum, Arsand, & Ribu, 2018) and asthma (Finkelstein, Hripcsak, & Cabrera, 1998; Gupta, Chang, Anyigbo, & Sabharwal, 2011; Rudin et al., 2017; Xiao et al., 2018), control of obesity (Callender & Thompson, 2018; Delisle Nystrom et al., 2018), smoke cesation (Ghorai, Akter, Khatun, & Ray, 2014; Ybarra, Holtrop, Prescott, & Strong, 2014), management of seizure (Pandher & Bhullar, 2014) and stress (Clarke et al., 2014), depression treatment (Burns et al., 2011; Miranda et al., 2018), parkinsons disease patient management (Tsiouris et al., 2017) among others.

The global market for mHealth is estimated at 37 billion dollars for 2019, while telehealth is estimated at 22 billion dollars (The Statistics Portal, 2018). The majority of mHealth applications are for fitness (43%) followed by health resource (15.0%) and diet/caloric intake (14.3%,), while the user engagement has the form of self-monitoring and training (74.8%) (Sama, Eapen, Weinfurt, Shah, & Schulman, 2014); in contrast, despite there are applications targeting patients, which sometimes show lack of adoption (Thies, Anderson, & Cramer, 2017); there are rather limited applications targeting physicians and doctor-patient interactions (T. Martin, 2012). From the clinical applications, pioneering in the field of mHealth is, as expected, radiology (Choudhri et al., 2012; Choudhri et al., 2013; European Society of, 2018; Johnson et al., 2012; Toomey et al., 2010) and ECG transmission (Guzik & Malik, 2016; Rachim & Chung, 2016; Sahoo, Thakkar, & Lee, 2017; Vaisanen, Makijarvi, & Silfvast, 2003). In relation to pathology, mHelath applications are rather limited, even less in cytopathology, despite both specialties deal largely with images, this may be attributed to the rather short number of served patients in pathology; However, concerning cytopathology, in countries that apply organized screening programs, a large proportion of women are examined usually every three or five years. The most reported uses of handhelds for pathology are limited to experimental settings in education and telemedicine (Park, Parwani, Satyanarayanan, & Pantanowitz, 2012). Especially in the field of cytopathology, the published articles or reports are rather limited. However, pathology and cytopathology share many common characteristics. Therefore, applications, concepts and ideas applied in pathology, can be, rather easily, useful in cytopathology; thus, applications can be transferred from one domain to the other.

Cytopathology is a medical sector/discipline that gained popularity when George Papanicolaou, the founder of cytopathology (Papanicolaou, 1928), proposed the famous test Papanicolaou (known as Pap test), about 80 years ago (Diamantis, Magiorkinis, & Koutselini, 2014; Papanicolaou & Traut, 1941). Nowadays Pap test is still proved the most valuable tool for cervical cancer screening and prevention and is the major reason for cytopathology popularity. Additionally, cytopathology has the advantage to obtain biological material by minimally invasive (or not invasive) techniques. Cytopathology is a discipline that the diagnosis is mainly based on the examination of cells via the microscope, histopathology (or pathology) does the same; however using complete tissues (obtained via a more invasive and usually painful technique, i.e. biopsy). The routine cytological examinations are performed, since the invention of the microscope, via the utilization of a glass slide and subsequent visual analysis.

Today, the modern cytopathology laboratory is continuously changing. Modern cytopathology laboratories perform additional examinations based on molecular techniques and immunocytochemistry methods (i.e. cell staining with special technique to reveal disease aspects, if exist). Today, the modern cytopathology laboratory is equipped with a plethora of modalities; these are capable of performing medical tests, and to exchange data via computer networks. Additionally, there are available imaging systems, capable of creating digital pictures of the slides or even virtual slides, which are complete slides, scanned and available in digital form. The volume of data, in a cytopathology laboratory, nowadays is enormous; consequently, there are many applications that are available and others that can be envisioned for facilitation of cytopathologists and the benefit of the patients. The recent advances in handheld hardware and software; in parallel, with concurrent advances in whole slide imaging (WSI) and cloud computing, offer new opportunities and challenges for cytopathology. Cloud computing (one of the important foundations for mHealth) has already been proposed as a useful platform for modern cytopathology (Pouliakis, Archondakis, Karakitsou, & Karakitsos, 2014; Pouliakis, Archondakis, Margari, & Karakitsos, 2016; Pouliakis, Margari, Archondakis, Karakitsou, & Karakitsos, 2016) as well as in other medical laboratories (Pouliakis, Spathis, et al., 2014).

In this chapter an update of mHealth application in cytopathology (Pouliakis, Archondakis, et al., 2016) is provided. We address the current state of the art in handheld hardware and software, analyze the history of handheld devices, with special focus on pathology and cytopathology, and present use cases that have the potential to be future applications. Various aspects of the modern cytopathology laboratory are analyzed as well, we present a thorough research of mobile applications, related to cytopathology and try to foresee applications, that, if enhanced with mobility and translated for mobile devices, may provide an important benefit to the modern cytopathology laboratory, as well as, for the patients. Wherever possible, we propose new mobile applications, having the potential to enhance the routine of the laboratory. Finally, we highlight issues, controversies and problems and propose solutions and recommendations.

BACKGROUND

An extensive search in PubMed can reveal that from the articles related in handheld computing, there are two groups: one group related to the usage of handhelds in medicine and a second group related to health risks caused by handheld devices (for example cancer risks due to radiation (microwaves), automobile accidents when texting or speaking via the mobile device, electromagnetic interference in hospital devices). The vast majority of research articles are published in the last 15 years; for example, two articles were published in 1983, and 61 articles in October 2011 alone (Park et al., 2012).

Focusing on pathology and cytopathology there is a limited number of articles that deal directly with handheld computing. Some conclusions may be extracted: almost half of the scientific articles deal with static telepathology using mobile phone cameras, and there are only two papers that discuss whole slide imaging and a large proportion of the articles deal with medical education. Nowadays, there are available applications, that exploit the built-in phone camera, mainly for taking photographs through the eyepiece of the microscope and interfacing the mobile phone directly (Breslauer, Maamari, Switz, Lam, & Fletcher, 2009; Roy et al., 2014) and recently were reported two evaluations on applications that create WSIs with the smart phone (Huang et al., 2018; Yu, Gao, Jiang, & Ma, 2017). In short, the scientific literature, related to mobile pathology and cytopathology is rather poor.

Cytopathology and pathology are not the sole medical specialties based heavily on images and other data, however considering images, can be ranked as the first medical specialty in the scale of imagery that must handle. It is considered that over 70% of the data in a typical electronic medical record are generated within the clinical pathology laboratory (Pantanowitz, Henricks, & Beckwith, 2007). In pathology, a Whole Slide Image can easily be in the range of gigabytes in size, even when heavy and lossy compression is applied such as JPEG and JPEG2000 (Pouliakis, Archondakis, et al., 2014). Comparing pathology with radiology, the latest being a medical specialty with extensive use of images as well, we can conclude that it is rather rare for radiology digital images to be more than a few hundred megabytes in size. Note that radiology uses mainly grayscale images (8-bit and in more advanced settings 12 or 16 bits) having resolutions in the thousands of pixels. In pathology color images are required (24-32 bit, thus the amount of data is tripled, simply due to the image depth [3 colors instead of gray scale]). Additionally, the resolution of images is in the range of tens to hundreds of thousands of pixels. Those "heavy" images simply pose requirements for high computational power, high-quality in terms of color reproduction and high-resolution screens with large bit depth (aka color range), fast networks with high bandwidth (sometimes with metropolitan or global aspects and not local for within building communications). Such characteristics were not available in handheld (and sometimes not even on desktop) computers until the evolution of processors, GPUs, 4G networks and high-resolution screens. These represented a barrier to the adoption of electronic data interchange in pathology and even worst in mobile pathology and cytopathology. Modern mobile devices have extremely good characteristics and performance. Therefore there is potential for mobile pathology and cytopathology.

The New Generation of Mobile Devices

Mobile telephony is in everyday use for more than 20 years, during the last decade, advances have converted the mobile phone to the smartphone; especially due to the sophisticated operating systems and the addition of numerous sensors supported by high-quality graphics and processing power. Mobile phones have been enriched with numerous new features:

- The battery that has the capacity to last for days and support computing intensive application and the addition of wireless charging
- CPU with processing power competing for desktop and laptops if we consider that users rarely use the full processing power, mobile phones nowadays can have up to 10 processing cores and support a smooth multitasking environment, while efficiency is improving and, designs to embed neural chips have been announced
- Excellent graphics capabilities with displays that nowadays are in the resolution of 3840x2160 pixels (Ultra high definition displays)
- Processor memory in the range of gigabytes to support applications with a large footprint
- Storage memory in the range of hundreds of Gigabytes if not terra bytes
- Embedded GPS chips for positioning and navigation
- 4G and 4G+ connectivity supporting high-speed wireless communications via the mobile operator networks
- Wi-Fi connectivity of advanced wireless protocols supporting 600 Mbps and competing for the standard (1,000 Mbps) LAN connectivity
- Bluetooth connectivity that supports the creation of personal area networks (PANs)

- USB connectivity for coupling the device to other devices
- NFC (Near Field Communications) to support financial transactions and RF identification
- Accelerometer, gyroscope and compass for enhancement of applications and user experience
- Temperature and light sensors
- One or more high-resolution cameras, higher than 20 million pixels, capable of capturing extremely detailed photographs
- Capacitive touch screen allowing rich user interaction with multi-touch capability
- Connectors to interface with displays on high-end models
- Specialized sensors, measuring vital signs such as heart rate and step counters for fitness measurements, as well as, fingerprint identification for security
- Voice recognition, gesture analysis, and integration of artificial intelligence for enhanced human-machine interface
- Ruggedized design and implementation to withstand harsh environmental conditions and accidents

All these features reversed the trend to shrink the telephone; mobile phones now are becoming larger due to the need for larger and denser displays. New generation smartphones compete for tablets and have the maturity for health sector applications.

CYTOPATHOLOGY AND THE SMARTPHONE

New types of cameras, microscopes, introduced during the last decades, made possible cytological image capture and transmission, aka telecytology (Pantanowitz, Hornish, & Goulart, 2009; Pinco, Goulart, Otis, Garb, & Pantanowitz, 2009). Such telemedical systems have been tested extensively and became a necessity due to the need for therapeutic decisions in real time (Briscoe et al., 2000; Jialdasani et al., 2006; Mun, Elsayed, Tohme, & Wu, 1995; Raab et al., 1996; Weinstein, Epstein, Edlow, & Westra, 1997; Yamashiro et al., 2004), as well as, for training of physicians (Stergiou et al., 2009). Telediagnosis and training are just two of the applications relevant to cytopathology, however, do exist other applications, including but not limited to everyday routine tasks of modern laboratories. For example: for reporting of results, routine laboratory management, WSI, patient-doctor communication, doctor-doctor communication among laboratory members or between separate laboratories and clinics, additionally quality control and assurance has become a necessity in modern laboratories with mHealth applications. In the sequel are presented existing mHealth applications, and, wherever possible, potential applications are pinpointed.

Training via the Mobile Device

In 2006, it was reported that medical students possessed, within their mobile phones, photographs of nearly all typical pathology specimens that could be encountered during examinations (Sharma & Kamal, 2006). Such photographs were considered by the medical department similar to note-taking and eventually was decided to allow the mobile device during examinations as a memory aid. This was perhaps one of the earliest applications of mobile pathology. Five years later (Collins, 2011), it was reported the use of iPads for online distribution of cytopathology textbooks. This application was based on the epub 3.0 standard, which is used to create electronic books (e-books). The authoring software was Adobe InDesign CS5, and the e-book contained both text and images and w accessible from a variety of different mobile platforms (due to the epub standard). In 2011, the 64 GB capacity of the mobile device was considered as ample storage space for such applications, today, cloud-based storage and the always-connected capability provides virtually unlimited storage (Pouliakis, Archondakis, et al., 2014; Pouliakis, Spathis, et al., 2014).

Electronic books have numerous advantages against paper books: a) e-book is searchable content b) interactive text and references can be followed by a click c) high-resolution cytopathology images d) capability to bookmark a page e) storage of user added references and text f) embedding of video and in general multimedia rich content g) instant access to medical references with a single touch. Moreover, images and text can be viewed in a stand-alone mode in full screen because, since iPad and some other mobile phones can be connected to external HDTV displays. Moreover, content could be copied, pasted, printed, and emailed.

Two other aspects of training are: a) the application of webcasts and b) the use of mobile phones to augment the education of remotely located lab technicians. For example, in developing countries, training of laboratory technicians by pathologists, thus they are competent to capture pathology images from the microscope for cytology of pathology (Livia Bellina et al., 2014; Hartman, 2016).

Training related applications on the mobile device is now a fact and not only for research. Nowadays, there are numerous commercial applications related to cytopathology: handbooks (Elsevier, 2015), medical atlases, e.g. Johns Hopkins Atlas of Pancreatic Cytopathology (Meszaros, 2014) and moreover the majority of cytopathology scientific journals.

In the first endeavors, applications were designed specifically taking to account the characteristics of the mobile device (such as image resolution). However browsers in smartphones, have turned such pioneering efforts almost obsolete. Today any web page can be viewed by the mobile phone browser, and the high resolution of the screen and the zoom capability facilitates this. Modern browsers are not anymore proprietary, in fact, all popular browsers are available for almost all smartphones and almost identical to the browsers of a desktop computer. Thus, there is no need to develop web-based training material and applications, specifically for the mobile device. Moreover, Web 2.0 technologies, are now directly available on the mobile phones as well.

In terms of connectivity capabilities, smartphones have numerous connectivity subsystems, and surprisingly there are integrated relational databases. Thus, the handheld device can be used both as server and client. In 2004,, the use of Internet search engines to find reference material for oral and maxillofacial pathology was reported (Ng & Yeo, 2004), and in 2004 it was proposed the caching of material on a PDA due to limits on communication capacity and local storage, nowadays caching is not a necessity as the mobile device is always connected.

Reporting Results via the Mobile Device

The appropriate reporting format for medical diagnosis can have consequences for patient management and treatment (Crowe et al., 2011; Hirsch, Robenshtok, Bachar, Braslavsky, & Benbassat, 2015). Frequently, laboratories produce medical reports that are incomplete, i.e. do not contain all the information required by clinical doctors; this may lead towards a suboptimal treatment or cause additional communication and between laboratory and clinic for resolution. In short, medical reports should be formulated and contain only the required information, which should be useful. Especially for cytopathology and pathology, whereas, descriptive answers can be provided; based on the microscopic and macroscopic findings. These medical reports are often described in a qualitative (rather than quantitative) manner, thus, it is crucial to formulate diagnoses based on cellular or tissue features, and to communicate the results in a useful manner for the clinical doctors. Additionally, cytopathology reporting systems (Field, Schmitt, & Vielh, 2017; Fulciniti et al., 2018; Margari et al., 2016; Nayar & Wilbur, 2015; Pusztaszeri et al., 2016) evolve continuously; thus, there a need for training and adaptation on how to report.

ReportSupport (Skeate, Wahi, Jessurun, & Connelly, 2007) was a software environment for the mobile phone that facilitated reporting. The researchers used ReportSupport and extracted a conclusion on its usage based on a PDA. They concluded that PDAs might improve resident learning as well as report completion as well. ReportSupport was relevant to the pathology discipline. However, similar outcomes are expected for cytopathology reporting, due to the fact that reporting has similar complexity in both specialties/disciplines. ReportSupport software was based on a navigable document, written in Hyper Text Mark-Up Language (HTML) by Macromedia's Dreamweaver 4, and was presented by a web browser. Users have to supply credentials to use the system, after a short introduction and instructions, it is possible to search for a diagnosis of interest (via a choice of organ/system or alphabetically), For tho diagnosis of choice is presented a list of possible responses. Subsequently is presented a list of the elements required for a report to be complete. Additional help is provided for each diagnosis component, for instance is a descriptionof the criteria used to determine and the possible values/choices for report element. Evaluation of ReportSupport was based on two groups or residents; one group used the software, while the second did not. The performance of the first group was evaluated three times: T0: before use of ReportSupport, T1: when ReportSupport was accessed and T2: after T1 but when users did not ha access to the software. According to the results, ReportSupport could not ensure report completeness, but, was associated with more complete reports and more accurate judgments for report completeness. Due to the introduction of T2 was possible to conclude that residents' performance was persistent even when ReportSupport was not accessible. In summary, the use of the PDA with the relevant software was a useful tool for user training and improved reporting.

It is well known that the vast majority of cytopathology reports are related to cervical cancer prevention (via the Papanicolaou test), i.e. screening. Consequentlly, and despite this chapter is related to laboratories, it is worth mentioning some clinical applications, especially for the gynecologist, since it is aspecialty closelly related to cytopathology. In a recent study (S. J. Martin, Chen, Dattilo, & Johnson, 2015), the baseline knowledge for mobile applications of trainees and practicing gynecologists and obstetricians focusing on their field of practice was assessed. An electronic questionnaire was filled by residents, and the responses were analyzed. More than 80% of practitioners were using a mobile phone in their practice for physician and student reference. The applications used were predominantly related to cervical cytology guidelines and obstetrics; more than 80% of the health care providers would like to see more applications on the mobile device. Thus, mobile applications for gynaecologists seems to be an expanding field, as such new technologies may provide benefits and advancement in obstetrics and gynecologic, both for health services providers, as well as for education.

Static Images on the Mobile Device for Diagnosis, Telepathology and Telecytology

The term conventional telecytology and telepathology is usually for a remotely controlled microscope providing a live view of a glass slide. Telecytology is usually employed for activities of low throughput, usually when a remote diagnosis is requested, as well as in the context of a second consultation review or for a preliminary diagnosis. This mainly applies to situations that on-site cytopathologists are not available.

Digital cytopathology had a period of exponential growth and expansion, and this was possible from catalytic changes in imaging hardware and an increase in computational processing. Telecytology (Della Mea, Cataldi, Pertoldi, & Beltrami, 2000; Markidou, Karakitsos, & Pouliakis, 1999; B. H. Williams, Mullick, Butler, Herring, & O'Leary T, 2001) is probably the most obvious application with potential for application directly on the mobile device. In the past, telecytology has been applied for reproducibility assessment (Archondakis, 2013; Archondakis, 2014; Archondakis et al., 2009; Tsilalis et al., 2012) and remote diagnosis (Breslauer et al., 2009; Briscoe et al., 2000; Jialdasani et al., 2006; Pantanowitz et al., 2009; Pinco et al., 2009; Raab et al., 1996; Ribu et al., 2013; Spat et al., 2013; Yamashiro et al., 2004) as already mentioned. However, desktop computers are used in all cases. Due to the advances on mobile devices, on communication bandwidth and speed, on display resolution and capability to use external monitors, it seems feasible to have mobile cytopathology. Applications can be very simple and even not require the development of special software. Images can be transmitted via e-mail or even uploaded on a secure web space since image viewers have already been embedded into the mobile device software.

For pathology, in 2009, two independent groups (L. Bellina & Missoni, 2009; McLean, Jury, Bazeos, & Lewis, 2009) published on the application of mobile phone cameras. The application was to snap static digital microscopy images through the eyepiece lens of the microscope and use them for telepathology. In teledermatopathology there are numerous applications (Borve, Terstappen, Sandberg, & Paoli, 2013; Chao, Loescher, Soyer, & Curiel-Lewandrowski, 2013; Janda, Loescher, Banan, Horsham, & Soyer, 2014; Manahan et al., 2015; Massone, Brunasso, Campbell, & Soyer, 2009; Massone, Brunasso, Hofmann-Wellenhof, Gulia, & Soyer, 2010; Wu et al., 2015), In this case mobile phones are used to take static dermatoscopic images and send them for teledermatopathologic consultation. In the field of cytopathology, image capture by the mobile phone camera, directly from the microscope is obviously a very important application, as reported recently (Huang et al., 2018).

Telecytology is a valuable tool to manage and promote interlaboratory collaboration, as better cytological data management and sharing can be achieved in a user-friendly and secure manner. Ideally, a mHealth application for cytopathology should be able to invite collaborators, share digital slides with just a few clicks and additionally put limitations on shared files and individual collaborators. Finally, users should be able to annotate images simultaneously with digital markers, with notes visible immediately to all collaborators. Of course, all this functionality should be available on the mobile device with simultaneous voice conferencing.

Whole Slide Imaging Can the Mobile Device Perform Whole Slide Imaging?

Nowadays, digitization of an entire glass slide can occur in minutes (depending on the optical resolution and slide area), in addition, it is possible to scan whole slides in fluorescence and by multispectral imaging cameras and moreover to use robotic systems capable of scanning hundreds of slides sequentially (see Figure 1). WSI (or Virtual Slides) have been reported to be used successfully in pathology; however, their application in cytology is not so popular (as resulted from the published studies). This perhaps can be attributed to the requirement for z-stack (i.e. scanning of the slide in various positions of the z-axis). This is due to focusing requirements since cytological samples in contrast to histological have a 3D structure. When z-stack capable systems appeared, the application of digital slides for cytology was boosted (Al-Janabi, Huisman, Willems, & Van Diest, 2012; Cucoranu, Parwani, & Pantanowitz, 2014;

Figure 1. Automated whole slide scanner equipped with loader capable of serving sequentially 200 slides

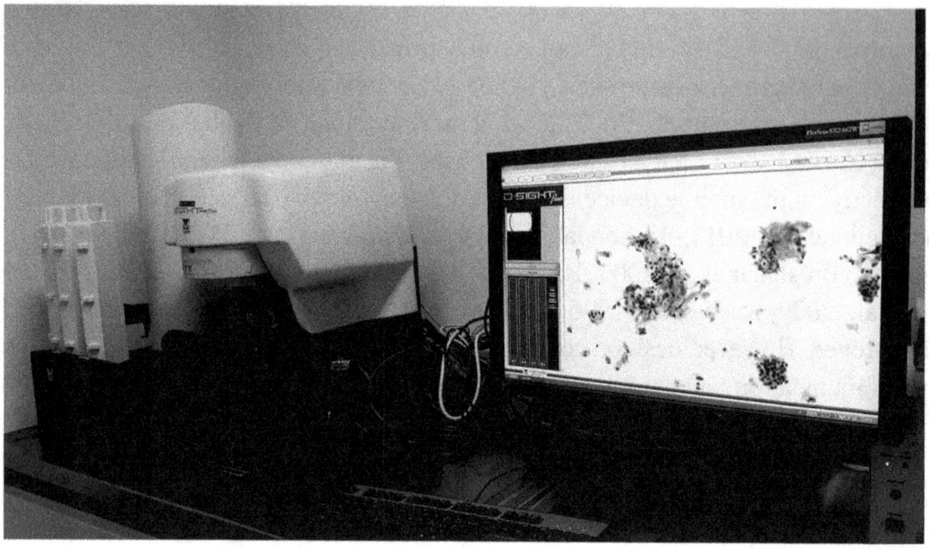

Fung et al., 2012; Ghaznavi, Evans, Madabhushi, & Feldman, 2013; Gutman et al., 2013; Hipp, Lucas, Emmert-Buck, Compton, & Balis, 2011; Huang et al., 2018; Krishnamurthy et al., 2013; Rudnisky et al., 2007; Tawfik et al., 2014; Taylor, 2011; B. J. Williams, Bottoms, & Treanor, 2017; Wright et al., 2013).

A PubMed search for WSI or digital slides reveals that there are about 210 references. However, there is just one directly relevant to cytopathology along with the use of the mobile device (and mainly for capturing the WSI through the eyepiece). However, the technology developments seem to support WSI viewing through the mobile device. Perhaps it is just a matter of time and resources to implement WSI viewing applications. Mapping and navigation applications for the mobile device do exist, and perhaps it is the starting point to develop such applications. Google Maps and Microsoft Bing Maps have functioned similarly to WSI. For example, the use of pyramidal images broken into tiles is light enough to serve satellite imagery (and of course WSIs) to a viewer application on the mobile device in real-time. Indeed, there are some efforts using the map Application Programming Interface (API) (from Google and Microsoft) used to create WSI viewers for the desktop (Triola & Holloway, 2011). Such applications can be transferred to the mobile device as in the case of mapping and navigation. Concerning the depth (aka z-axis) of WSIs, the already available capability of APIs, to display numerous information layers, seems to be able to solve this requirement. Finally, the multi-touch user interface of the mobile device screen along with the zoom capability with an incremental detail is an advantage of the mobile device and can provide a high-quality user experience.

WSI is simply the tool or the enabling technology, the most important aspect is applications, those include: a) long or short-term archiving of the slides b) use for onsite diagnosis c) use for remote consultation and diagnosis d) providing the examination media to the patient e) training f) quality control and proficiency testing.

In a study performed in 2012, it was used an application (for the iPad device), for the online distribution of WSIs, to be used for teaching (Fontelo, Faustorilla, Gavino, & Marcelo, 2012). The study was performed with therd and fourth-year medical students. Since networking for the mobile device was not very efficient in 2012 two web servers were employed to feed the WSIs to the students, one server for remote access and a second with mirrored content for local area network access. According to the results, since the speed of serving the WSIs via the local server was much faster, it was preferred by the students. This role of telecommunication infrastructures is critical for the acceptance of such a "heavy" mHealth application.

The Mobile Device Capturing Images and for WSI Creation

Microscopes are readily available on the cytopathologist desk, however usually they are not equipped with a camera to snap images. In parallel, the mobile phone has a camera, usually with very high resolution and is at the side of the doctors. Adding a digital camera on the microscope comes at a high cost, especially if a computer is not available nearby. In contrast, the mobile phone has become a computer with processing capability and numerous communication channels. It seems that all required components to capture images from the microscope are in place! However, they are not interfaced to do the job!

Consequently, the concept is straightforward, and indeed, there are numerous efforts to use the nearby mobile phone as an image capturing device. In a more advanced application, a WSI system may cost on average between $30,000 and $300,000 (Auguste & Palsana, 2015), this cost is not affordable in low resource environments, and thus WSI cannot be available in the majority of laboratories. Cleverly, there are efforts to use the mobile phone not only as an image capturing device but for the more elaborate task of WSI creation.

Typical applications for image capturing involves interfacing of the mobile phone camera to the microscope eyepiece, a task requiring an adaptor usually of very low price (on average a few euros or a couple of decades). An alternative method involves a device equipped with optics and sometimes a light source, being capable of holding the slide, in this case, no microscope is required (Orth, Wilson, Thompson, & Gibson, 2018). Thus the microscope becomes not mobile and additionally digital and with capabilities for telemedicine! Such interfacing devices come at an extremely low cost since they are a small piece of plastic. In a recent study (Orth et al., 2018) the authors describe the procedure for a 3D printed add-on clip for microscopy with the mobile phone. This clip enabled both bright field and dark field microscopy without additional light source or optics, since by design the integrated flash of the mobile device along with a diffuse reflection enabled lighting of the microscopy slide. Moreover, the 3D designs were made publicly available. Image quantification was possible by the mobile phone in rather older report (Skandarajah, Reber, Switz, & Fletcher, 2014). By such low-cost settings, it was possible to capture and measure images and perform telemedicine; the major concern could be the diagnostic accuracy and perhaps the risk of misdiagnoses. Several studies in various fields have been performed using such mobile microscopes and all report relatively accurate results (Bogoch et al., 2017; D'Ambrosio et al., 2015; Orth et al., 2018; Pirnstill & Cote, 2015; Skandarajah et al., 2014; Sun & Hu, 2018; Yoon et al., 2017).

In the WSI arena, in 2015, it was reported a WSI system called Open Mobile Telepathology System (OMT). This was a combination of two components, namely the Pocket Electronic Health Record (pEHR) and the Mobile Whole Slide Imaging (mWSI) application (). The authors used custom design and constructor adaptor to interface the phone to the eyepiece. The technology to create the WSI was based on a panorama technique, and the first diagnostic slide was feasible using an objective magnification of 10x coupled with an eyepiece magnification 15x. The conclusion was that the system could be deployed at a fraction of the cost of commercial WSI systems, the images were easily transportable since their average size was less than 500 MBs. Additionally any non-medical grade technician could perform the scans, and thus all components for low-cost telepathology and telecytology were feasible. In a more recent study () was reported a similar concept targeted to pathology frozen sections. The very low-cost system had an estimated cost for setup approximately $100 and for scanning a slide from $1-$10, thus was possible to have a WSI cost-effective for infrequent or low-throughput use. The authors additionally performed a clinical evaluation of the diagnostic reliability. The average accuracy was rather low for a pathology laboratory since it ranged from 78% to 50% depending on the organ (breast, uterine corpus, thyroid, and lung). The same system was reported to be used recently in cytopathology applications (). The authors tested the capabilities of 200 different android- based smartphones and concluded that there are technical issues, especially due to the smartphone software capabilities to export uncompressed images when captured by the camera. This leads to high CPU usage and power consumption issues. In the medical evaluation. The produced ThinPrep cytology WSI had similar and high quality when captured by Android or iOS (iPhone) based devices, as commented by the medical team. The correct diagnosis was achieved on 87.5% (175/200) of the cases when using the virtual slides. Moreover the agreement among various medical experts was substantial as the kappa value was in the range 0.70-0.82. Finally, participating doctors considered the quality of the WSI created by the mobile phones adequate for routine usage.

Laboratory Management, Quality Control and the Smartphone

Day to day laboratory management requires accurate operations since the product of the laboratory is a diagnosis or a test result, which it should be produced and transmitted within a specific time (turnaround time TAT). The laboratory results are critical to the clinical doctors. Thus they provide timely intervention and prevent adverse outcomes (Lam, Ajzner, Campbell, & Young, 2016). Definitely, the TAT is strongly linked to the provisioning of quality health services (Pouliakis, Athanasiadi, et al., 2014; Pouliakis, Margari, et al., 2014; Shen & Yang, 2001) and is described as a requirement in ISO 15189 (International Organization for Standardization, 2012). Risk management is a part of this process (Sciacovelli, Secchiero, Zardo, D'Osualdo, & Plebani, 2007); it can be applied within the pre-analytical phase (Vacata, Jahns-Streubel, Baldus, & Wood, 2007; Westbrook, Georgiou, & Rob, 2008) or in the analytical phase (i.e. during sample analysis) or during the post-analytical phase. Laboratories use computerized systems (Laboratory Information Systems-LIS) (Pearlman, Wolfert, Miele, Bilello, & Stauffer, 2001; Pouliakis, Athanasiadi, et al., 2014; Pouliakis, Margari, et al., 2014) to facilitate such workflow and to enable automation; thus reduction of TAT and errors.

Reporting of critical results is a crucial part since laboratories should report them within a strict timeframe to clinicians. Thus, mobile devices could not be kept outside of this process. Actually mobile phones have been already used in reporting of such critical results, and are ideal for such applications, due to the fact that they are always connected and always by the side of the user (aka the clinical doctor in this case). In a study about 15 years ago (Saw, Loh, Ang, Yip, & Sethi, 2011), was reported the experience with a setting employing Short Message Service (SMS) in reporting critical results of examinations. SMSs were used to notify clinicians in a teaching hospital for critical results; this application was used to provide the service and in addition to meet both documentation and auditing requirements of critical result reporting, as these were described by regulatory agencies and/or ISO 15189. The service was called Critical Reportable Result Health care Messaging System (CRR-HMS) and was simply sending a text message that allowed the receiver to acknowledge or reject the critical result by replying to the SMS. If there was no response or no confirmation within 10 minutes, a new procedure was activated, and escalation was performed by sending the SMS to another physician (according to a predefined roster). Finally, the procedure was stopped when confirmation was received. The process was possible to run unattended, and therefore no personnel was employed, thus was affordable! When the experiments and the measurements were finished, it was concluded that CRR-HMS reduced the required time for a response from 7.3 minutes to 2 minutes (almost four times reduction). The CRR-HMS was a useful tool to communicate critical results rapidly. Eventually this enabled timely therapeutic or patient management interventions.

Choice of SMS in this study was based on the following: a) users are familiarized with the software b) messages are delivered almost instantly c) has an adequate word limit that can be expanded d) it is a two way communication channel e) it can be stored electronic audit trail for the communication history (thus there are the records for quality requirements and f) the hardware is available and is in common use among the users, thus there is no need for additional cost for a new portable device (Saw et al., 2011). Nowadays, there are numerous applications that allow two way communications. However, these are based on IP networking capabilities and the ability of the smartphone to connect to Wi-Fi or a 3G/4G data network; since IP connectivity is not ensured and additionally can be disabled by the end users, SMS, despite the small overhead in costs, seems to be still the preferred technology for text-based critical results reporting.

According to ISO 15189:2012 requirements for medical laboratories, one of the most important tasks for cytopathology laboratories is the conformance with a board certified external quality assessment (EQA) program (i.e. proficiency testing). The role of this conformance is to ensure that tests performed by the cytology laboratory are accurate and that the findings are correctly identified and interpreted by physicians or other membres of a laboratory (e.g. biologists). Moreover, the results should be archived and communicated properly towards the clinicians or patients (Archondakis, 2013; Archondakis, 2014; Friedman & Wyatt, 2006; E. S. Lee et al., 2003; Nagy & Newton, 2006; Vooijs et al., 1998). Telecytology has already applications for EQA schemes, as virtual slides are served by web servers towards cytopathology laboratory participating in certification schemes (i.e. no physical slides are sent to the cytopathology laboratories. Instead there is remote diagnosis via WSIs). A promising application in this field can be enabled if WSI viewing will be possible through the mobile device. This can facilitate immediate quality control and moreover collaboration among cytopathology teams.

Other applications related to the use of mHealth for quality control and assurance have already been proposed (Laktabai et al., 2018; Y. Lee et al., 2015), some especially focusing on cytopathology and cervical cancer screening (Archondakis, Vavoulidis, & Nasioutziki, 2016; Athanasiadi et al., 2014; Pouliakis, Athanasiadi, et al., 2014; Pouliakis, Margari, et al., 2014). Especially for screening programs, women conformance can be increased if there are reminders of appointments through the smartphone.

The Smartphone as a Communication Channel Between Patient and Doctor or With the Health System

Today, it is unlikely to imagine people without a mobile phone nearby, especially in the developed and developing countries mobile phones are always connected with high-speed networks (3G/4G or Wi-Fi). Therefore, the device can easily have a role of a terminal point of a communication channel. Patients can be informed for various cytology related aspects. Women can a) be immediately informed for the availability of cytological result, i.e. that their test Papanicolaou is completed and the result is available, a notification could be sent via SMS or email b) women may receive a reminder for their appointment related to cytological sampling and subsequent examination c) women may receive a reminder to book a meeting for test Pap or confirm a predefined meeting, depending on the screening strategy (Athanasiadi et al., 2014; Moumtzoglou & Pouliakis, 2015).

Doctors and patients have to communicate in other circumstances as well. For example, for consulting; often patients do have questions on their test results, especially when they are abnormal and they have not already consulted a clinician. Cytopathology usually provides services to other medical specialties; however, in clinical cytopathology, the patients are treated directly by cytopathologists. Thus, when examination results, eventually are known by the patients, and there is contact information of the laboratory, patients communicate with cytopathologists to be informed for the details reported, and especially directly from the microscopist rather from the clinical doctor (for example the gynecologist). Since the mobile device is always on the patient side, it is the obvious media for such communications, by voice or messages, in real time or asynchronously. Number recognition systems can immediately pop the medical history of the patient on the screen and thus facilitate patient-doctor interactions. However, specialized and complex applications should be developed.

The Smartphone as a Communication Channel Between Doctors

The standardized workflow of a cytopathology laboratory starts with the sample reception along with a referral form; ends with the production, release and dispatching of the cytological report (Pouliakis, Athanasiadi, et al., 2014); these two are the major interaction points of the laboratory with the "external" world. Cytopathology laboratories may produce reports printed on paper or reports in digital form, which can be distributed by secured e-mail or retrieved electronically by the requesting clinician via access to a remote system managed by the laboratory. The next step towards this automation is to use the smartphone capabilities and send SMS or emails. Thus, clinicians are immediately informed of the availability of results and get a link inviting them to login into their account and retrieve the reports from a web server via secured communication protocols. another doctor to doctor communication may involve requests of the laboratory for additional data related to a patient under examination.

In a similar manner to the patient-doctor interactions being reported previously, clinicians may have a plethora of options to consult cytopathologists. For example, interpretation of Papanicolaou test results. However, gynecology is not the sole specialty related to cytopathology, despite interactions between gynecologists and cytopathologists are the most frequent. The majority of medical specialties may request examinations from the cytopathology laboratory, and the group of users can become very large. Consequently the need for services provided by cytopathology laboratories becomes more interesting.

The Smartphone as a Communication Channel for Laboratory Personnel

Exchanging information among cytopathology laboratory members is the third axis relevant to mobile communications. It involves laboratory doctors' requests for ancillary tests or preparations (for example, immunocytochemistry), towards biologists or technicians or urgent requests to repeat an examination. Usually, such requests are issued verbally, or written in a book of requests, and in the case, there is available a LIS, they are recorded via the use of a desktop workstation. Mobile technology is an attractive technology that has the potential to streamline such everyday routine. Laboratory personnel can be independent of desktop computers located in fixed physical locations and alternatively can be on the move. A single mobile phone adapted to their preferences can serve such purposes, in more details, since the mobile phone is nowadays so powerful that it can replace the desktop computer.

One issue could be the use of a second mobile device. However, users are not in favor to take care and carry more than one device. Since modern devices are capable of having more than one commercial communication channel (i.e. SIM cards), it is relatively easy to serve private and job-related tasks simultaneously. The mobile phones are configurable and can get optimization related to user personal needs/tasks, and preferences related to the laboratory tasks. Therefore, mHealth technology, if integrated into the daily laboratory y workflow, can provide exceptional opportunities. mHealth technology has the capability to improve the professional skills of the medical staff and consequently make them feel more confident in their daily work tasks.

ISSUES, CONTROVERSIES AND PROBLEMS

Early adopters of emerging technologies, usually encounter issues not foreseen in advance. Mobile cytopathology could be outside of this rule, in the sequel we try to foresee potential problems that may arise from such applications.

Considering WSI, systematic reviews show some evidence for the accuracy of the method. However there is no high quality of evidence since most studies are small. In a review of 1,155 abstracts, 38 papers were analyzed systematically (Goacher, Randell, Williams, & Treanor, 2017). The diagnostic concordance between WSI and conventional microscopy according to this study ranged from 63% to 100% (kappa values: 0.29 - 1.00), while the mean diagnostic concordance of light microscopy alone is 93.4%. Thus, WSI is not a confirmed technique even when using desktop computing; specifically images appear with high fidelity and visually pleasing on a computer screen, but medical information may be lacking due to contrast issues in important parts that can affect image interpretation. Such issues have never been considered for use WSI on a smartphone (Park et al., 2012); another issue is the smartphone screen size (i.e. physically small), in contrast, resolution of the mobile phone is excellent and competes or sometimes is higher than the resolution of desktop screens. However, a physically large display is important when viewing and interpreting a WSI; moreover, image colors and brightness should be calibrated; in the radiology domain there are guidelines governing the use and assessment of displays (Hirschorn, Krupinski, & Flynn, 2014; Samei et al., 2005) however when dealing with digital cytopathology there are not established requirements of displays (Brettle, 2007).

A second issue related to WSI and smartphones proprietary (vendor specific) data formats, these inhibit universal viewing in mobile phones and desktops. Note that WSI manufacturers use different and sometimes proprietary file formats, as the accompanying software is in the line of business for each manufacturer and it is supplied along with the scanners. This fragmentation complicates the efforts to create universal software for remote viewing of WSI and this has more emphasis on smartphones since there are numerous incompatible operating systems. There are a few efforts to create pathology oriented image viewers for handhelds, but, they are vendor specific (Leica Microsystems, 2011). The final issue related to WSI is the information size, a WSI ranges from tenths and thousands of Mbytes and up to GBytes, and this is dependent on magnification, scanned area and z-axis scanning (wherever available). Large file sizes of WSIs introduce important requirements for broadband communication channels and device memory as well, which is associated with costs and advanced infrastructures.

Another important issue of mHealth is related to security, especially since the General Data Protection Regulation (GDPR) became effective in EU (Krzysztofek, 2017; WikiPedia, 2018) but with a global effect. The mobile device is connected to numerous types of networks, mostly being public. On the other hand, patient data is stored remotely on secured sites and have to be communicated via non-secure networks. Thus many vulnerabilities and security issues arise such as virus threats, hacker attacks or data storage in non-secure mobile devices. Therefore, special measures should be taken to ensure data encryption and access to data in cases of device loss.

SOLUTIONS AND RECOMMENDATIONS

There are three important issues for WSI on the mobile device: screen size (not resolution), non-standard file formats and large data volume.

Flexible screens, small projectors and easy connectivity of mobile phones with large displays can be the solutions. Experimental prototypes of flexible and easy to carry screens were produced, more than 15 years ago, by Sony (SONY, 2010); the flexible screens are so thin that can be easily rolled around a pencil. The application of projectors with very small size can facilitate digital slide presentation on a wall. Finally, availability of embedded connectors or wireless connections on smartphones, such as miniature HDMI connectors or Bluetooth, can be useful to use nearby large displays.

Towards the resolution of the second issue (incompatible WSI image formats); nowadays exists a vendor-neutral open source software library for WSI [OpenSlide (Goode A, 2008)]. Although such software libraries are desktop computer specific, porting to the mobile platform seems feasible, since they are open source and software libraries do exist for the mobile platforms. Since OpenSlide is designed as a device driver, then can be ported into all operating systems. Moreover, OpenSlide supports remote [over the Internet] viewing and implementation is based on bindings with the OpenSeaDragon viewer (OpenSlide, 2015b). Thus it is expected to be operational on the mobile platform. WSIs, nowadays, can be viewed over any network using a smartphone browser available at the OpenSlide demo site (OpenSlide, 2015a) (see Figure 2). However adoption of the technology in the everyday routine is not straightforward.

The final WSI related issue is the enormous image size. The cloud perhaps is the solution towards this direction, as the cloud can provide affordable and unlimited storage space, expandable easily and with storage assurance, and no local personnel is required by the laboratory for maintenance. However, transferring of such large data from the server to the mobile device can be an issue. The most obvious solution is to transfer to the mobile device just the virtual slide parts requested to be viewed by the user.

Figure 2. Screen shot of whole slide image viewed horizontally, within the FireFox web browser on an Android-based mobile phone display (resolution: 1920x1080), zooming, panning, scale and slide information are feasible. Left side: slide part within browser interface, right side: another slide detail in full-screen mode (immuno-staining)

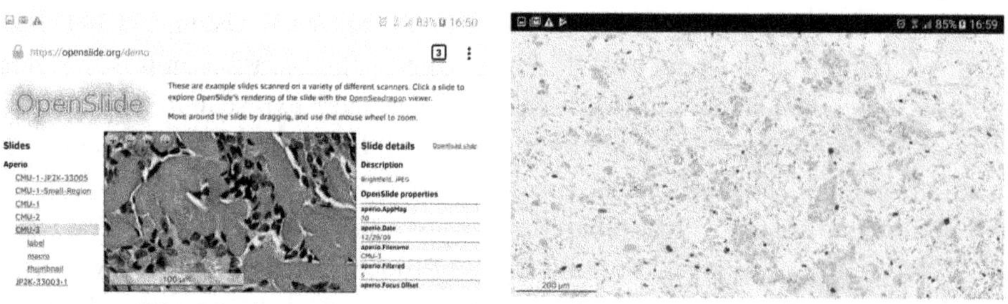

Tiles and pyramidal image formats along with multiple layers, is a solution to reduce the data volume required to be transmitted, WSI viewing on the mobile device should be similar to navigation and mapping applications such as Google Earth that uses satellite imagery, and that is already available today.

Finally, security issues raised by exposing data to the wireless networks and by exposing databases and servers to the edge of the networks, or requirements to open ports on servers/firewalls, some solutions are proposed. Cloud computing is probably the solution of choice (Pouliakis, Archondakis, et al., 2014; Pouliakis, Spathis, et al., 2014):

- Data should be encrypted during storage, and during their transmission, server to server connections should also be encrypted. More advanced methods, such as multi-cloud with key sharing (Mouli & Sesadri, 2013) or use of patient identification cross reference IDs (Kondoh, Teramoto, Kawai, Mochida, & Nishimura, 2013) are an option, especially due to GDPR requirements to separate identification from sensitive data.
- Unauthorized access can be controlled via strong passwords and password control mechanisms and in extreme cases via biometric checks; nowadays, mobile devices have the capability for biometric security: fingerprint, face and voice recognition, for example.
- Database safety, long-term archiving and failure overcome, perhaps can be ensured by:
    - **Server Failures:** By maintaining mirror servers and/or load/ balancing on the cloud
    - Multiple communication channels with multiple Internet service providers may prevent disruption of services.
    - Increased load can be handled by additional processing power into existing virtual servers or by splitting applications in order to run on multiple servers. Load balancing and multi-tier architectures and more than one application servers and database servers can be of help (MySQL, 2018; The Apache Software Foundation, 2018).

CONCLUSION

Mobile phone hardware and software are now mature and powerful and seem ready to be used in cytopathology applications. mHealth technology has a tremendous advantage to provide equal access for medical services patients as it enables the use of services in difficult to access areas, or in regions that are not financially viable to provide such services. mHealth is capable as well of providing new medical services in areas that it is rare to be needed. Additionally, mHealth enables immediate collaboration among medical professionals.

The most elegant and challenging application is mobile WSI. However, it does not represent an application that will be mostly used in the domain of cytopathology. Simple and lightweight services seem to be more practical and easier to implement, these include automation-related tasks such as notifications, transmission of results, education and on the spot access to medical information. Moreover, laboratory management tasks, related to smooth operations and compliancy with quality requirements are attractive. Finally, all types of interactions (such as voice, SMS, e-mail, conferences etc.) among stakeholders in the health chain are important.

The two major characteristics of the mobile device are related to time and place. The mobile phone can provide **freedom from the time** since asynchronous communications, such as e-mail, SMS, voice and video mail can be stored and consumed as information by the users on their own pace. Of course, it is always possible to have synchronous communications to serve urgent tasks. **Freedom from the place** is the second characteristic since the mobile device is personal, it is usually always on and always connected. Simultaneously it is available in every place as it follows the owner. As a result, people involved in the cytopathology ecosystem are not required to be at specific places and a specific time to perform their tasks.

In summary mHealth technology can provide important benefits that health organizations would like to take advantage:

- Low cost for the devices and dropping costs for the services, such as networking costs
- Flexibility: since mHealth technology is much more handy than other computing methods
- Mobility, mHealth users can access information irrelevant of time and place, and health professionals can perform their tasks in a more flexible manner

Research on mobile computing focusing in cytopathology is still scarce, probably due to the strong relation with pathology. However, the potential and the benefits seem important. Although more developments may be required: standards for practicing and guidelines for validation are required, security issues concerns should be ceased by proper implementations and more importantly experimental settings with applications in routine should be tested and the results communicated. Mobile computing seems to play an important role as it has the potential to change the picture of future cytopathology.

REFERENCES

Adibi, S. (2015). Mobile Health A Technology Road Map. Academic Press.

Al-Janabi, S., Huisman, A., Willems, S. M., & Van Diest, P. J. (2012). Digital slide images for primary diagnostics in breast pathology: A feasibility study. *Human Pathology*, *43*(12), 2318–2325. doi:10.1016/j.humpath.2012.03.027 PMID:22901465

Archondakis, S. (2013). The Use of Static Telemedical Applications of Cytopathology for Proficiency Testing. *International Journal of Reliable and Quality E-Healthcare*, *2*(2), 47–53. doi:10.4018/ijrqeh.2013040104

Archondakis, S. (2014). Static Telecytological Applications for Proficiency Testing. In A. Information Resources Management (Ed.), Nanotechnology: Concepts, Methodologies, Tools, and Applications (pp. 556-568). Hershey, PA: IGI Global. doi:10.4018/978-1-4666-5125-8.ch023

Archondakis, S., Georgoulakis, J., Stamataki, M., Anninos, D., Skagias, L., Panayiotides, I., ... Karakitsos, P. (2009). Telecytology: A tool for quality assessment and improvement in the evaluation of thyroid fine-needle aspiration specimens. *Telemedicine Journal and e-Health*, *15*(7), 713–717. doi:10.1089/tmj.2009.0037 PMID:19694595

Archondakis, S., Vavoulidis, E., & Nasioutziki, M. (2016). The Use of Mobile Health Applications for Quality Control and Accreditational Purposes in a Cytopathology Laboratory. In M. Anastasius (Ed.), *M-Health Innovations for Patient-Centered Care* (pp. 262–283). Hershey, PA: IGI Global.

Athanasiadi, E., Pouliakis, A., Bilirakis, E., Fragoulakis, V., Bilirakis, C., & Karakitsos, P. (2014). Quality Indicators for Cervical Cancer Screening Programs: The Role of Computerized Systems. *International Journal of Reliable and Quality E-Healthcare*, *3*(4), 19–37. doi:10.4018/ijrqeh.2014100102

Auguste, L., & Palsana, D. (2015). Mobile Whole Slide Imaging (mWSI): A low resource acquisition and transport technique for microscopic pathological specimens. *BMJ Innovations*, *1*(3), 137–143. doi:10.1136/bmjinnov-2015-000040

Banitsas, K., Perakis, K., Koutsouris, D., Konis, G., & Tachakra, S. (2005). Ambulance 3G. *Conference Proceedings; ... Annual International Conference of the IEEE Engineering in Medicine and Biology Society. IEEE Engineering in Medicine and Biology Society. Conference*, *1*, 371–374. doi:10.1109/IEMBS.2005.1616422 PMID:17282191

Banitsas, K. A., Perakis, K., Tachakra, S., & Koutsouris, D. (2006). Use of 3G mobile phone links for teleconsultation between a moving ambulance and a hospital base station. *Journal of Telemedicine and Telecare*, *12*(1), 23–26. doi:10.1258/135763306775321335 PMID:16438775

Bellina, L., Azzolina, G., Nucatola, I., Maggio, A., Consiglio, F., Ingrassia, R., ... Carrabino, R. (2014). M-phone impact on practical training: Role of m-phone as part of the educative method for training local health workers of rural areas of developing countries. *Health and Technology*, *4*(3), 289–294. doi:10.100712553-013-0073-4

Bellina, L., & Missoni, E. (2009). Mobile cell-phones (M-phones) in telemicroscopy: Increasing connectivity of isolated laboratories. *Diagnostic Pathology*, *4*(1), 19. doi:10.1186/1746-1596-4-19 PMID:19545373

Bogoch, I. I., Koydemir, H. C., Tseng, D., Ephraim, R. K. D., Duah, E., Tee, J., ... Ozcan, A. (2017). Evaluation of a Mobile Phone-Based Microscope for Screening of Schistosoma haematobium Infection in Rural Ghana. *The American Journal of Tropical Medicine and Hygiene*, *96*(6), 1468–1471. doi:10.4269/ajtmh.16-0912 PMID:28719262

Borve, A., Terstappen, K., Sandberg, C., & Paoli, J. (2013). Mobile teledermoscopy-there's an app for that! *Dermatology Practical & Conceptual*, *3*(2), 41–48. doi:10.5826/dpc.0302a05 PMID:23785643

Breslauer, D. N., Maamari, R. N., Switz, N. A., Lam, W. A., & Fletcher, D. A. (2009). Mobile phone based clinical microscopy for global health applications. *PLoS One*, *4*(7), e6320. doi:10.1371/journal.pone.0006320 PMID:19623251

Brettle, D. S. (2007). Display considerations for hospital-wide viewing of soft copy images. *The British Journal of Radiology*, *80*(955), 503–507. doi:10.1259/bjr/26436784 PMID:17704314

Briscoe, D., Adair, C. F., Thompson, L. D., Tellado, M. V., Buckner, S. B., Rosenthal, D. L., & O'Leary, T. J. (2000). Telecytologic diagnosis of breast fine needle aspiration biopsies. Intraobserver concordance. *Acta Cytologica*, *44*(2), 175–180. doi:10.1159/000326357 PMID:10740603

Burns, M. N., Begale, M., Duffecy, J., Gergle, D., Karr, C. J., Giangrande, E., & Mohr, D. C. (2011). Harnessing context sensing to develop a mobile intervention for depression. *Journal of Medical Internet Research*, *13*(3), e55. doi:10.2196/jmir.1838 PMID:21840837

Callender, C., & Thompson, D. (2018). Family TXT: Feasibility and Acceptability of a mHealth Obesity Prevention Program for Parents of Pre-Adolescent African American Girls. *Children (Basel), 5*(6). doi:10.3390/children5060081 PMID:29921811

Chao, J. T. II, Loescher, L. J., Soyer, H. P., & Curiel-Lewandrowski, C. (2013). Barriers to mobile teledermoscopy in primary care. *Journal of the American Academy of Dermatology, 69*(5), 821–824. doi:10.1016/j.jaad.2012.10.039 PMID:24124819

Choudhri, A. F., Carr, T. M. III, Ho, C. P., Stone, J. R., Gay, S. B., & Lambert, D. L. (2012). Handheld device review of abdominal CT for the evaluation of acute appendicitis. *Journal of Digital Imaging, 25*(4), 492–496. doi:10.100710278-011-9431-9 PMID:22146833

Choudhri, A. F., Norton, P. T., Carr, T. M. III, Stone, J. R., Hagspiel, K. D., & Dake, M. D. (2013). Diagnosis and treatment planning of acute aortic emergencies using a handheld DICOM viewer. *Emergency Radiology, 20*(4), 267–272. doi:10.100710140-013-1118-8 PMID:23525945

Clarke, J., Proudfoot, J., Birch, M. R., Whitton, A. E., Parker, G., Manicavasagar, V., ... Hadzi-Pavlovic, D. (2014). Effects of mental health self-efficacy on outcomes of a mobile phone and web intervention for mild-to-moderate depression, anxiety and stress: Secondary analysis of a randomised controlled trial. *BMC Psychiatry, 14*(1), 272. doi:10.118612888-014-0272-1 PMID:25252853

Collins, B. (2011). iPad and cytopathology: Content creation and delivery. *CytoJournal, 8*(16c). http://www.ncbi.nlm.nih.gov/pmc/articles/PMC3230889/

Crowe, A., Linder, A., Hameed, O., Salih, C., Roberson, J., Gidley, J., & Eltoum, I. A. (2011). The impact of implementation of the Bethesda System for Reporting Thyroid Cytopathology on the quality of reporting, "risk" of malignancy, surgical rate, and rate of frozen sections requested for thyroid lesions. *Cancer Cytopathology, 119*(5), 315–321. doi:10.1002/cncy.20174 PMID:21751427

Cucoranu, I. C., Parwani, A. V., & Pantanowitz, L. (2014). Digital whole slide imaging in cytology. *Archives of Pathology & Laboratory Medicine, 138*(3), 300. doi:10.5858/arpa.2013-0270-LE PMID:24576021

D'Ambrosio, M. V., Bakalar, M., Bennuru, S., Reber, C., Skandarajah, A., Nilsson, L., ... Fletcher, D. A. (2015). Point-of-care quantification of blood-borne filarial parasites with a mobile phone microscope. *Science Translational Medicine, 7*(286), 286re284. doi:10.1126citranslmed.aaa3480 PMID:25947164

Delisle Nystrom, C., Sandin, S., Henriksson, P., Henriksson, H., Maddison, R., & Lof, M. (2018). A 12-month follow-up of a mobile-based (mHealth) obesity prevention intervention in pre-school children: The MINISTOP randomized controlled trial. *BMC Public Health, 18*(1), 658. doi:10.118612889-018-5569-4 PMID:29793467

Della Mea, V., Cataldi, P., Pertoldi, B., & Beltrami, C. A. (2000). Combining dynamic and static robotic telepathology: A report on 184 consecutive cases of frozen sections, histology and cytology. *Analytical Cellular Pathology, 20*(1), 33–39. doi:10.1155/2000/734943 PMID:11007436

Diamantis, A., Magiorkinis, E., & Koutselini, H. (2014). 50 years after the death of George Nicholas Papanicolaou (1883-1962): Evaluation of his scientific work. *Acta Medico-Historica Adriatica: AMHA, 12*(1), 181–188. PMID:25310617

Elsevier. (2015). *Robbins Pathology Flash Cards*. Retrieved 15 April, 2015, from https://itunes.apple.com/us/app/robbins-pathology-flash-cards/id367031323?mt=8

European Society of R. (2018). ESR paper on the proper use of mobile devices in radiology. *Insights Imaging, 9*(2), 247-251. doi:10.100713244-017-0589-7

Field, A. S., Schmitt, F., & Vielh, P. (2017). IAC Standardized Reporting of Breast Fine-Needle Aspiration Biopsy Cytology. *Acta Cytologica, 61*(1), 3–6. doi:10.1159/000450880 PMID:27806362

Finkelstein, J., Hripcsak, G., & Cabrera, M. (1998). Telematic system for monitoring of asthma severity in patients' homes. *Studies in Health Technology and Informatics, 52*(Pt 1), 272–276. PMID:10384460

Fontelo, P., Faustorilla, J., Gavino, A., & Marcelo, A. (2012). Digital pathology - implementation challenges in low-resource countries. *Analytical Cellular Pathology (Amsterdam), 35*(1), 31–36. doi:10.1155/2012/125695 PMID:22233702

Friedman, C. P., & Wyatt, J. (2006). *Evaluation methods in medical informatics* (2nd ed.). New York: Springer.

Fulciniti, F., Yanoh, K., Karakitsos, P., Watanabe, J., Di Lorito, A., Margari, N., ... Hirai, Y. (2018). The Yokohama system for reporting directly sampled endometrial cytology: The quest to develop a standardized terminology. *Diagnostic Cytopathology, 46*(5), 400–412. doi:10.1002/dc.23916 PMID:29479846

Fung, K. M., Hassell, L. A., Talbert, M. L., Wiechmann, A. F., Chaser, B. E., & Ramey, J. (2012). Whole slide images and digital media in pathology education, testing, and practice: The Oklahoma experience. *Analytical Cellular Pathology (Amsterdam), 35*(1), 37–40. doi:10.1155/2012/103857 PMID:21965282

Ghaznavi, F., Evans, A., Madabhushi, A., & Feldman, M. (2013). Digital imaging in pathology: Whole-slide imaging and beyond. *Annual Review of Pathology, 8*(1), 331–359. doi:10.1146/annurev-pathol-011811-120902 PMID:23157334

Ghorai, K., Akter, S., Khatun, F., & Ray, P. (2014). mHealth for Smoking Cessation Programs: A Systematic Review. *Journal of Personalized Medicine, 4*(3), 412–423. doi:10.3390/jpm4030412 PMID:25563359

Goacher, E., Randell, R., Williams, B., & Treanor, D. (2017). The Diagnostic Concordance of Whole Slide Imaging and Light Microscopy: A Systematic Review. *Archives of Pathology & Laboratory Medicine, 141*(1), 151–161. doi:10.5858/arpa.2016-0025-RA PMID:27399211

Goode, A. S. M. (2008). *A vendor-neutral library and viewer for wholeslide images* (Vol. Tech Rep CMU-CS-08-136.). Pittsburgh, PA: School of Computer Science, Carnegie Mellon University.

Gupta, S., Chang, P., Anyigbo, N., & Sabharwal, A. (2011). mobileSpiro: accurate mobile spirometry for self-management of asthma. *Proceedings of the First ACM Workshop on Mobile Systems, Applications, and Services for Healthcare*.

Gutman, D. A., Cobb, J., Somanna, D., Park, Y., Wang, F., Kurc, T., ... Cooper, L. A. (2013). Cancer Digital Slide Archive: An informatics resource to support integrated in silico analysis of TCGA pathology data. *Journal of the American Medical Informatics Association, 20*(6), 1091–1098. doi:10.1136/amiajnl-2012-001469 PMID:23893318

Guzik, P., & Malik, M. (2016). ECG by mobile technologies. *Journal of Electrocardiology*, *49*(6), 894–901. doi:10.1016/j.jelectrocard.2016.07.030 PMID:27524474

Hartman, D. J. (2016). Mobile Technology for the Practice of Pathology. *Advances in Anatomic Pathology*, *23*(2), 118–124. doi:10.1097/PAP.0000000000000093 PMID:26849818

Hipp, J. D., Lucas, D. R., Emmert-Buck, M. R., Compton, C. C., & Balis, U. J. (2011). Digital slide repositories for publications: Lessons learned from the microarray community. *The American Journal of Surgical Pathology*, *35*(6), 783–786. doi:10.1097/PAS.0b013e31821946b6 PMID:21552111

Hirsch, D., Robenshtok, E., Bachar, G., Braslavsky, D., & Benbassat, C. (2015). The Implementation of the Bethesda System for Reporting Thyroid Cytopathology Improves Malignancy Detection Despite Lower Rate of Thyroidectomy in Indeterminate Nodules. *World Journal of Surgery*, *39*(8), 1959–1965. doi:10.100700268-015-3032-6 PMID:25809059

Hirschorn, D. S., Krupinski, E. A., & Flynn, M. J. (2014). PACS displays: How to select the right display technology. *Journal of the American College of Radiology*, *11*(12), 1270–1276. doi:10.1016/j.jacr.2014.09.016 PMID:25467904

Huang, Y. N., Peng, X. C., Ma, S., Yu, H., Jin, Y. B., Zheng, J., & Fu, G. H. (2018). Development of Whole Slide Imaging on Smartphones and Evaluation With ThinPrep Cytology Test Samples: Follow-Up Study. *JMIR mHealth and uHealth*, *6*(4), e82. doi:10.2196/mhealth.9518 PMID:29618454

International Organization for Standardization. (2012). *ISO 15189:2012. Medical laboratories – Requirements for quality and competence*. Geneva: International Organization for Standardization.

Janda, M., Loescher, L. J., Banan, P., Horsham, C., & Soyer, H. P. (2014). Lesion selection by melanoma high-risk consumers during skin self-examination using mobile teledermoscopy. *JAMA Dermatology*, *150*(6), 656–658. doi:10.1001/jamadermatol.2013.7743 PMID:24522284

Jialdasani, R., Desai, S., Gupta, M., Kothari, A., Deshpande, R., Shet, T., ... Chinoy, R. (2006). An analysis of 46 static telecytology cases over a period of two years. *Journal of Telemedicine and Telecare*, *12*(6), 311–314. doi:10.1258/135763306778558132 PMID:17022840

Johnson, P. T., Zimmerman, S. L., Heath, D., Eng, J., Horton, K. M., Scott, W. W., & Fishman, E. K. (2012). The iPad as a mobile device for CT display and interpretation: Diagnostic accuracy for identification of pulmonary embolism. *Emergency Radiology*, *19*(4), 323–327. doi:10.100710140-012-1037-0 PMID:22450843

Kiselev, A. R., Gridnev, V. I., Shvartz, V. A., Posnenkova, O. M., & Dovgalevsky, P. Y. (2012). Active ambulatory care management supported by short message services and mobile phone technology in patients with arterial hypertension. *Journal of the American Society of Hypertension*, *6*(5), 346–355. doi:10.1016/j.jash.2012.08.001 PMID:22995803

Kondoh, H., Teramoto, K., Kawai, T., Mochida, M., & Nishimura, M. (2013). Development of the Regional EPR and PACS Sharing System on the Infrastructure of Cloud Computing Technology Controlled by Patient Identifier Cross Reference Manager. *Studies in Health Technology and Informatics*, *192*, 1073. PMID:23920847

Krishnamurthy, S., Mathews, K., McClure, S., Murray, M., Gilcrease, M., Albarracin, C., ... Liang, K. (2013). Multi-Institutional Comparison of Whole Slide Digital Imaging and Optical Microscopy for Interpretation of Hematoxylin-Eosin-Stained Breast Tissue Sections. *Archives of Pathology & Laboratory Medicine*, *137*(12), 1733–1739. doi:10.5858/arpa.2012-0437-OA PMID:23947655

Krzysztofek, M. (2017). *Post-reform personal data protection in the European Union: general data protection regulation (EU) 2016/679*. EU.

Laktabai, J., Platt, A., Menya, D., Turner, E. L., Aswa, D., Kinoti, S., & O'Meara, W. P. (2018). A mobile health technology platform for quality assurance and quality improvement of malaria diagnosis by community health workers. *PLoS One*, *13*(2), e0191968. doi:10.1371/journal.pone.0191968 PMID:29389958

Lam, Q., Ajzner, E., Campbell, C. A., & Young, A. (2016). Critical Risk Results - An Update on International Initiatives. *EJIFCC*, *27*(1), 66–76. PMID:27683507

Lee, E. S., Kim, I. S., Choi, J. S., Yeom, B. W., Kim, H. K., Han, J. H., ... Leong, A. S. (2003). Accuracy and reproducibility of telecytology diagnosis of cervical smears. A tool for quality assurance programs. *American Journal of Clinical Pathology*, *119*(3), 356–360. doi:10.1309/7YTVAG4XNR48T75H PMID:12645336

Lee, Y., Shin, S. Y., Kim, J. Y., Kim, J. H., Seo, D. W., Joo, S., ... Bates, D. W. (2015). Evaluation of Mobile Health Applications Developed by a Tertiary Hospital as a Tool for Quality Improvement Breakthrough. *Healthcare Informatics Research*, *21*(4), 299–306. doi:10.4258/hir.2015.21.4.299 PMID:26618037

Leica Microsystems. (2011). *Leica Microsystems Launches Free Digital Pathology App for iPad and iPhone*. Retrieved 10 April, 2015, from http://www.leica-microsystems.com/news-media/news/news-details/article/leica-microsystems-launches-free-digital-pathology-app-for-ipad-and-iphone/

Manahan, M. N., Soyer, H. P., Loescher, L. J., Horsham, C., Vagenas, D., Whiteman, D. C., ... Janda, M. (2015). A pilot trial of mobile, patient-performed teledermoscopy. *British Journal of Dermatology*, *172*(4), 1072–1080. doi:10.1111/bjd.13550 PMID:25418126

Margari, N., Pouliakis, A., Anoinos, D., Terzakis, E., Koureas, N., Chrelias, C., ... Karakitsos, P. (2016). A reporting system for endometrial cytology: Cytomorphologic criteria-Implied risk of malignancy. *Diagnostic Cytopathology*, *44*(11), 888–901. doi:10.1002/dc.23605 PMID:27653446

Markidou, S., Karakitsos, P., & Pouliakis, A. (1999). Telecytology. In O. Ferrer-Roca & M. Sosa-Iudicissa (Eds.), *Handbook of Telemedicine* (Vol. 54). Amsterdam: IOS press.

Martin, S. J., Chen, G., Dattilo, J., & Johnson, C. T. (2015). Physicians' Knowledge Regarding Tablet- and Handheld-Based Applications in Gynecology and Obstetrics. *Obstetrics and Gynecology*, *125*(Suppl 1), 119S–120S. doi:10.1097/01.AOG.0000463206.49148.98

Martin, T. (2012). Assessing mHealth: Opportunities and barriers to patient engagement. *Journal of Health Care for the Poor and Underserved*, *23*(3), 935–941. doi:10.1353/hpu.2012.0087 PMID:24212144

Massone, C., Brunasso, A. M., Campbell, T. M., & Soyer, H. P. (2009). Mobile teledermoscopy--melanoma diagnosis by one click? *Seminars in Cutaneous Medicine and Surgery*, *28*(3), 203–205. doi:10.1016/j.sder.2009.06.002 PMID:19782945

Massone, C., Brunasso, A. M., Hofmann-Wellenhof, R., Gulia, A., & Soyer, H. P. (2010). Teledermoscopy: Education, discussion forums, teleconsulting and mobile teledermoscopy. *Giornale Italiano di Dermatologia e Venereologia, 145*(1), 127–132. PMID:20197751

McLean, R., Jury, C., Bazeos, A., & Lewis, S. M. (2009). Application of camera phones in telehaematology. *Journal of Telemedicine and Telecare, 15*(7), 339–343. doi:10.1258/jtt.2009.090114 PMID:19815902

Meszaros, L. (2014). *Johns Hopkins Atlas of Pancreatic Cytopathology*. Retrieved 10 February, 2015, from http://www.mdlinx.com/endocrinology/mobile-app-center/mobile-app-detail.cfm?app_id=1221

Miranda, J. J., Moscoso, M. G., Toyama, M., Cavero, V., Diez-Canseco, F., & Ovbiagele, B. (2018). Role of mHealth in overcoming the occurrence of post-stroke depression. *Acta Neurologica Scandinavica, 137*(1), 12–19. doi:10.1111/ane.12832 PMID:28901543

Miyamoto, S., Dharmar, M., Fazio, S., Tang-Feldman, Y., & Young, H. M. (2018). mHealth Technology and Nurse Health Coaching to Improve Health in Diabetes: Protocol for a Randomized Controlled Trial. *JMIR Research Protocols, 7*(2), e45. doi:10.2196/resprot.9168 PMID:29449200

Modzelewski, K. L., Stockman, M. C., & Steenkamp, D. W. (2018). Rethinking the Endpoints of mHealth Intervention Research in Diabetes Care. *Journal of Diabetes Science and Technology, 12*(2), 389–392. doi:10.1177/1932296817733007 PMID:28952379

Mouli, K. C., & Sesadri, U. (2013). Single to Multi Clouds for Security in Cloud Computing by using Secret Key Sharing. *International Journal of Computers and Technology, 10*(4), 1539–1545. doi:10.24297/ijct.v10i4.3254

Moumtzoglou, A., & Pouliakis, A. (2015). Mapping Population Health Management Roadmap into Cervical Cancer Screening Programs. *International Journal of Reliable and Quality E-Healthcare, 4*(3), 1–18. doi:10.4018/IJRQEH.2015070101

Mun, S. K., Elsayed, A. M., Tohme, W. G., & Wu, Y. C. (1995). Teleradiology/telepathology requirements and implementation. *Journal of Medical Systems, 19*(2), 153–164. doi:10.1007/BF02257066 PMID:7602247

MySQL. (2018). *MySQL NDB Cluster: High Availability*. Retrieved December 6th, 2017, from https://www.mysql.com/products/cluster/availability.html

Nagy, G. K., & Newton, L. E. (2006). Cytopathology proficiency testing: Where do we go from here? *Diagnostic Cytopathology, 34*(4), 257–264. doi:10.1002/dc.20361 PMID:16544329

Nayar, R., & Wilbur, D. (2015). *The Bethesda system for reporting cervical cytology: definitions, criteria, and explanatory notes* (2nd ed.). New York: Springer.

Ng, C. H., & Yeo, J. F. (2004). The role of Internet and personal digital assistant in oral and maxillofacial pathology. *Annals of the Academy of Medicine, Singapore, 33*(4Suppl), 50–52. PMID:15389308

OpenSlide. (2015a). *OpenSlide Demo Site*. Retrieved 25 May, 2015, from http://www.openslide.org/demo

OpenSlide. (2015b). *OpenSlide homepage*. Retrieved 10 April, 2015, from http://www.openslide.org/

Orth, A., Wilson, E. R., Thompson, J. G., & Gibson, B. C. (2018). A dual-mode mobile phone microscope using the onboard camera flash and ambient light. *Scientific Reports*, *8*(1), 3298. doi:10.103841598-018-21543-2 PMID:29459650

Pandher, P. S., & Bhullar, K. K. (2014). Smartphone applications for seizure management. *Health Informatics Journal*. doi:10.1177/1460458214540906 PMID:25038202

Pantanowitz, L., Henricks, W. H., & Beckwith, B. A. (2007). Medical laboratory informatics. *Clin Lab Med, 27*(4), 823-843. doi:10.1016/j.cll.2007.07.011

Pantanowitz, L., Hornish, M., & Goulart, R. A. (2009). The impact of digital imaging in the field of cytopathology. *CytoJournal*, *6*(1), 6. doi:10.4103/1742-6413.48606 PMID:19495408

Papanicolaou, G. (1928). *New Cancer Diagnosis.* Paper presented at the 3rd Race Bettrment Conference, Battle Creek.

Papanicolaou, G., & Traut, H. (1941). The diagnostic value of vaginal smears in carcinoma of the uterus. *American Journal of Obstetrics and Gynecology*, *42*(2), 193–206. doi:10.1016/S0002-9378(16)40621-6

Park, S., Parwani, A., Satyanarayanan, M., & Pantanowitz, L. (2012). Handheld computing in pathology. *Journal of Pathology Informatics*, *3*(1), 15–15. doi:10.4103/2153-3539.95127 PMID:22616027

Pavlopoulos, S., Kyriacou, E., Berler, A., Dembeyiotis, S., & Koutsouris, D. (1998). A novel emergency telemedicine system based on wireless communication technology--AMBULANCE. *IEEE Transactions on Information Technology in Biomedicine*, *2*(4), 261–267. doi:10.1109/4233.737581 PMID:10719536

Pearlman, E. S., Wolfert, M. S., Miele, R., Bilello, L., & Stauffer, J. (2001). Utilization management and information technology: Adapting to the new era. *Clinical Leadership & Management Review*, *15*(2), 85–88. PMID:11299910

Pinco, J., Goulart, R. A., Otis, C. N., Garb, J., & Pantanowitz, L. (2009). Impact of digital image manipulation in cytology. *Archives of Pathology & Laboratory Medicine*, *133*(1), 57–61. doi:10.1043/1543-2165-133.1.57 PMID:19123737

Pirnstill, C. W., & Cote, G. L. (2015). Malaria Diagnosis Using a Mobile Phone Polarized Microscope. *Scientific Reports*, *5*(1), 13368. doi:10.1038rep13368 PMID:26303238

Pouliakis, A., Archondakis, S., Karakitsou, E., & Karakitsos, P. (2014). Cloud Computing for Cytopathologists. In A. Moumtzoglou & A. Kastania (Eds.), *Cloud computing applications for quality health care delivery* (pp. 250–271). Hershey, PA: IGI Global. doi:10.4018/978-1-4666-6118-9.ch013

Pouliakis, A., Archondakis, S., Margari, N., & Karakitsos, P. (2016). From telecytology to mobile cytopathology: Past, present and future. In A. Moumtzoglou (Ed.), *M-Health Innovations for Patient-Centered Care*. Hershey, PA: IGI Global. doi:10.4018/978-1-4666-9861-1.ch012

Pouliakis, A., Athanasiadi, E., Karakitsou, E., Archondakis, S., Mourtzikou, A., Stamouli, M., ... Karakitsos, P. (2014). ISO 15189:2012 Management Requirements for Cytopathology Laboratory Information Systems. *International Journal of Reliable and Quality E-Healthcare*, *3*(3), 37–57. doi:10.4018/ijrqeh.2014070103

Pouliakis, A., Margari, N., Archondakis, S., Karakitsou, E., & Karakitsos, P. (2016). Emerging Technologies Serving Cytopathology. Big Data, the Cloud and Mobile Computing. In I. E. Naqa (Ed.), Handbook of Research on Emerging Developments and Practices in Oncology. Hershey, PA: IGI Global.

Pouliakis, A., Margari, N., Spathis, A., Kottaridi, C., Stamouli, M., Mourtzikou, A., ... Karakitsos, P. (2014). ISO 15189:2012 Technical Requirements for Cytopathology Laboratory Information Systems. *International Journal of Reliable and Quality E-Healthcare*, *3*(3), 58–80. doi:10.4018/ijrqeh.2014070104

Pouliakis, A., Spathis, A., Kottaridi, C., Mourtzikou, A., Stamouli, M., Archondakis, S., & Karakitsos, P. (2014). Cloud Computing for BioLabs. In A. Moumtzoglou & A. Kastania (Eds.), *Cloud computing applications for quality health care delivery* (pp. 228–249). Hershey, PA: IGI Global. doi:10.4018/978-1-4666-6118-9.ch012

Pusztaszeri, M., Rossi, E. D., Auger, M., Baloch, Z., Bishop, J., Bongiovanni, M., . . . Faquin, W. C. (2016). The Bethesda System for Reporting Thyroid Cytopathology: Proposed Modifications and Updates for the Second Edition from an International Panel. Acta Cytol, 60(5), 399-405. doi:10.1159/000451020

Raab, S. S., Zaleski, M. S., Thomas, P. A., Niemann, T. H., Isacson, C., & Jensen, C. S. (1996). Telecytology: Diagnostic accuracy in cervical-vaginal smears. *American Journal of Clinical Pathology*, *105*(5), 599–603. doi:10.1093/ajcp/105.5.599 PMID:8623769

Rachim, V. P., & Chung, W. Y. (2016). Wearable Noncontact Armband for Mobile ECG Monitoring System. *IEEE Transactions on Biomedical Circuits and Systems*, *10*(6), 1112–1118. doi:10.1109/TBCAS.2016.2519523 PMID:27214910

Ribu, L., Holmen, H., Torbjornsen, A., Wahl, A. K., Grottland, A., Smastuen, M. C., ... Arsand, E. (2013). Low-intensity self-management intervention for persons with type 2 diabetes using a mobile phone-based diabetes diary, with and without health counseling and motivational interviewing: Protocol for a randomized controlled trial. *JMIR Research Protocols*, *2*(2), e34. doi:10.2196/resprot.2768 PMID:23978690

Rosales Saurer, B., Mueller-Gorchs, M., & Kunze, C. (2009). Scenario-based design of an ICT platform for mobile information services in ambulatory care nursing. *Studies in Health Technology and Informatics*, *146*, 64–68. PMID:19592810

Roy, S., Pantanowitz, L., Amin, M., Seethala, R. R., Ishtiaque, A., Yousem, S. A., ... Hartman, D. J. (2014). Smartphone adapters for digital photomicrography. *Journal of Pathology Informatics*, *5*(1), 24. doi:10.4103/2153-3539.137728 PMID:25191623

Rudin, R. S., Fanta, C. H., Predmore, Z., Kron, K., Edelen, M. O., Landman, A. B., ... Bates, D. W. (2017). Core Components for a Clinically Integrated mHealth App for Asthma Symptom Monitoring. *Applied Clinical Informatics*, *8*(4), 1031–1043. doi:10.4338/ACI-2017-06-RA-0096 PMID:29241243

Rudnisky, C. J., Tennant, M. T., Weis, E., Ting, A., Hinz, B. J., & Greve, M. D. (2007). Web-based grading of compressed stereoscopic digital photography versus standard slide film photography for the diagnosis of diabetic retinopathy. *Ophthalmology*, *114*(9), 1748–1754. doi:10.1016/j.ophtha.2006.12.010 PMID:17368543

Sahoo, P. K., Thakkar, H. K., & Lee, M. Y. (2017). A Cardiac Early Warning System with Multi Channel SCG and ECG Monitoring for Mobile Health. *Sensors (Basel)*, *17*(4), 711. doi:10.339017040711 PMID:28353681

Sama, P. R., Eapen, Z. J., Weinfurt, K. P., Shah, B. R., & Schulman, K. A. (2014). An evaluation of mobile health application tools. *JMIR mHealth and uHealth*, *2*(2), e19. doi:10.2196/mhealth.3088 PMID:25099179

Samei, E., Badano, A., Chakraborty, D., Compton, K., Cornelius, C., Corrigan, K., ... Aapm, T. G. (2005). Assessment of display performance for medical imaging systems: Executive summary of AAPM TG18 report. *Medical Physics*, *32*(4), 1205–1225. doi:10.1118/1.1861159 PMID:15895604

Saw, S., Loh, T. P., Ang, S. B., Yip, J. W., & Sethi, S. K. (2011). Meeting regulatory requirements by the use of cell phone text message notification with autoescalation and loop closure for reporting of critical laboratory results. *American Journal of Clinical Pathology*, *136*(1), 30–34. doi:10.1309/AJCPUZ53XZWQFYIS PMID:21685029

Sciacovelli, L., Secchiero, S., Zardo, L., D'Osualdo, A., & Plebani, M. (2007). Risk management in laboratory medicine: Quality assurance programs and professional competence. *Clinical Chemistry and Laboratory Medicine*, *45*(6), 756–765. doi:10.1515/CCLM.2007.165 PMID:17579529

Sharma, P., & Kamal, V. (2006). A novel application of mobile phone cameras in undergraduate pathology education. *Medical Teacher*, *28*(8), 745–746. PMID:17642089

Shen, Z., & Yang, Z. (2001). The problems and strategy relevant to the quality management of clinical laboratories. *Clinical Chemistry and Laboratory Medicine*, *39*(12), 1216–1218. doi:10.1515/CCLM.2001.194 PMID:11798079

Skandarajah, A., Reber, C. D., Switz, N. A., & Fletcher, D. A. (2014). Quantitative imaging with a mobile phone microscope. *PLoS One*, *9*(5), e96906. doi:10.1371/journal.pone.0096906 PMID:24824072

Skeate, R. C., Wahi, M. M., Jessurun, J., & Connelly, D. P. (2007). Personal digital assistant-enabled report content knowledgebase results in more complete pathology reports and enhances resident learning. *Human Pathology*, *38*(12), 1727–1735. doi:10.1016/j.humpath.2007.05.019 PMID:17949779

SONY. (2010). *Sony Develops a "Rollable" OTFT*1-driven OLED Display that can wrap around a Pencil.* Retrieved 24 May, 2015, from http://www.sony.net/SonyInfo/News/Press/201005/10-070E/

Spat, S., Holl, B., Petritsch, G., Schaupp, L., Beck, P., & Pieber, T. R. (2013). Automatic system testing of a decision support system for insulin dosing using Google Android. *Studies in Health Technology and Informatics*, *186*, 187–191. PMID:23542995

Stergiou, N., Georgoulakis, G., Margari, N., Aninos, D., Stamataki, M., Stergiou, E., ... Karakitsos, P. (2009). Using a web-based system for the continuous distance education in cytopathology. *International Journal of Medical Informatics*, *78*(12), 827–838. doi:10.1016/j.ijmedinf.2009.08.007 PMID:19775933

Sun, D., & Hu, T. Y. (2018). A low cost mobile phone dark-field microscope for nanoparticle-based quantitative studies. *Biosensors & Bioelectronics*, *99*, 513–518. doi:10.1016/j.bios.2017.08.025 PMID:28823976

Tawfik, O., Davis, M., Dillon, S., Tawfik, L., Diaz, F. J., & Fan, F. (2014). Whole Slide Imaging of Pap Cell Block Preparations versus Liquid-Based Thin-Layer Cervical Cytology: A Comparative Study Evaluating the Detection of Organisms and Nonneoplastic Findings. *Acta Cytologica*, *58*(4), 388–397. doi:10.1159/000365046 PMID:25033897

Taylor, C. R. (2011). From microscopy to whole slide digital images: A century and a half of image analysis. *Applied Immunohistochemistry & Molecular Morphology*, *19*(6), 491–493. doi:10.1097/PAI.0b013e318229ffd6 PMID:22089486

The Apache Software Foundation. (2018). *Apache Tomcat web site*. Retrieved May 8, 2018, from http://tomcat.apache.org/

The Statistics Portal. (2018). *Global digital health market from 2015 to 2020, by major segment (in billion U.S. dollars)*. Retrieved July 27, 2018, from https://www.statista.com/statistics/387867/value-of-worldwide-digital-health-market-forecast-by-segment/

Thies, K., Anderson, D., & Cramer, B. (2017). Lack of Adoption of a Mobile App to Support Patient Self-Management of Diabetes and Hypertension in a Federally Qualified Health Center: Interview Analysis of Staff and Patients in a Failed Randomized Trial. *JMIR Human Factors*, *4*(4), e24. doi:10.2196/humanfactors.7709 PMID:28974481

Toomey, R. J., Ryan, J. T., McEntee, M. F., Evanoff, M. G., Chakraborty, D. P., McNulty, J. P., ... Brennan, P. C. (2010). Diagnostic efficacy of handheld devices for emergency radiologic consultation. *AJR. American Journal of Roentgenology*, *194*(2), 469–474. doi:10.2214/AJR.09.3418 PMID:20093611

Torbjornsen, A., Smastuen, M. C., Jenum, A. K., Arsand, E., & Ribu, L. (2018). Acceptability of an mHealth App Intervention for Persons With Type 2 Diabetes and its Associations With Initial Self-Management: Randomized Controlled Trial. *JMIR mHealth and uHealth*, *6*(5), e125. doi:10.2196/mhealth.8824 PMID:29784635

Triola, M. M., & Holloway, W. J. (2011). Enhanced virtual microscopy for collaborative education. *BMC Medical Education*, *11*(1), 4. doi:10.1186/1472-6920-11-4 PMID:21269474

Tsilalis, T., Archondakis, S., Meristoudis, C., Margari, N., Pouliakis, A., Skagias, L., ... Karakitsos, P. (2012). Assessment of Static Telecytological Diagnoses' Reproducibility in Cervical Smears Prepared by Means of Liquid-Based Cytology. *Telemedicine Journal and e-Health*, *18*(7), 516–520. doi:10.1089/tmj.2011.0167 PMID:22856666

Tsiouris, K. M., Gatsios, D., Rigas, G., Miljkovic, D., Korousic Seljak, B., Bohanec, M., ... Fotiadis, D. I. (2017). PD_Manager: An mHealth platform for Parkinson's disease patient management. *Healthc Technol Lett*, *4*(3), 102–108. doi:10.1049/htl.2017.0007 PMID:28706727

Vacata, V., Jahns-Streubel, G., Baldus, M., & Wood, W. G. (2007). Practical solution for control of the pre-analytical phase in decentralized clinical laboratories for meeting the requirements of the medical laboratory accreditation standard DIN EN ISO 15189. *Clinical Laboratory*, *53*(3-4), 211–215. PMID:17447659

Vaisanen, O., Makijarvi, M., & Silfvast, T. (2003). Prehospital ECG transmission: Comparison of advanced mobile phone and facsimile devices in an urban Emergency Medical Service System. *Resuscitation*, *57*(2), 179–185. doi:10.1016/S0300-9572(03)00028-5 PMID:12745186

Vooijs, G. P., Davey, D. D., Somrak, T. M., Goodell, R. M., Grohs, D. H., Knesel, E. A. Jr, ... Wilbur, D. C. (1998). Computerized training and proficiency testing. International Academy of Cytology Task Force summary. Diagnostic Cytology Towards the 21st Century: An International Expert Conference and Tutorial. *Acta Cytologica*, *42*(1), 141–147. doi:10.1159/000331539 PMID:9479333

Weinstein, L. J., Epstein, J. I., Edlow, D., & Westra, W. H. (1997). Static image analysis of skin specimens: The application of telepathology to frozen section evaluation. *Human Pathology*, *28*(1), 30–35. doi:10.1016/S0046-8177(97)90275-6 PMID:9013828

Westbrook, J. I., Georgiou, A., & Rob, M. I. (2008). Computerised order entry systems: Sustained impact on laboratory efficiency and mortality rates? *Studies in Health Technology and Informatics*, *136*, 345–350. PMID:18487755

WikiPedia. (2018). *General Data Protection Regulation*. Retrieved 11 February, 2018, from https://en.wikipedia.org/wiki/General_Data_Protection_Regulation

Williams, B. H., Mullick, F. G., Butler, D. R., Herring, R. F., & O'Leary, T. J. (2001). Clinical evaluation of an international static image-based telepathology service. *Human Pathology*, *32*(12), 1309–1317. doi:10.1053/hupa.2001.29649 PMID:11774162

Williams, B. J., Bottoms, D., & Treanor, D. (2017). Future-proofing pathology: The case for clinical adoption of digital pathology. *Journal of Clinical Pathology*, *70*(12), 1010–1018. doi:10.1136/jclinpath-2017-204644 PMID:28780514

Wright, A. M., Smith, D., Dhurandhar, B., Fairley, T., Scheiber-Pacht, M., Chakraborty, S., ... Coffey, D. M. (2013). Digital slide imaging in cervicovaginal cytology: A pilot study. *Archives of Pathology & Laboratory Medicine*, *137*(5), 618–624. doi:10.5858/arpa.2012-0430-OA PMID:22970841

Wu, X., Oliveria, S. A., Yagerman, S., Chen, L., DeFazio, J., Braun, R., & Marghoob, A. A. (2015). Feasibility and Efficacy of Patient-Initiated Mobile Teledermoscopy for Short-term Monitoring of Clinically Atypical Nevi. *JAMA Dermatology*, *151*(5), 489. doi:10.1001/jamadermatol.2014.3837 PMID:25629626

Xiao, Q., Wang, J., Chiang, V., Choi, T., Wang, Y., Sun, L., & Wu, Y. (2018). Effectiveness of mHealth Interventions for Asthma Self-Management: A Systematic Review and Meta-Analysis. *Studies in Health Technology and Informatics*, *250*, 144–145. PMID:29857410

Yamashiro, K., Kawamura, N., Matsubayashi, S., Dota, K., Suzuki, H., Mizushima, H., ... Azumi, N. (2004). Telecytology in Hokkaido Island, Japan: Results of primary telecytodiagnosis of routine cases. *Cytopathology*, *15*(4), 221–227. doi:10.1111/j.1365-2303.2004.00147.x PMID:15324451

Ybarra, M. L., Holtrop, J. S., Prescott, T. L., & Strong, D. (2014). Process evaluation of a mHealth program: Lessons learned from Stop My Smoking USA, a text messaging-based smoking cessation program for young adults. *Patient Education and Counseling*, *97*(2), 239–243. doi:10.1016/j.pec.2014.07.009 PMID:25103183

Yoon, T., Shin, D. M., Kim, S., Lee, S., Lee, T. G., & Kim, K. (2017). Precise observation of C. elegans dynamic behaviours under controlled thermal stimulus using a mobile phone-based microscope. *Journal of Microscopy*, *266*(1), 28–34. doi:10.1111/jmi.12513 PMID:28066886

Yu, H., Gao, F., Jiang, L., & Ma, S. (2017). Development of a Whole Slide Imaging System on Smartphones and Evaluation With Frozen Section Samples. *JMIR mHealth and uHealth*, *5*(9), e132. doi:10.2196/mhealth.8242 PMID:28916508

Zerth, J., Besser, J., & Reichert, A. (2012). Effectiveness and efficiency for ambulatory care assisted by mobile technological devices. *Biomedizinische Technik. Biomedical Engineering*, *57*(Suppl 1.). doi:10.1515/bmt-2012-4062 PMID:23096280

KEY TERMS AND DEFINITIONS

Cytopathology: A specialty of medicine related to the study and diagnosis of diseases by the examination of cells.

E-Health: Is the healthcare supported by electronics, informatics and tele-communications.

E-Learning: Is a broad concept referring to the application of information and communication technologies (ICT) for learning purposes.

Laboratory Information System (LIS): Or laboratory information management system (LIMS) is a software-based system for the support of operations in a modern laboratory, such as workflow, sample tracking, data exchange interfaces, LIS systems are often capable to be connected with medical analyzers for automated extraction and storage of measurements.

Mobile Health (mHealth): The practice of medicine and public health supported by mobile devices.

Pathology: From Greek *pathos* (πάθος), meaning "suffering" and -logia (-λογία), meaning study, a medical diagnosis and research field, studying cause of diseases, traditionally by tissue, cells or body fluid analysis via the microscope. Cytopathology is considered a sub specialty of pathology in many countries.

Quality Control: The set of processes by which entities review the quality of all factors involved in product, service or activity, during QC processes, the products, services and activities are tested or validated in order to reveal defects and problems, before their release.

Telecytology: The application of cytopathology from distance.

Telediagnosis: Is the determination of a disease at a site remote from the patient based on transmitted data.

Virtual Slide: or whole slide imaging, a virtual slide is created when a glass slide is entirely scanned digitally.

Chapter 8
Mobile Health Applications and Cloud Computing in Cytopathology:
Benefits and Potential

Stavros Archondakis
401 Military Hospital, Greece

Angelos Daniilidis
Thessaloniki Medical School, Greece

Eleftherios Vavoulidis
Thessaloniki Medical School, Greece

Anastasia Vatopoulou
Thessaloniki Medical School, Greece

Maria Nasioutziki
Thessaloniki Medical School, Greece

Alexios Papanikolaou
Thessaloniki Medical School, Greece

Ourania Oustampasidou
401 Military Hospital, Greece

Konstantinos Dinas
Thessaloniki Medical School, Greece

ABSTRACT

Modern cytopathology labs offer an outstanding portfolio of important testing services that must be of high quality and credibility. Over the last decade, clinical cytopathology was influenced by the wide implementation of computer sciences. Cytopathology labs wishing to achieve a seamless workflow process have successfully adopted automation and information management systems. Innovative information technologies, including e-health, constitute a valuable tool for interlaboratory collaboration and quality improvement. Cloud computing will enhance the opportunities in cytological data management and sharing. The authors present thorough research of mobile applications related to cytopathology and try to foresee applications that may benefit modern cytopathology. Also, the feasibility of such applications for inter-laboratory comparisons, proficiency testing, and diagnostic accuracy validation is examined. Finally, the role of mobile applications for providing and/or enhancing the laboratory capabilities through educational training and other research activities is investigated.

DOI: 10.4018/978-1-5225-8021-8.ch008

Copyright © 2019, IGI Global. Copying or distributing in print or electronic forms without written permission of IGI Global is prohibited.

INTRODUCTION

During the last decades, medical data deriving from the analysis of patient samples were stored in medical laboratories and was provided to physicians manually (Brender & McNair, 1996). The absence of an integrated laboratory information system was making medical data transfer slow and possibly ineffective while results inquiry/control and quality control (QC) was a rather expensive and time-consuming process (Kubono, 2004).

Over the last decade, the practice of clinical cytopathology was dramatically influenced by the wide implementation of informatics and computer sciences in the everyday laboratory workflow. The wide implementation of laboratory information systems became a necessity dictated by the need for real-time results and the increasing role of laboratory medicine in therapeutic decisions (Georgiou & Westbrook, 2006).

Laboratory information systems have been implemented in many medical laboratories wishing to improve their quality standards. A laboratory information system (LIS) is a valuable tool for medical professionals in order to manage complex processes, ensure regulatory compliance, promote collaboration between departments of the same or different laboratories, deliver detailed reports, and enhance the laboratory networking capabilities. That results in better data management and sharing between the laboratory and its clients (laboratories, clinicians or examinees) (Brender & McNair, 1996).

Cytopathology laboratory services are essential for patient care and include arrangements for examination requests, patient preparation and identification, collection, transportation, storage, processing and evaluation of clinical samples, together with subsequent interpretation, reporting and advice.

The main cytological examination, the well-known Papanicolaou test consists of a widely applied, cost-effective screening method for the early detection of cervical dysplasia and cancer. A well-written and well-implemented LIS software can improve the diagnostic accuracy of this method by introducing new emerging technologies. Pap smears screening, and cytological diagnosis provision for the vast majority of the female population requires a large number of skilled cytotechnologists and cytopathologists. Since the number of these professionals is still inadequate, the development of automated laboratory instruments and screening systems may provide a practical and satisfactory solution. Laboratory informatics are regarded nowadays as an essential tool for the laboratory's quality assurance (QA) and improvement due to its key role in the pre-analytical, analytical and post-analytical diagnostic phases. A well-written and well-implemented LIS software can use medical data for the documentation of QC measures and the improvement of the laboratory's performance.

Mobile Health technology is changing the way enterprises, institutions and people understand and use current software systems. It allows imaging flexibility and may be used for creating a virtual mobile workplace. Security and privacy issues have to be addressed in order to ensure the wide implementation of Mobile Health technology shortly.

Cloud services (in modern tech jargon often referred as "the cloud") refers to a network of servers connected by the Internet or another network that enables users to combine and use computing power on an as-needed basis. Cloud computing is a novelty that rapidly showed tremendous opportunities for application in medicine and health care improvement (Eugster, Schmid, Binder, & Schmidberger, 2013; Glaser, 2011; Kuo, 2011; Lupse, Vida, & Stoicu-Tivadar, 2012; Mirza & El-Masri, 2013; Patel, 2012; Rosenthal et al., 2010; Waxer, Ninan, Ma, & Dominguez, 2013; Webb, 2012). It is forecasted that there will be an increase in the US cloud computing market for medical images from \$56.5m in 2010 by 27% in 2018 at a Compounded Annual Growth Rate (CAGR). That is mainly due to the growing volume of medical images and the increasing costs of the ownership for owning Picture Archiving and Communication Systems (PACS) (GlobalData, 2012).

The purpose of this chapter is to present our experience on the application of Mobile Health technology to Cytopathology Laboratories, and on the possible ways Mobile Health technology can encourage or facilitate the wide implementation of ISO 15189:2012 specific requirements concerning every laboratory aspect and process.

Within this chapter we analyze state of the art related to the application of cloud computing services and infrastructure for cytopathology, identify and propose potential applications, explore possible solutions for potential problems and finally promote the benefits of transforming traditional application of the cytopathology lab into cloud-based services.

Furthermore, we examine the feasibility of applying Mobile Health technology for laboratory information systems data sharing and handling, for medical inter-laboratory comparisons, proficiency testing and for validating the accuracy of cytological diagnoses.

Also, we examine the role of Mobile Health applications to provide or/and enhance the existing laboratory capabilities for educational training and other research activities.

Finally, we give clear and comprehensive guidance concerning various financial, legal, professional, and ethical problems in this field.

BACKGROUND

Laboratory automation has been propelled during the last decade by the advantages of greater productivity, cost efficacy and the capacity of integration with modern instrumental equipment that has Internet Connection (Vacata, Jahns-Streubel, Baldus, & Wood, 2007; Westbrook, Georgiou, & Rob, 2008). Laboratory information systems provide better functionality through automation in parts of the inspection procedures, permitting the lab to achieve maximum efficiency (Vacata et al., 2007; Westbrook et al., 2008). Such systems also improve service to physicians and other stakeholders and ultimately reduce the probability of human errors. It is widely accepted that error-prone activities can be substantially reduced, but not eliminated. However, information technology systems can provide reasonable, accurate and reliable standardized procedures of QC for the assessment procedure as well as sophisticated quality indices for all the control system of the medical laboratory (Vacata et al., 2007; Westbrook et al., 2008). Medical laboratory computers may be used in various ways. They may be used for preparing and administering the management handbook and standard operation procedures, for personnel training, for providing and archiving documents via a network. They may also be used for creating customer databases, for evaluating test results, for online connecting with external sources of information, for contacting with customers, or as a typewriter as well. A computing system contains at least one computer unit, some peripheral devices and some software packages.

Computing systems operating parameters require custom verification and validation. Verification is the confirmation that specified requirements have been fulfilled. Computing system monitoring, user acceptance testing and code reviews are some verification tools. Validation is the confirmation that the requirements for the specific use are fulfilled. Electronic records contain any combination of digital data that is created, modified, archived, or distributed by a computer system. Electronic records must be protected from exposure to accidental or malicious alteration or destruction (record security).

Computing systems may be open or closed. In closed computing systems, individuals responsible for the content of the electronic records control access to medical archives. On the contrary, in open computing systems, people not responsible for the content of the electronic records (Vacata et al., 2007) control access to medical archives.

The computing systems software may be used for testing, calibration and sampling purposes (testing software) or for managing document control (document software) (Vacata et al., 2007; Westbrook et al., 2008). The integrity of electronic records must be checked periodically (file integrity check) while the computing system must be tested periodically to determine if it meets specific requirements (acceptance test). Finally, according to the European Federation of National Associations of Measurement (2006), the software of the laboratory computing system must be periodically tested.

The ISO 15189:2012 requirements cover all aspects of the laboratory activities, including the laboratory information system (LIS) (Pouliakis et al., 2014a, 2014b; Vacata et al., 2007; Westbrook et al., 2008). ISO 15189:2012 suggests specific measures for the protection of electronic laboratory records (Pouliakis et al., 2014a, 2014b; Vacata et al., 2007; Westbrook et al., 2008). The proposed measures comprise a valuable tool for quality improvement in the field of electronic documentation of medical records. It is worthwhile mentioning that the ISO 15189:2012 requirements do not apply to desktop calculators, small programmable technical computers, computers used only for office applications by one single user, or microprocessors integrated in assessment instruments (Kubono, 2004; Pouliakis et al., 2014a, 2014b; Westbrook et al., 2008).

The laboratory information system (LIS) functions include workflow management, specimen tracking, data entry and reporting, assistance with regulatory compliance, code capture, interfacing with other systems, archiving, inventory control, security, and providing billing information. The LIS components include hardware (e.g. servers), peripherals (e.g. instruments, printers, cameras, monitors and scanners), a network, interfaces (e.g. links to other information systems), database(s) and software (e.g. database management system).

In the field of Cytopathology, laboratory information systems have enabled cytotechnologists and cytopathologists to achieve efficient, streamlined workflows, regulatory compliance, and superior reporting capabilities. A well-written and well-implemented cytopathology LIS, when integrated to Electronic Medical Records (EMRs) can provide full lab automation through connections to instrumentation and clinicians' offices, minimize human errors and achieve detailed test order entry and efficient results retrieval.

Early software programs in the field of Cytopathology included reporting, data storage, and elementary data mining. During the past ten years, laboratory information systems capabilities have been dramatically increased by automated enhancements, such as specimen tracking, barcode labelling, reflex testing, automated and customized report delivery and billing system interfaces.

Laboratory information systems in the field of Cytopathology may be autonomous or may consist a part of an integrated anatomic pathology system, or a part of a larger hospital information system.

National or international regulatory agencies are nowadays specifying the minimum period cytopathology laboratories should record and retrieve specimen information and patient reports. The information system applied, should permit easy access to all cytology reports and, if possible, to related surgical pathology reports, in order to make the possible cytologic/histologic correlation. Older records should be archived and stored offsite as long as retrieval does not hinder patient care or delay regulatory inspections. Laboratory information systems should be able to correlate or merge records when there is an alteration in patient identifiers without altering the data in the original records. It is advisable for laboratory information systems in cytopathology departments to use unique identifiers, such as the patient's record number, in order to achieve more accurate matching.

QC defines the service's quality, imparting to it the credibility needed for its intended purpose, while QA activities measure the degree to which desired outcomes are successful (Archondakis, 2015). QC may be internal or external. QC in the field of Cytology is mainly achieved by slide rescreening or by clinical-histological correlation of cytological diagnoses (Archondakis, 2015). Many slide rescreening procedures have been proposed for QA purposes, such as rapid reviewing of smears initially reported as negative or inadequate, rapid preview/prescreening of all smears, random rescreening, targeted rescreening of specific patient groups, seeding abnormal cases into the screening pools, retrospective rescreening of negative cytology specimens from patients with a current high-grade abnormality and automated rescreening of smears initially reported as negative (Archondakis, 2015). The laboratory managers are responsible for the selection of the most appropriate method for QA purposes, according to the specific needs of their laboratories (Archondakis, 2015).

The practice of diagnostic cytopathology performed on digital images is a novel process that can be used for obtaining expert opinions on difficult cases from remote laboratories (telecytology) (Archondakis et al., 2009).

Telecytological diagnosis can be achieved either with the use of cytological pictures viewed in real time with the microscope (dynamic telecytological systems), or with the use of cytological pictures that are first captured in a digital format and then transmitted to distant observers (static telecytological systems) (Archondakis et al., 2009; Stamataki et al., 2008). The static telecytology systems have the advantage of considerably lower cost, but they only allow the capture of a selected subset of microscopic fields (Pantanowitz, Hornish, & Goulart, 2009). The dynamic telecytology systems permit evaluation of the cytological material present on a slide (Yamashiro et al., 2004). These systems may be hampered by high network traffic and their high cost of purchase and maintenance that makes them unaffordable for small laboratories wishing to participate in proficiency testing programs.

The use of digital images in quality control/assurance programs eliminates the need for glass slides retrieval from the laboratory's registry (at least at the point of examination), allows annotations to be added to images, enhances the ability to rapidly transmit and remotely share images electronically for several purposes (telecytology, conferences, education, quality assurance, peer review) and protects more efficiently patient anonymity (Archondakis, 2013, 2014).

Moreover, the use of digital images for QA programs is more practical and time-efficient, although the conversion process of glass slides into digital image files may require some additional time. Static telecytology systems are preferred due to their low cost by laboratories that cannot afford the high cost of purchasing and maintaining dynamic systems (Archondakis, 2013, 2014).

The limitations and diagnostic errors related to telecytology that are already mentioned by some authors may cause misinterpretation of digital images by less experienced participants (Briscoe et al., 2000). Appropriate field selection, sufficient image quality and especially diagnostic expertise are the most crucial parameters ensuring the proper function of a static telecytological system (Archondakis, 2013, 2014).

The most common manifestations of the inter-observer discrepancy are upgrading of the telecytological diagnosis to a definitive carcinoma diagnosis or downgrading of a suspicious telecytological diagnosis to a rather benign lesion because of image deficiencies (Archondakis et al., 2009).

Proficiency testing (PT) is a well-recognized method for evaluating actual laboratory performance usually using inter-laboratory comparisons (Archondakis, 2013, 2014). Proficiency testing results can be used as an independent indication of a laboratory's diagnostic competence and can be integrated into the ordinary process of the laboratory's assessment and accreditation (Archondakis, 2013, 2014). According to ISO 15189:2007, all accredited laboratories must conduct proficiency tests by their normal patient testing and reporting procedures (Pantanowitz et al., 2009, Archondakis et al., 2011). A recent revision of ISO 15189, published in 2012 proposes the additional use of alternative methods for the evaluation of laboratories technical competence, where accredited PT schemes are not available. The practice of diagnostic cytopathology performed on digital images is a process by which remote laboratories can obtain expert opinions on difficult cases (telecytology) (Archondakis et al., 2009, Pouliakis et al., 2014a, 2014b). Telecytological diagnosis can be achieved either with the use of cytological pictures viewed in real time from the microscope (dynamic telecytological systems), or with the use of cytological pictures that are first captured in a digital format and then transmitted to distant observers (static telecytological systems) (Archondakis, 2013, 2014; Stamataki et al., 2008). Hybrid systems have also been developed. The majority of relevant articles have focused on the possible use of telecytology for diagnostic and consultation purposes (Archondakis, 2013, 2014).

Diagnostic agreement and reproducibility between the same (intra-observer) and different (inter-observer) observers are the main parameters monitored and recorded during telecytology programs (Stamataki et al., 2008; Pantanowitz et al., 2009). The agreement is the total or a comparable number of cases in which the same diagnosis was issued between or within observers, including the part of the agreement that may be attributed to chance (Landis & Koch, 1977). Reproducibility, which is part of the agreement that cannot be explained purely by chance (Landis & Koch, 1977) is measured by the kappa statistic. Within the positive kappa values and in accordance with the study by Landis and Koch (1977), the agreement was interpreted as follows: a range of 0.00– 0.20 indicates slight agreement, a range of 0.21–0.40 indicates fair agreement, a range of 0.41–0.60 indicates moderate agreement, a range of 0.61–0.80 indicates very good agreement, while a range of 0.81–1.00 indicates excellent or almost perfect agreement (Landis & Koch, 1977).

QA in the field of Cytopathology is achieved mainly by monitoring diagnostic discrepancies, through cytological and histological correlation. The improvement of information systems and LIS in most pathology laboratories allows such correlations to be performed just immediately after the release of the examination results. Additionally, data mining either online or in a later stage may produce important knowledge for trends and problematic areas in the processes and, therefore, to initiate corrective actions for quality improvement. Also, image-based systems to evaluate the quality of classification systems such as the Bethesda System 2001 for reporting the results of cervical cytology (Solomon et al., 2002) have already been reported in the literature (Sherman, Dasgupta, Schiffman, Nayar, & Solomon, 2007). Mobile Health technology obviously can be of help for QC&QA, as the related application may be developed for such an environment, storage and application load will not be an issue, and additional benefits may be obtained as the QC&QA application can be shared among numerous laboratories and rare cytological cases can be used by all participating labs.

Until now, Mobile Health technology is not widely used for the various tasks related to Cytopathology. However, there are numerous fields in which it could be applied. The envisioned advantages for the everyday practice of laboratories workflow and eventually for the patients are significant.

Mobile Health technology, in the field of cytopathology, may provide a valuable web-based service, which may be incorporated in the LIS and become part of a web-based Electronic Health Record (EHR).

A cytopathology laboratory wishing to store a large number of images and patient information files is nowadays obliged to install one or more servers and accompanying disk arrays, having poor or no earlier experience in its upkeep. A possible server crash may result in severe data loss. Furthermore, the server may require constant upgrades. These two reasons are good enough for a modern cytopathology laboratory to shift its data to the Mobile Health. By doing so, the laboratory reduces dramatically all costs related to server software and hardware as well as the costs for maintenance and licenses. In such a scenario, the Mobile Health acts as LIS, telecytology software, and billing unit at the same time. A patient may perform a cytological examination at a hospital or a private laboratory. Representative images of the case may be stored on a hybrid Mobile Health. If the patients perform another cytological examination after some time, in another laboratory, the cytopathologists can retrieve and merge images that were stored previously in the Mobile Health directly from their offices. This way, the final diagnosis is made after having reviewed the images of the first cytological examination.

MOBILE HEALTH APPLICATIONS FOR QUALITY ASSURANCE PURPOSES IN A CYTOPATHOLOGY LABORATORY: BENEFITS AND CURRENT POTENTIAL

Mobile Health applications provide many advantages regarding scalability, maintainability, and massive data processing. They can provide exceptional consultation opportunities to distant cytopathology laboratories. Also, they can improve the professional skills and boost the confidence of the participating medical staff.

Mobile Health technology, when applied in the field of Cytopathology, has some main benefits, such as innovative dashboard for easy use, report formatted custom for each participant's lab with images, automatic versioning history, secure access to records that removes backup concerns, faster cytopathologist approval process, easy to use browser-based system, automatic spell-checking, images integration into reports, faster "voice-to-file" process, HL7 interface availability, safe storage, safe records transmission, low cost of record retrieval, labor, copying, filing and storage, easy PDF documents production for easy integration to EMR systems and use of digital signatures for document control and compliance with standards.

Using Mobile Health applications, cytopathology laboratories can avoid huge spending on maintenance of costly applications and image storage and sharing. Mobile Health technology allows imaging flexibility and may be used for creating a virtual mobile workplace. Security and privacy issues have to be addressed in order to ensure Mobile Health applications wide implementation shortly.

The main components of Cloud computing in the field of Cytopathology are the following:

1. **Applications:** The Cloud applications are hosted on servers that are remote from the user and can be run in real time from a thin client that hosts the application through a web browser. The majority of Cloud applications are accessible via browsers. Thus, there is no installation of the application, no maintenance required, and support issues are resolved because the software is hosted on a machine that is dedicated to that software, so there is no danger that the thin client could influence the software. Cloud applications may be run as software as a service (SaaS), software plus service or data as a service. In Cloud applications, used by cytopathologists, the end users take advantage of some kind of "Software as a Service" for image reviewing, creating diagnostic reports or patient billing.
2. **Client:** It is usually a web browser such as Mozilla Firefox. In the mobile telephone environment, Apple's iPhone or Google's Android platforms some applications can be considered to run from the

cloud. A client may also be a certain website such as Facebook, where there are many applications available for use. Cloud client, in the field of Cytopathology, is the medium which cytopathologists use to access the Cloud via the Internet. Cloud client may be a computer or a Smartphone.

3. **Infrastructure:** Cloud infrastructure includes all computer hardware and the buildings containing it. The hardware consists of mass-produced server technology. The server environment may be running partial or complete virtualization, grid computing or paravirtualization technologies. Cloud infrastructure, in the field of Cytopathology, includes computer hardware and servers used for software running and data storage.
4. **Platform:** The cloud platform is referring to the way that applications can be deployed. In the field of Cytopathology, a well-designed platform is an essential parameter for efficient application of laboratory's Cloud applications.
5. **Service**: Service refers to what users can reap from their cloud experience. To date, there is a great number of services for users wishing to take advantage of. Some of these services are unique, while others enhance services that were already available. A cloud service, in the field of Cytopathology, can be, without having to be limited to, either a web-based image archiving system or a web-based image gallery.
6. **Storage:** Storage devices are the often first to fail on a computer. By using cloud technology, companies assure their data safety. In case there is an emergency situation, the chances of complete failure of all systems are very slim, due to a large number of computers working in the cloud environment. Cloud computing, in the field of Cytopathology, enables, for example, the storage of large medical laboratory databases in the form of documents and image libraries, instead of physical storage at the site (hospital or imaging center) which is much more expensive and difficult to maintain.
7. **Processing Power:** The processing power that cloud computing is capable of has no boundaries. Cloud companies are willing to scale up their infrastructure if needed, so when there is a need for more processing power, it will be available on the fly. Due to Cloud computing immense processing power, companies do not have to worry about infrastructure purchasing or costs. Cloud computing, in the field of Cytopathology, can provide infinite processing power to all cytopathology laboratories at a very low cost.

The power of Mobile Health technology combined with the convenience of web applications can improve significantly the collaboration among cytology labs participating in image or data sharing QA programs.

Storing, archiving, sharing and accessing images in the Mobile Health allows a modern cytopathology laboratory to manage data more efficiently and cost-effectively while overcoming many of the legal, regulatory and technical challenges that data requirements pose.

This technology enables a modern cytopathology laboratory to handle large bandwidth images efficiently, to use non-proprietary, standards-based, vendor-neutral architecture, to expand or contract storage capacity easily as needed, to manage authentication, encryption and security protocols, to conduct efficient system-wide application upgrades and finally to extend the life of existing infrastructure/investments.

As there is pressure to reduce costs, many laboratories nowadays are exploiting virtualization capabilities that are essential characteristics of Mobile Health technology.

The servers applied for image or data sharing QA programs need to support most digital slide formats and to be easily integrated with various scanners for single-click slide upload for on-premises deployment.

A Mobile Health-based infrastructure for digital cytology can analyze whole slides on special image servers from each professional's web browser with just a few clicks. Each cytopathologist simply has to select analysis, template settings and parameters with interactive visual preview, and let the server run complete slide analysis using the scalable power of the Mobile Health.

All professionals, although possessing different imaging equipment, can use Mobile Health-based software to integrate seamlessly with imaging hardware. Software like that permits the digital slide to be uploaded to the user workspace via the Mobile Health server automatically.

A modern cytopathology laboratory and the network of cooperating cytopathology laboratories have no obligation to conform to any single unified corporate IT policy. A modern cytopathology laboratory and the network of cooperating cytopathology laboratories can use a variety of computers, operating systems, and browsers. The special web interface can work with all the commercially available operating systems like Windows, iOS, Android and Linux that are used in modern tablets, smartphones, and personal computers without exceptions. Each professional (whether cytotechnologist or cytopathologist) can view digital slides online without having to download, install or update anything. A simple log-in to the browser is enough for establishing a connection with the Mobile Health platform.

Integrated Flexible Database module can create powerful knowledge database from each cytopathologist's digital slide collection. Mobile Health-based software can use flexible attributes, quick tags, comments and attachments for cases and slides to organize images and keep track of all available medical data.

Cytopathology professionals should be able to separate shared and private images. A modern cytopathology laboratory and the network of cooperating cytopathology laboratories can invite collaborators and share digital slides via email, by using a Mobile Health-based software.

No need to mention once more that digital cytology images storage and transmission must follow strict regulations to avoid any unauthorized alteration or improper use. Current standards of electronic medical data handling are still informative, yet the need for a secure electronic environment continues to grow.

A modern cytopathology laboratory has already established a system where images and virtual slides are available online, and all cytopathologists can report remotely. By using the laboratory's server, the users experienced many difficulties because of frequent local network disruptions. By shifting the data to the Mobile Health, the cytopathologists are now able to access the web-based cytopathology software. Here, the Mobile Health enables the implementation of teleconsultation applications.

Mobile Health technology can be used for making the entire medical record of a patient accessible for review by a remote cytopathologist. All cytopathologists can review admission notes for all cases, seek prior data from other laboratories that are mentioned in these notes and review all available imaging material to make all applicable correlations.

Further evaluation and development of intelligent Mobile Health based search engines exploiting artificial intelligence appear worthwhile.

Another aspect of primary diagnosis is related to homeworker cytopathologists. Virtual slide technology enables the digitization of complete slides. Thus, the diagnostic data can be now stored and transmitted, the barrier, in this case, is a large amount of data. Eventually, Mobile Health technology provides unlimited storage and fast communication channels, in this aspect; the remote primary diagnosis could be a reality.

A modern cytopathology laboratory is electronically tracking QC/QA indicators which can be done either within the LIS and/or by exporting data from the LIS (via spreadsheet software).

Mobile Health applications can be used for monitoring laboratory requisition completeness, problems documented by the users, occurrences and trends with any particular physicians' office sending specimens to the laboratory. Identification of such problems could prompt a redesign of requisition forms. Specimen rejection incidents and labelling errors are also electronically documented, and specimen rejection frequency is regularly reported to all physicians' offices. Comments entered within available QA fields are included in the final cytological report. Electronic monitoring of lost specimens is accomplished with a simple spreadsheet log.

A cytopathology laboratory information system is monitoring electronic data integrity and is taking all available security measures, which may include regular back-up of data, password protection, data encryption, antivirus software, firewalls, and audit trails. Mobile Health applications can be used for assigning users different levels of privileges so that only certain individuals can finalize and sign out abnormal cytological diagnoses ensuring the integrity of finalized reports.

Mobile Health applications can be used for recording workloads for each cytopathologist. That is achieved by evaluating the diagnostic accuracy in comparison with productivity.

A modern cytopathology laboratory information system prohibits screening of more than 200 conventional slides over an 8-hour period. Non-gynecologic and gynecologic liquid-based preparation slides also count as half-slides in such daily counts.

Mobile Health applications can be used for designating cases as high risk, based on database searches for particular entries within specific fields. In a modern cytopathology laboratory, computer-assisted designation of high-risk cases greatly increases the likelihood that high-risk cases are correctly identified to be a part of a detailed review process before signing out.

These applications can be used for creating pivot tables, which are useful tools to cross-reference diagnoses by cytopathologists and for analyzing diagnostic correlations and discrepancies. In a cytopathology laboratory, software systems allow for individual cases to be easily retrieved for continuing education purposes.

Potential Applications of Cloud Computing in Cytopathology

Modern Cytopathology laboratories deal mainly with images as the routine cytological examinations are performed via the use of a glass slide and analysis with the microscope. However, modern cytopathology laboratories perform additional examinations based on molecular techniques and immunocytochemistry methods. The modern cytopathology laboratory is equipped with numerous modalities capable of performing medical tests and exchange data via networks, imaging systems capable of creating digital pictures of the slides or even virtual slides, which are complete slides in electronic format. The volume of data in a cytopathology lab nowadays is enormous. The major cloud-based applications that can be envisioned for the benefit of cytopathologists and the patients as well may be as follows:

Data Storage

Storing, archiving, sharing and accessing images in the cloud allows the industry to manage data more efficiently and cost-effectively while overcoming many of the legal, regulatory and technical challenges that data requirements pose (AT&T, 2012). The cloud enables hospitals to:

- Efficiently handle large bandwidth images
- Use non-proprietary, standards-based, vendor-neutral architecture
- Expand or contract storage capacity easily as needed
- Manage authentication, encryption and security protocols
- Conduct efficient system-wide application upgrades
- Extend the life of existing infrastructure/investments

A cytopathology laboratory wishing to store a large number of images and patient information files is nowadays obliged to install one or more servers and accompanying disk arrays, having poor or no earlier experience in its upkeep. A possible server crash may result in severe data loss.

Furthermore, the server may require constant upgrades. These two reasons are good enough for a modern cytopathology laboratory to shift its data to the Cloud. By doing this, the laboratory reduces dramatically all costs related to server software and hardware as well as the costs for maintenance and licenses. Here the cloud acts as LIS, telecytology software, and billing unit. A patient may perform a cytological examination at a hospital or a private laboratory. Representative images of the case may be stored on a hybrid Cloud. If the patient performs another cytologic examination after some time, in another (and possibly distant), he can provide the reporting cytopathologists direct access to the images stored in the Cloud. The cytopathologists can retrieve and merge the images on his/her workstation. The cytopathologists can make his final diagnosis after having reviewed the images of the first cytological examination.

Laboratory Information Systems

Laboratory information systems (LIS) are used to supervise many varieties of inpatient and outpatient medical tests. The major features that laboratory information systems have include management of sample check-in, order entry, specimen processing, result entry and patient demographics as well as medical history. A LIS tracks and stores all the information related to a patient from arrival until he/she leaves and stores the data for future retrieval. LISs also produce reports for the tests that handle and statistics related to various aspects of a laboratory such as time for execution of examinations, sample volumes etc. Therefore, a (LIS) can be defined as a series of computer programs that process, store and manage data from all stages of medical processes and tests. Modern LISs are networked and the various modern modalities (biomedical analyzers) having networking capabilities can automatically send examination results directly for storage. Additionally, barcode technology automates sample and patient identification.

Usually, large laboratories have internal information technology (IT) personnel to handle hardware, software and provide technical expertise and support, and take care in cases of infrastructure lack as well as to optimize the systems to run mission-critical applications. However, cloud computing is changing this picture. As there is pressure to meet timelines, to reduce costs for example by spreading costs associated with infrastructure ownership and support, many laboratories nowadays are exploiting virtualization capabilities that are basic characteristics of cloud computing, virtualization provides convenient and on-demand network access to a shared pool of configurable resources such as networks, servers, storage and applications, and in the modern world the cost for owning and managing in-house the equipment and personnel. In addition to cost reduction, the set-up and configuration time for a laboratory wishing to adopt a new LIS is minimal. Therefore, a cytopathology laboratory that does not have an LIS, but wants to start using a Cloud-based LIS, may purchase an LIS system hosted in the cloud, configure it according to the needs, train the users and launch the application within a short time. Using a community Cloud, many hospitals can share standard software and save large amounts of money.

Screening Programs

Cervical cancer is one of the most common women mortality reasons in the world (Jemal et al., 2011). However, it is a well-studied disease with known natural history and can be prevented and treated if diagnosed in early stage. The key to prevention is the regular check of all women fulfilling specific criteria with Papanikolaou test; this process is called population-based cervical cancer screening program. As the involved population is very large, critical to the success of the program is the organization and quality control and assurance. Unavoidable a computerized information system supporting the program must be in place (Pouliakis, Iliopoulou, & Karakitsou, 2012; Pouliakis & Karakitsos, 2011). There are several important issues related to the software systems supporting screening programs where the application of cloud computing can be a solution:

- **Availability:** it is the ability to cope with, and if necessary recover from failures of the host server either due to hardware reasons or due to the failure of the operating system and the application software, and to cope with hardware and maintenance activities that may cause downtime. The system availability is crucial for the program smooth operation; if the system is not operational the consequences range from missing appointments to cancelled treatments. Hosting of such systems in a cloud ensures the high availability of servers; moreover, as cloud services providers have multisite hosting and multiple internet connections, the availability of connectivity is ensured as well.
- **Scalability:** refers to the ability to spread both the system software and the load across multiple servers. Hosting the application in a cloud provider ensures that there will be plenty of CPU power available. Virtual machines offered by cloud services providers are fault tolerant and utilize many servers that appear to the end user as a single machine.Additionally, escalation of the application is easily performed by using additional servers both for the application and the database as well.
- **Deployment and Problem Resolution:** Deploying the traditional application in end user computers is not anymore a choice for IT systems supporting screening programs. The chosen solution is central hosting of the applications and preferably web-based applications hosted in the cloud. The benefits from this architecture are evident: the maintenance is easier and applied in a single place, and bug fixes and improvements when applied immediately are available to the other users.

Quality Control and Assurance

There are many aspects related to the quality in cytology, and how to control and assess. One of the fundamental methods is the correlation of the cytologic and histologic answers (Izadi-Mood, Sarmadi, & Sanii, 2013). The concept is to evaluate the discrepancies, determine why occurred, and to ensure the appropriate patient care. The way Cytologic and histologic correlation is performed changed over time. Years ago, it was to collect all cases every few months and go through them. That is not any more acceptable method because patients would not like to learn about a mistake a few months after it especially if this could have been corrected (Renshaw, 2011). The improvement of information systems and LIS in most cytologic and histologic laboratories, allows such correlations to be performed just immediately after the release of the examination results.

Additionally, data mining either on-line or in a later stage may produce important knowledge for trends and problematic areas in the processes and therefore to initiate corrective actions for quality improvement. Additionally, image-based systems on evaluating the quality of classification systems such as the Bethesda System 2001 for reporting the results of cervical cytology (Solomon et al., 2002) have already been reported in the literature (Sherman, Dasgupta, Schiffman, Nayar, & Solomon, 2007). The cloud obviously can be of help for QC&QA as the related application may be developed and operate for such an environment, storage and application load will not be an issue and additional benefits may be obtained as the QC&QA application can be shared among numerous laboratories, and rare cytological cases can be used by all participating labs.

Proficiency Testing

Proficiency testing is not a new concept. European countries have tested a variety of areas in pathology. In the United Kingdom, there are quality-assurance testing programs for a variety of areas called National External Quality Assessments Schemes; whereas, in the European Union, there is an aptitude test for cervical cytology that was created by the Committee for Quality Assurance, Trading, and Education (QUATE)(Demichelis, Della Mea, Forti, Dalla Palma, & Beltrami, 2002). The objective of the QUATE committee is to test each individual using the same slides to ensure equity of examination. Today there is available published evidence that the results of proficiency testing by virtual slides are comparable to those of glass slides, thus computer-based testing can be equivalent.

Additionally, according to the International Academy of Cytology Task Force (Vooijs et al., 1998), the training programs for cytotechnologists and cytopathologists should provide instruction and experience in new technologies. Advantages of digital images for training include standardization of teaching sets and interactive capabilities, allowing educational feedback.

The position of the International Academy of Cytology Task Force in 1998: "Diagnostic Cytology Towards the 21st Century" is highlighted by the following:

- Computerized support/assistance devices aid the complete screening of the slide during training and provide feedback to cytologists on screening techniques.
- The subjective nature of cytologic analysis poses many challenges for implementation.
- There is a concern for the value and validity of any large-scale formal testing programs.
- Locator and diagnostic skills are both critical in cytology, but assessment of each skill may occur in different ways using digital technologies.
- Assessments should provide educational feedback to participants.
- The reliability or consistency of the testing event is critical.
- A valid and reliable correlation between work performance and performance on a proficiency test needs to be established.
- Any cytology proficiency test program should also be considered in the context of other laboratory quality assurance tools and the entire cervical cancer screening program.
- Regulatory agencies should evaluate entire laboratory performance, while each laboratory director should assume primary responsibility for evaluating and documenting the competency and daily performance of each practising cytologist.

- Professional scientific organizations should take the lead in recommending methods and standards of performance assessment.
- A reliable method of correlating daily competency with results on PT is not yet established.
- Methods may evolve ever time using new technologies.
- The use of computerized techniques and images for assessment will require careful deliberation by experts as well as validation by practising cytologists.
- Variables include diagnostic categories for testing, numbers of challenges per testing event, types of slide preparations and characteristics of the digital images.
- Availability of equipment and staff will affect the introduction of new technologies in different regions.

Definitely 15 years ago the International Academy of Cytology had foreseen, concluded and recommended the application of information technology in the proficiency testing field, as a promising solution to numerous issues. The trend for proficiency testing today is based on whole slide imaging, the advantages of cloud computing for storing and transmitting such large data is obvious.

Digital/Virtual Slides

Digital imaging in pathology has undergone an exponential period of growth and expansion catalyzed by changes in imaging hardware and gains in computational processing. Today, digitization of entire glass slides at near the optical resolution limits of light can occur in a few minutes. Additionally, whole slides can be scanned in fluorescence or by multispectral imaging systems. Whole slide imaging has been successfully used in surgical pathology, but its usefulness and clinical application have been limited in cytology for several reasons, mainly the lack of availability of z-axis depth focusing as cytological samples in contrast to histological have a 3D structure. However, nowadays, there are available systems capable of whole slide imaging with z-axis control. This boosted the application of digital slides for cytology (Al-Janabi, Huisman, Willems, & Van Diest, 2012; Fung et al., 2012; Ghaznavi, Evans, Madabhushi, & Feldman, 2013; Gutman et al., 2013; Hipp, Lucas, Emmert-Buck, Compton, & Balis, 2011; Krishnamurthy et al., 2013; Rudnisky et al., 2007; Taylor, 2011; Wright et al., 2013).

Digital imaging is unlocking the potential to integrate primary image features into high-dimensional genomic assays by moving microscopic analysis into the digital age. That creates the opportunity for the application and use of these methods in clinical care and research settings. Digital whole slide imaging seems to be the future of cytopathology, probably sign-out of glass slides will be replaced by the whole slide scanned images.

Virtual slide sizes are enormous, ranging from more than 500 Megabytes and up to 1 Gigabyte, depending on the magnification and the scanned slide area. The use of cloud has similar advantages regarding the storage of standard cytological images. The cloud can provide affordable storage space, easily expandable and offering data storage assurance. Additionally, no local maintenance by laboratory technicians is required. Transfer of such data volumes from/to the lab and the cloud is an issue, however, the revolution in telecommunication networks, nowadays may provide the required bandwidth. Additionally, automated slide scanning workstations may operate overnight and store unattended the virtual slide data.

Continuous Medical Education, E-Learning

Over the past decades, education has met the introduction of the Internet; this has changed radically the way humans learn and teach. As the evolution of information technologies, and telecommunications, made the World Wide Web (WWW) a low cost and easily accessible tool for the dissemination of information and knowledge, education could not be left outside. Various researchers have proved that the traditional learning theories can be applied in a web-based learning system and moreover web-based distance education may improve education and support new educational systems, radically changed in comparison to traditional learning, (Garrison, Schardt, & Kochi, 2000). Medical science and medical education represent a major category of lifelong learning, as it is one of the most rapidly evolving sciences and new media offer an advantage for improvement. Therefore, the new developments and the constant growth of existing knowledge make continuous education vital for continuous medical education. In the field of cytopathology, teaching usually takes place in front of the microscope, supplemented by real-case presentations, didactic lectures and audiovisual materials. However, it is not possible for all hospitals to provide microscopes dedicated for educational purposes and a smaller number of them possess multi-user microscopes, permitting simultaneous access to a high number of trainees.

A common technique for teaching cytopathology is via the exploration of ambiguous cases. In this case, trainees attempt to provide a diagnosis in a situation where the patient outcome would be unaffected. Pitfalls during this type of training, i.e. false negative or a false positive answers, give a value to the trainees, as they experience problems that should never happen in the clinical practice and affect patients. The cytolopathogy lab is the environment where training takes place in front of the microscope, being the means of knowledge delivery. Web-based training programs appear to be a promising solution; as the financial barriers, workplace and time restrictions, experienced by the traditional educational methods in cytopathology, can be eliminated. Additionally, web-based learning systems can involve traditional learning methods and skills such as decision making, reasoning and problem solving, can be developed (Casebeer et al., 2003; Stergiou et al., 2009). Such skills are critical for the everyday medical practice of professionals.

Cloud computing seems that can become the means to give additional value, to the already available digital age education. Rich information becomes crucial for training. Still, images captured by the microscope do have limitations. The trainee experiences only a small part of the glass slide and areas selected by experts. That constitutes a bias for the trainees of the digital era. The solution is obvious completely digitized slides; however, the storage and transmission of such large amount of data, despite being possible nowadays, faces many difficulties. The rise and spread of cloud computing facilitate the elimination of both barriers, as storage is virtually unlimited, has low price and telecommunication infrastructure has a large capacity and is cheap as it is shared. Thus cloud computing and virtual slides seem to be the future of continuing medical education and eLearning for cytopathologists.

Tele-Cytology, Teleconsultation

Telecytology is the interpretation of cytological material at a distance via the use of digital images. Historically there are numerous attempts to implement telecytology (Khurana, 2012; O'Brien et al., 1998; Thrall, Pantanowitz, & Khalbuss, 2011; Tsilalis et al., 2012). Telecytology is ideally suited to situations that often encounter transportation problems, such as countries with lots of mountains, islands or many dispersed cities and villages. In these situations due to weather conditions vehicles, ships or planes are unable to move and in many cases due to extreme weather conditions (snow, rain, winds) cities and villages are cut-off. However, telecytology has still limited applications and acceptance. That is mainly due to the challenges of making digital images of acceptable quality reproducing the biological material available on the glass slides. Therefore, minimizing diagnostic errors due to the poor quality of the digital representation.

Primary Diagnosis

Cytopathologists traditionally perform diagnostic tasks with minimal information. Thus they are using other sources of information in order to improve the accuracy of their diagnoses (the triple test in breast fine-needle aspiration cytology, immunocytochemistry or molecular tests such as flow cytometry for cervical cancer detection). The cloud represents a system of interconnected information systems. Therefore, disconnected medical data sources will be possible to be integrated. As more and more of patients' medical record could be available, the amount of information available to cytopathologists will increase. Cloud computing has the potential to make the entire medical record of a patient accessible for review by a cytopathologist. However, the obligation of the cytopathologist to review such records is questionable and a subject for discussion (Renshaw, 2011), because at present there is no standard or a recommendation. Some questions are: should cytopathologist review admission notes for all cases? Should cytopathologists seek prior material from other laboratories that are mentioned in these notes if they were not sent for review by the clinicians? Should cytopathologists review imaging material? For example, reviewing mammograms to ensure that the radiographic and pathologic lesions are correlated and from the same tissue that is diagnosed.

Despite the questions mentioned in the previous paragraph, it is a fact that there will be increasing access to more and more information, probably using cloud computing technology. Accessing all these data is time to consume and in the most of the cases of no value, and this is the major reason for the previous questions related to the obligations of cytopathologists in the digital era. The answer is not clear. However, cloud systems can exploit advanced and intelligent search engines that may automatically identify important information and alert cytopathologists. These capabilities will remove the time barriers for the adoption of extensive health record examination. Further evaluation and development of intelligent cloud-based search engines exploiting artificial intelligence appear worthwhile. Computing power intensive algorithms seem to be easily a reality with cloud-based services on demand.

Another aspect of primary diagnosis is related to home worker cytopathologists. Virtual slide technology enables the digitization of complete slides. Thus, the diagnostic data can be now stored and transmitted, the barrier, in this case, is a large amount of data. Eventually, cloud computing provides unlimited storage and fast communication channels. In this aspect, remote primary diagnosis could be a reality.

RESEARCH

The potential applications of cloud computing for research in cytopathology seem endless, due to the storage and mainly for the availability of processing power. The major research fields envisioned are:

Cytogenetics

Large comparative genomics studies and tools require increasing computational power mainly because the number of available genome sequences continually rises. Local computing infrastructures are likely to become not capable of coping with the demand for increased computational power and the associated cost. Therefore, alternative parallel computing architectures, toolboxes (Drozdov, Ouzounis, Shah, & Tsoka, 2011; Konganti, Wang, Yang, & Cai, 2013; Shannon et al., 2003) and in particular cloud computing systems, seem to be the solution to alleviate this increasing pressure. Nowadays, many efforts and implementations are already available in the literature: existing similar genomics algorithms (specifically the Reciprocal Smallest Distance-RSD algorithm) from local computing infrastructures have been redesigned for cloud environments and in order to exploit their speed and flexibility (Wall et al., 2010). The results indicated that cloud computing environments might provide a substantial boost for the algorithm execution time and problem-solving with a manageable cost. However, the design and transformation of the TSD algorithm into a cloud application was not a trivial task. Technological advances for DNA sequencing have lowered the price for a personal genome sequence (the 3 billion letters in our DNA) to under $1,000 (Davies, 2010). That creates a new challenge for scientists, the analysis of cohorts of cancer research and treatment. However, large databases are required due to the increased data volume and extreme CPU power for their analysis. Cloud computing seems to be the solution for both issues. A side effect of low costs in DNA sequencing comes from the offered opportunity that allows scientists to collect and analyze whole genomes for genome-wide association studies. As such genetic data do have the potential to be more informative than standard medical records and in addition to the capability offered by cloud computing to access and analyze such data sets supplied by scientific groups around the planet, necessitates either a paradigm shift in the way that the science is done, and/or revised understandings of privacy and informed consent. A proposal by some researchers is to promote both shifts (Greenbaum & Gerstein, 2011).

Proteomics

Proteomics techniques can be used to identify markers for cancer diagnosis because the proteome reflects both the intrinsic genetic program of the cells as well as the impact of the environment. Proteome analysis has been used in cytopathology for the identification of tumors in various organs: thyroid (Torres-Cabala et al., 2006), breast (Li, Zhao, & Cui, 2013; Sohn et al., 2013), gastric (Fowsantear, Argo, Pattinson, & Cash, 2013; Lee et al., 2013; Uppal & Powell, 2013) and cervix (Yim & Park, 2006) among others as well as for response to treatment (Madden et al., 2009), One of the most promising developments from the study of human proteins is the identification of new drugs for the treatment of diseases.

Proteome research is mainly based on the assignment of unidentified spectra to peptides. These methods, including tag-based and de novo searches, have a high computational cost and involve processing of large volumes of experimental spectra thus requiring computers with large storage capacity. These exhaustive identification attempts are rarely carried out in laboratories, due to the lack of computational power, and limited support by information technology specialists to run identification algorithms. Cloud computing is the ideal environment to perform such a type of research. Recently, several attempts have been proposed and conducted by various researchers (Halligan, Geiger, Vallejos, Greene, & Twigger,

2009; Leprevost et al., 2013; Mohammed et al., 2012; Muth, Peters, Blackburn, Rapp, & Martens, 2013). Cloud computing allows laboratories to pay for computing time as per requirements, rather than investing in local server clusters.

Artificial Intelligence

The application of artificial intelligence in cytopathology is not new (Karakitsos, Stergiou, et al., 1996). During the last decades, various classification techniques have been used in medicine and especially in diagnostic cytology, involving either classical statistical models or more advanced techniques, such as neural networks (Astion & Wilding, 1992; Cochand-Priollet et al., 2006; Karakitsos, Cochand-Priollet, Guillausseau, & Pouliakis, 1996; Marchevsky, Tsou, & Laird-Offringa, 2004; C. Markopoulos et al., 1997; Pantazopoulos et al., 1998). More specifically, concerning cytology, these techniques have been applied to various organs, among others stomach(Karakitsos et al., 2004; Yamamura et al., 2002), breast (Dey, Logasundaram, & Joshi, 2013), urinary system(Schaffer, Simon, Desper, Richter, & Sauter, 2001; Vriesema et al., 2000), cervix(Boon & Kok, 1993; Giovagnoli, Cenci, Olla, & Vecchione, 2002) and thyroid(Haymart, Cayo, & Chen, 2009; Varlatzidou et al., 2011).

One of the major artificial intelligence technique/science is related to Artificial Neural Networks (ANNs). A typical cycle for the creation of a useful ANN system involves:

- **Data Collection:** Obtaining the data that will be used to create the intelligent system
- **Data Preprocessing:** Depending on the type of the ANN system and algorithm that is selected (data preprocessing may be required)
- **ANN Model Selection:** Choice of a suitable ANN type for the problem requiring a solution
- **Parameter Selection:** Configuration of the selected ANN parameters
- ANN training: identification of the ANN parameters that compose the solution to the problem
- **Evaluation:** Check the performance of the produced system on known and unknown data

If the performance of the system is satisfactory, then the produced ANN system can be used in a production environment otherwise the procedure should start again from an earlier stage. This type of complexity and the requirement to run numerous systems and combinations of ANN types, architectures and parameters increases the required number of experiments geometrically and thus the required computing resources and computing time. Additionally, the training procedure for several ANN types is computing "hungry", as it is not unusual that training of some ANNs can take weeks of computer time. Cloud computing can provide a pool of shared resources available on demand thus can facilitate the production of the ANN system both by increasing the number of experiments that can run and by decreasing the time of each experiment.

IMPACT OF CLOUD COMPUTING ON CYTOPATHOLOGY DAILY WORKFLOW

- **Knowledge of IT:** Until now, cytopathologists had total responsibility for the laboratory's IT infrastructure, by having the authority to decide which IT element could improve daily laboratory workflow. In the Cloud computing era, cytopathologists are expected to use IT services without having to take control over the infrastructure that supports it.

- **Costing:** Cloud computing permits cytopathology end users to use hardware and software stored remotely over the Cloud-based systems, without having to purchase them, but rather to apply a pay-per-use model.
- Using cloud computing, various cytology and medical applications are delivered as a service over the Internet, which is named software as a service (SaaS software).
- **Integration:** Cloud computing can provide a software platform for laboratory information systems, remote image review software (telecytology) and billing software to cytopathologists, having remote access to all applications by using computers or tablets over the Internet.

How Does Cloud Computing Benefit the Cytopathology Department?

Cloud computing allows administrators of cytopathology departments to take advantage of virtual imaging possibilities without having to maintain any software or hardware. Cytopathologists only have to maintain a single central processing unit.

This system permits cytopathologists to focus on their diagnostic practice and not how or where the service is hosted or processed.

FEW CASES ILLUSTRATING THE ROLE OF CLOUD COMPUTING IN CYTOPATHOLOGY

Advantages of Cloud Computing in Cytopathology

Cytopathology laboratories can benefit from the Cloud by using it in order to:

- Store data
- Increase productivity
- Make new software and extra storage available as and when required
- Provide access to patient data, billing, insurance, reports outside the hospital
- Archive studies
- Maintain directories
- Conduct examinations
- Maintain access control, manage the bill, and keep an audit trail for telecytology purposes
- Decrease costs on infrastructure
- Ensure system maintenance, performance, and security by professional agencies

Shortcomings in Cloud Computing

Cloud computing protected patient data is stored remotely and is sent and received through the Internet. That makes the data vulnerable to security violations. However, solutions may be proposed. The main threats Cloud computing is facing are:

- New threats of data security and privacy, these threats may be anticipated by data encryption during storage and transfer and connecting with the server using an encryption protocol.

- Unauthorized access may be anticipated by passwords and password control mechanisms and via mandatory biometric checks.
- Database safety and long-term archival process in case of emergencies and natural disasters have to be discussed with the Cloud computing service provider in detail.
- Server failures may be avoided by maintaining mirror servers.
- The efficiency of service, related to broadband speed may be ensured by the hospital cooperation with multiple Internet service providers to prevent disruption of service.
- The increased load can be easily handled by adding more processing power to existing virtual servers and/or by splitting the application to run on multiple servers, either via load balancing or by the exploitation of multi-tier architectures and by splitting to one or more separate application servers and database servers.

THE USE OF MOBILE HEALTH APPLICATIONS FOR ACCREDITATION PURPOSES IN A PRIVATE CYTOPATHOLOGY LABORATORY

Safety and Input Optimization of Clinical Information

A modern cytopathology laboratory's information system is secured from unauthorized internal and external access and preserves the confidentiality of health records, according to national law and regulations. Different levels of security are available.

Mobile Health applications will be used for remote log-in access to ordering and reporting systems via a secure web browser and will also allow reliable electronic signatures for data authentication.

Regarding test ordering, Mobile Health applications will be used for providing immediate feedback to all users. They will be used for guiding clinicians on how to order the appropriate cytological examinations while the clinicians are allowed and encouraged to enter the order directly into the system.

In the future, Mobile Health applications will be used for receiving inputs from clinicians that will have to include the following information:

- Ordering physician information (name, specialty, address, contact media for routine notification, contact information for critical result notification)
- Patient information (patient demographics, including date of birth/age, sex, location, results of laboratory and non-laboratory tests, medications, medical procedures applied to the patient, gynecologic and obstetric information, other pertinent clinical information)

Management of Biological Specimens and Laboratory Orders

In the future, Mobile Health applications will possess a user-friendly display of the test catalog with available alternative groupings. They will be used for relaying orders to different interfaced systems without manual intervention so that tests ordered in one facility can enable specimens to be collected and accessioned at another location. Also, they will be used for keeping a list of the reference laboratories available to the ordering provider and for generating a report with sender, receiver and shipping information. Furthermore, they will be able to split clinicians' orders, track the progress and report the status of each component separately under one order.

In addition, new aspects for optimizing specimen collection and processing will be gradually introduced into the Mobile Health applications, such as:

- Specimen collection lists as appropriate to laboratory operation
- Printed and electronic guidelines to the specimen collectors with a comprehensive display of proper instructions
- List of pending laboratory orders
- Automatic generation of unique barcoded labels
- Automatic recording of patient information, location, date and time of collection, and collector identity

In the future, Mobile Health applications will be used for interfacing with laboratory automation management software to ensure that all the pre-analytic requirements stipulated in the ordering process are transmitting to the specimen-processing system. These applications will be used for tracking the specimen location throughout the pre-analytic, analytic, and post-analytic phases, including transportation to various sections of the laboratory or external sites, and management of specimen storage.

Regarding optimizing the analytic phase, future Mobile Health applications will support:

- Tracking of all the components necessary for testing and association with individual testing records
- Generation of printed and electronic versions of appropriate standardized operating procedures for each test upon request by the cytopathologist
- Generation of laboratory-specific workload lists
- Generation of "Incomplete Lists" of tests that have been accessioned but not completed, highlighting those that have exceeded the stated time for the category of the request
- Generation of lists of incomplete or unfulfilled orders

Management of Testing Results and Diagnostic Reports

Mobile Health applications will be gradually involved in optimizing the result entry and validation through the integration of:

- Ability to record results in various data formats
- Automated and manual entry and correction of results of tests, with appropriate security levels applied
- Application of different levels of result certification
- Reception of results in a variety of formats from other laboratories, including external reference laboratories, through electronic interfaces
- Utilization of advanced expert decision support for auto-validation of results. Inputs used to arrive at an auto-validation decision include comparison with results of previous tests in the patient record, comparison with results of other related tests in the same or closely related specimens, statistical data on result distribution)

Regarding optimizing result reporting, future Mobile Health applications will support:

- Generation of reports with information on both laboratory staff and recipients (clinicians, patients) of the test
- Generation of reports available by user-configurable automated secure faxing and e-mailing
- Sophisticated graphing of laboratory results
- Ability to incorporate, in the result, comments hyperlinks to pages containing further test information
- Ability to append appropriate interpretative comments on test results

These applications will be used for optimizing notification management through the addition of new services such as:

- Possession of a sophisticated "significant result" notification system that includes multiple tiers of urgency for significant result notification
- Utilization of dynamic rules to determine whether a result is critical
- Utilization of a rule-based notification of appropriate third parties
- Rapid update and notification about any changes or corrections to laboratory results

Also, these will efficiently optimize data mining and cross-sectional reports through:

- Ability to perform queries into the laboratory and clinical databases
- Search functions for combinations of laboratory results and clinical information
- Production of laboratory testing turn-around time reports with the ability to consolidate or split the various components
- Online reporting of surveillance data to public health agencies in their required format, using the appropriate standards

Optimization of Laboratory Quality Management and Other Functionalities

In the future, Mobile Health applications will be used for optimizing Quality management, by using a module that supports accreditation requirements, including International Organization for Standardization (ISO) 15189:2012 standards and includes the following functionalities:

- QC protocols and alerting mechanisms that use thresholds for acceptability
- Linkage of each patient test result to the relevant QC results in an easily retrievable record
- Automated alerts to appropriate staff to perform QC tasks
- Active QC rules and reports customizable by test
- Ability to document corrective actions resulting from QC failure in real time
- Ability to remove outliers and erroneous results from QC calculations
- Ability to provide user-definable QC summary reports for review by supervisory and management staff
- Ability to manage proficiency-testing (PT) programs, from inventory control of PT materials to documenting PT results and investigation of PT failures
- Ability to manage accreditation requirements online, including preparation of appropriate documents

Regarding incorporating advanced administrative and financial functionalities, future Mobile Health applications will support:

- Ability to generate and transmit the necessary forms and notifications for reimbursement of tests
- Intelligent generation of online and printed regulatory forms associated with laboratory testing, billing, compliance, and accreditation
- Tracking of costs of laboratory operation
- Analysis of profitability, pricing and outreach client management capabilities
- Ability to produce periodic reports of laboratory productivity and management efficiency, by using aggregate numbers and individual cost and productivity analysis per test
- Automated ordering from selected suppliers and real-time tracking of budget
- Tracking of human resource databases, labor-cost accounting, and credentials, competency, continuing education training, and performance appraisals

ISSUES, CONTROVERSIES, PROBLEMS

The implementation of ISO 15189:2012 guidelines in medical laboratories information systems presents some problems that need further analysis. Medical data that is stored and retrieved from a laboratory information system contains valuable information that needs to remain confidential. The widespread use of computers makes access to classified documents easier than ever. The use of electronic signature in medical reports may diminish bureaucratic problems but, on the other hand, makes the laboratory information system more vulnerable. The laboratory management has to implement specific policies that will protect medical data from unauthorized access but will not endanger cooperation between medical and laboratory information systems (Shen & Yang, 2001; Vacata et al., 2007).

Laboratory personnel training in informatics is necessary for ensuring the efficient function of the laboratory information system. The laboratory management has to plan personnel training in such a way that the main laboratory function will not be put in danger (Shen & Yang, 2001; Vacata et al., 2007). Poor hardware maintenance or improper use by inadequately trained personnel may cause a laboratory information system failure. Laboratory reports may be lost or deteriorated due to malignant software (virus programs), while LIS hardware may be damaged by adverse environmental conditions, such as heat, humidity or a possible fire, due to the vulnerability of wires and cables to unfavorable environmental conditions (Vacata et al., 2007; Westbrook et al., 2008). Finally, medical data stored only in electronic mediums may be easily lost due to a system's unexpected failure (Vacata et al., 2007). All these possible threats of a laboratory information system require the implementation of specific measures and policies that may have a considerable economic impact, or may even prove non-affordable. The laboratory management handles the development of an economic plan, after taking into account the specific laboratory resources and needs (Shen & Yang, 2001; Westbrook et al., 2008).

The implementation of Mobile Health technology in medical laboratories information systems causes some problems that need further evaluation. The main threats Mobile Health technology is anticipating in the field of Medical Informatics are:

- New threats of data security and privacy, these threats may be anticipated by data encryption during storage and transfer and connecting with the server using encryption protocols

- Unauthorized access may be anticipated by passwords and password control mechanisms and via mandatory biometric checks
- Database safety and long-term archival process in case of emergencies and natural disasters have to be discussed with the Mobile Health technology service provider in detail
- Server failures may be avoided by maintaining mirror servers
- The efficiency of service, related to broadband speed may be ensured by the hospital cooperation with multiple Internet service providers to prevent disruption of service
- The increased load can be easily handled by adding more processing power to existing virtual servers and/or by splitting the application to run on multiple servers

The implementation of telemedical applications for proficiency testing purposes in medical laboratories wishing accreditation presents some problems that need further analysis. In conventional cytology, specific diagnostic criteria and pitfalls are already described. During static telecytological diagnosis, the cytopathologist has to use the same diagnostic criteria and to avoid the same pitfalls. What makes the telecytological diagnosis more demanding is the uncertainty about the real specimen's adequacy or the representativity of the selected images (Archondakis et al., 2009). Static digital images suffer from representing only limited portions of the specimen, and hence there is a potential bias of the image acquirer relative to the image observer. The inability of image focusing and image manipulating (contrast, brightness, and color) may cause additional problems.

Cytology slides used for digital images must be validated in order to make sure that the initial cytological diagnosis was correct and did not differ significantly from the final histological diagnosis.

Reporting terminology is well-established for some categories of cytological specimens such as thyroid fine needle aspiration specimens and cervicovaginal smears. Still, cytological diagnosis for the majority of specimens remains descriptive, and no specific diagnostic categories have been established and implemented in the everyday laboratory practice. The absence of a universally accepted and adopted reporting terminology is a serious problem for the correct statistical elaboration of cytological diagnoses provided by participants in a proficiency testing scheme. A widely accepted reporting terminology would make easier the implementation of scoring systems, validating participants' performance and improvement.

Participation in proficiency testing programs is still weak. Many large Cytological Departments are reluctant to implement such practices as a measure of continuous improvement and quality assurance. Even when a proficiency testing program is ordered, only one or two certified cytopathologists are participating.

Last but not least, digital images storage and transmission must follow strict regulations to avoid any unauthorized alteration or improper use (Mun, Elsayed, Tohme, & Wu, 1995). Current standards of electronic medical data handling are still informative, yet the need for a secure electronic environment, especially in the field of static telecytology, continues to grow.

SOLUTIONS AND RECOMMENDATIONS

A modern cytopathology laboratory may need to cooperate in real time with a cytopathology laboratory in a remote location. In order to send or receive images in real time, a modern cytopathology laboratory can push the images into a Mobile Health application, enabling the cytopathologists to review images at nodal centers, without having to buy additional software and hardware. Here, the Mobile Health application works as a gateway to the peripheral center where all its information is available on the Mobile Health.

Mobile Health applications are affordable for all cytopathology departments and give the opportunity to all scientific personnel to participate in proficiency testing programs, even when there is a significant time difference among participating laboratories. Moreover, laboratory management should encourage personal participation of all scientific personnel in such proficiency testing programs (Pinco, Goulart, Otis, Garb, & Pantanowitz, 2009).

Proper Education and Training of Laboratory Personnel

Before new software or hardware is introduced in a laboratory, the risk connected with such an introduction should be assessed (Vacata et al., 2007). A risk assessment should include identification of possible events, which may result in non-compliance, estimation of their likelihood, identification of their consequences, and ways of avoiding them, costs, drawbacks, and benefits (Vacata et al., 2007). Good knowledge of computer software and hardware details is also essential for maintenance, troubleshooting, and update. Medical laboratory personnel have to be periodically trained in the use of new computer facilities and new software products. Their training may be extremely difficult. Therefore, the laboratory director has to encourage these training sessions and continuously motivate its personnel (Pearlman, Wolfert, Miele, Bilello, & Stauffer, 2001; Westbrook, Georgiou, & Rob, 2008).

Moreover, we have to take into account that computer facilities maintenance is of paramount importance in the workflow of a medical laboratory. Therefore, the laboratory personnel should take specific measures for protecting the hardware (Markin & Whalen, 2000; Sciacovelli, Secchiero, Zardo, D'Osualdo, & Plebani, 2007). These measures should be documented in specific procedures to include aspects of:

- How to operate a computer
- How to maintain and clean the computer and its hardware components and peripherals
- What programs are required for specific computer labor and how to install and use them
- How to manage specific files and data-sets
- How to handle internet security programs

Hardware-Related Implemented Laboratory Procedures

The hardware should also be fully protected from any actual damages, and especially fire (Markin & Whalen, 2000; Sciacovelli et al., 2007; Vacata et al., 2007). The measures should be documented in specific procedures, and might include:

- Installation and periodical testing of smoke alarms and fire extinguishers
- Storage and use of heating sources and flammable items
- Control of electrical wires and cables regarding connection networking and proper maintenance

The provision of an uninterruptible power supply will protect the computer from crashing during power outages, or from low and high voltage occurrences (Markin & Whalen, 2000; Sciacovelli et al., 2007). A UPS is much better than a surge protector and can save the laboratory computer facilities from virtually any type of power failure.

Medical records and computer facilities should also be well protected from unauthorized access (Markin & Whalen, 2000; Sciacovelli et al., 2007). The laboratory should establish guidelines for the protection of medical data from unauthorized access, which should:

- Protect all laboratory data and information
- Analyze access methods based on standards
- Use the standard application methods wherever possible
- Designate personnel responsible for the integrity of specific data-sets
- Restrict access to data and information and relative editing privileges to authorized individuals only

The laboratory should also obtain a complete record of all preventive actions concerning computer maintenance (Markin & Whalen, 2000; Sciacovelli et al., 2007). Hardware preventive maintenance is the best way to reduce all factors threatening or shortening the computer's life dramatically. The laboratory should implement specific procedures referring to many issues, such as:

- Excessive heat prevention
- Dust removal
- Magnetism radiated electromagnetic interference and static electricity prevention
- Power surges, incorrect line voltage, and power outages handling
- Water and corrosive agents prevention

Software-Related Implemented Laboratory Procedures

Software preventive maintenance is achieved by using anti-virus applications, defragmentation software and testing utility programs (Markin & Whalen, 2000; Sciacovelli et al., 2007). The laboratory should/must implement specific procedures referring to many issues, such as:

- Proper activation/deactivation and utilization of computer and installed programs
- Systematic backup recovery and proper management of files and data-sets
- Scheduled hardware cleaning and maintenance and periodical software security and integrity verification by authorized personnel. System's maintenance should be scheduled in such a way that it will not interrupt patient-care service

Every modification of the system hardware and software should be documented and verified while all computer problems and malfunctions should be analytically reported. Corrective action must be taken in order to avoid these problems in the future.

Specific Scoring Systems and Reporting Terminologies for Cytological Specimens

In the field of telecytology applied for accreditation purposes, the role of the person appointed to image capture and transmission is of paramount importance for the success of a static telecytology system. In our study, the person who captures and transmits the digital images is an already certified cytopathologist with adequate experience in conventional cytological diagnosis. Less specialized personnel, such as inexperienced screeners, may endanger the acquisition of representative images from each cytological slide (Archondakis et al., 2009).

Besides the histological examination, other measures for cytology slides validation must be adopted in order to avoid possible indiscriminate failure of qualified, competent personnel (Nagy & Newton, 2006). Such measures may be verification of cytological diagnosis by a board certified, well-trained, scientific personnel, the establishment of specific scoring system and reporting terminology for all kinds of cytological specimens and finally capturing of a significant number of representative images by certified well-trained personnel (Nagy & Newton, 2006).

The scoring system and reporting terminology may be simplified. Specific scoring systems and reporting terminologies should be established for each kind of cytological specimens in order to ensure that the cytological diagnoses reflect the clinical implications associated with this terminology in modern practice, particularly regarding recommended follow-up (Williams, Mullick, Butler, Herring, & O'Leary T, 2001).

Participation of Laboratory Staff in Proficiency Testing Schemes

Cytology scientific societies should focus on cytology proficiency testing particularities and define particular technical aspects such as images' size and analysis, suggested testing intervals, diagnostic categories and methodology used for statistical evaluation of the proficiency testing results (Nagy & Newton, 2006).

Static telecytological systems are affordable by all cytopathology departments and give the opportunity to all scientific personnel to participate in proficiency testing programs, even when there is a significant time difference among participating laboratories (Raab et al., 1996). Laboratory management should encourage personal participation of all scientific personnel in such proficiency testing programs (Pinco et al., 2009). Laboratory management must have in mind that proficiency testing programs proffered by static digital images can improve the professional skills of the participating medical staff and make them feel more confident in their daily work.

Proficiency testing providers should ensure that the personnel appointed to image capture and transmission has adequate experience in both conventional and image-based diagnosis. Previous experience in that field should be well-documented and recorded (Nagy & Newton, 2006).

It is expected that Cloud computing will be further exploited by cytopathology laboratories wishing to improve their quality standards. One of the major challenges of Cloud computing will be to resolve possible problems regarding data safety and security. A possible solution could be a multi-cloud approach with a key sharing mechanism (Mouli & Sesadri, 2013) and patient identification cross reference numbers (Kondoh, Teramoto, Kawai, Mochida, & Nishimura, 2013).

In the distant future, it is expected that the cytopathology departments will witness a large-scale migration to Cloud-based LIS due to ease of availability and low cost of ownership and maintenance.

In relation to the research activities, as sequencing costs are continuously becoming lower, nowadays it is not only possible but extremely easier for genomics researchers to have large amounts of data. The increasing availability of computational power according to Moore's low and the falling overhead for data storage, give the scientists the opportunity not only to create and store large genetic data sets over the course of their research but it is possible to process them. However, the majority of the laboratories, have already become, or will soon become, oversubscribed and underpowered about the exploitation of data. Unavailable software and lack of computational power to run exhaustive search algorithms, eventually, will lead many researchers towards cloud computing to conduct their research. Alternatively, much of the minable information may remain untouched, underutilized and not adequately explored. As a bonus, cloud computing provides the means for data sharing among research teams; thus, larger data sets can be exploited, more robust results and conclusions related to rear diseases can be obtained.

FUTURE RESEARCH DIRECTIONS

Telecytology, when integrated into the daily workflow, can provide exceptional consultation and professional testing opportunities to distant laboratories. Static telecytology systems are preferred by laboratories that cannot afford the high cost of buying and maintaining dynamic systems. In any case, the cost of participation in a running telecytology program is inexpensive for small cytopathology departments (Archondakis et al., 2009; Nagy & Newton, 2006). Provincial hospitals, where immediate scientific collaboration and support is necessary, can take advantage of this excellent opportunity to improve their cytology services (Archondakis et al., 2009).

It is expected that Cloud computing will be further exploited by cytopathology laboratories wishing to improve their quality standards. The primary challenge of Cloud computing will be to resolve possible problems regarding data safety.

In the distant future, it is expected that the cytopathology departments will witness a large-scale migration to Cloud-based LIS due to its easy availability and its low cost.

Future research must focus on the details of the implementation of a low-cost Mobile Health based application for proficiency testing purposes, that is determining the required testing interval, elucidating the validation criteria applied to the electronic material used for proficiency testing purposes and possibly changing the focus of the test from individuals to laboratory level testing.

The diagnostic reliability of telecytology provides the potential for the further amelioration of the laboratory services, by producing digital educational material for use in web-based training systems (Stergiou et al., 2009). Those programs can improve the professional skills of the participating medical staff and make them feel more confident in their daily work (Stergiou et al., 2009).

The use of ISO 15189:2012 requirements in electronic data storage and retrieval are expanding, and many informative clauses of the standard are expected to become normative shortly. A net of accredited laboratories is globally expanding (Kubono, 2007; Pearlman et al., 2001). Many more countries will incorporate ISO 15189 requirements in their national or local regulations. Medical laboratories that will develop the most innovative and up to date procedures for electronic medical reporting and storage will become referral laboratories for their countries or regions (Kubono, 2007; Murai, 2002; Okada, 2002, Pouliakis et al., 2014a, 2014b).

All laboratories notices concerning the implementation of the ISO 15189:2012 are collected by an international working group, which handles the revision of the standards when necessary. Problems that might be reported to this international working group are examined, and suitable solutions will be incorporated in the standard's future editions or specific guidelines (Kubono, 2007; Murai, 2002; Okada, 2002, Pouliakis et al., 2014a, 2014b).

Future research must focus on the details of the implementation of a static telecytological application for proficiency testing purposes, that is, determining the required testing interval, elucidating the validation criteria applied to the electronic material used for proficiency testing purposes and possibly changing the focus of the test from individuals to laboratory level testing.

Considering the future of Mobile Health technology in Cytopathology, it is expected that Mobile Health technology will be further exploited by cytopathology laboratories wishing to improve their quality standards. One of the major challenges of Mobile Health technology will be to resolve possible problems regarding data safety and security. A possible solution could be a multi-Mobile Health approach with a key sharing mechanism (Mouli & Sesadri, 2013) and patient identification cross reference numbers (Kondoh, Teramoto, Kawai, Mochida, & Nishimura, 2013).

In the distant future, it is expected that the cytopathology departments will witness a large-scale migration to Mobile Health-based LIS due to ease of availability and low cost of ownership and maintenance.

In relation to the research activities, as sequencing costs are continuously becoming lower, nowadays it is not only possible but extremely easier for genomics researchers to have large amounts of data. The increasing availability of computational power according to Moore's Law and the falling overhead for data storage, give the scientists the opportunity not only to create and store large genetic data-sets over the course of their research but it is possible to process them. However, the majority of the laboratories, have already become, or will soon become, oversubscribed and underpowered about the exploitation of data. Unavailable software and lack of computational power to run exhaustive search algorithms, eventually, will lead many researchers towards Mobile Health technology to conduct their research. Alternatively, much of the minable information may remain untouched, underutilized and not properly explored. As a bonus, Mobile Health technology provides the means for data sharing among research teams. Thus, larger data-sets can be exploited, more robust results and conclusions related to rear diseases can be obtained.

Shortly, cytopathology laboratory information systems will be able to record large data-sets and interface with legacy systems to capture historical laboratory data, with the goal of storing life-long results for each patient. Capabilities for handling large genomic data-sets will be increasingly necessary for future LIS.

Shortly, cytopathology laboratory information systems will have to capture industry standards for coding, billing, document generation, and interface formats, such as CDC, HL7 CDA1/2, XML, ASC X12, LOINC, SNOMED-CT, ICD-9, or ICD-10, as appropriate for each data type. The user interface and navigation will become more user-friendly. The LIS will minimize the number of keystrokes required for all activities and will be uniform for similar tasks within the software.

In addition, all screens and reports will be printed and exported in the appropriate document text, spreadsheet, or graphics formats, while fully functional text editors will be used in text entry fields.

Moreover, cytopathology laboratory information systems will use interfaces that will be flexible in data formats and fully functional with appropriate routines available for testing the functionality of the interfaces before using them to meet end-user expectations.

The cytopathology laboratory information systems will be able to integrate instant messaging, forum, online meeting, and social-networking capabilities while they will become powerful enough to perform multiple functions simultaneously with an imperceptible impact on their speed.

CONCLUSION

The standard ISO 15189:2012 includes direct and indirect references to the requirements concerning the implementation of laboratory information systems in medical laboratories. These requirements constitute a powerful tool for medical laboratories wishing to improve the quality of their laboratory information system because they diminish the possibility of human error or unexpected hardware or software failure dramatically. Laboratories should only specify the procedures to be followed according to their needs.

Laboratory informatics is critical to meet current and future challenges. Many of these challenges can be met by advancing technologies, such as improving the integration of disparate information systems, automation, specimen tracking, electronic document management systems, and streamlining procedures.

Telecytology can be used as an economical method for the implementation of QA programs in the everyday laboratory practice, provided that representative images be taken, standard diagnostic criteria are applied, and the participants have already acquired sufficient experience in the evaluation of digital images. The use of static telecytology systems for proficiency testing provision is possible, and the first steps towards this direction are already made in Greece.

Mobile Health technology promotes the concept of bedside, point-of-care, and instant cytopathology. It gives the cytopathologists, pathologists, physicians, and even patients the possibility to review images and medical data via any display device with Internet connection. Furthermore, Mobile Health technology will play a significant role in the patient-centered healthcare since each patient can be associated with a unique individual EMR, that once created, could be easily accessible by numerous physicians and doctors (if needed or required) so as to promote efficient professional collaboration in the effort to define and apply the most ideal clinical healthcare and management plan suitable to the unique medical profile of each patient making a way towards the concept of "personalized medicine".

Mobile Health technology is expected to provide flexibility to all cytopathology services and has the potential to revolutionize the way cytopathology data will be stored, accessed, and processed.

REFERENCES

Al-Janabi, S., Huisman, A., Willems, S. M., & Van Diest, P. J. (2012). Digital slide images for primary diagnostics in breast pathology: A feasibility study. *Human Pathology*, *43*(12), 2318–2325. doi:10.1016/j.humpath.2012.03.027 PMID:22901465

Archondakis, S. (2013). The Use of Static Telemedical Applications of Cytopathology for Proficiency Testing. *International Journal of Reliable and Quality E-Healthcare*, *2*(2), 47–53. doi:10.4018/ijrqeh.2013040104

Archondakis, S. (2014). *Static Telecytological Applications for Proficiency Testing. In Nanotechnology: Concepts, Methodologies, Tools, and Applications* (pp. 556–568). Hershey, PA: Information Science Reference. doi:10.4018/978-1-4666-5125-8.ch023

Archondakis, S. (2015). The Use of Information Systems in a Modern Cytopathology Laboratory. In A. Moumtzoglou, A. Kastania, & S. Archondakis (Eds.), *Laboratory Management Information Systems: Current Requirements and Future Perspectives* (pp. 208–236). Hershey, PA: Medical Information Science Reference. doi:10.4018/978-1-4666-6320-6.ch011

Archondakis, S., Georgoulakis, J., Stamataki, M., Anninos, D., Skagias, L., Panayiotides, I., & Karakitsos, P. (2009). Telecytology: A tool for quality assessment and improvement in the evaluation of thyroid fine-needle aspiration specimens. *Telemedicine Journal and e-Health*, *15*(7), 713–717. doi:10.1089/tmj.2009.0037 PMID:19694595

Archondakis, S., Stathopoulou, A., & Sitaras, I. (2011). ISO 15189:2007: Implementation in a Laboratory Information System. In A. Moumtzoglou & A. Kastania (Eds.), *E-Health Systems Quality and Reliability: Models and Standards* (pp. 64–72). Hershey, PA: Medical Information Science Reference. doi:10.4018/978-1-61692-843-8.ch006

Astion, M. L., & Wilding, P. (1992). Application of neural networks to the interpretation of laboratory data in cancer diagnosis. *Clinical Chemistry*, *38*(1), 34–38. PMID:1733603

Boon, M. E., Kok, L. P., & Under, J. (1993). Neural network processing can provide means to catch errors that slip through human screening of pap smears. *Diagnostic Cytopathology*, *9*(4), 411–416. doi:10.1002/dc.2840090408 PMID:8261846

Brender, J., & McNair, P. (1996). User requirements on the future laboratory information systems. *Computer Methods and Programs in Biomedicine*, *50*(2), 87–93. doi:10.1016/0169-2607(96)01738-Q PMID:8875016

Briscoe, D., Adair, C. F., Thompson, L. D., Tellado, M. V., Buckner, S. B., Rosenthal, D. L., & O'Leary, T. J. (2000). Telecytologic diagnosis of breast fine needle aspiration biopsies. Intraobserver concordance. *Acta Cytologica*, *44*(2), 175–180. doi:10.1159/000326357 PMID:10740603

Casebeer, L. L., Strasser, S. M., Spettell, C. M., Wall, T. C., Weissman, N., Ray, M. N., & Allison, J. J. (2003). Designing tailored Web-based instruction to improve practicing physicians' preventive practices. *Journal of Medical Internet Research*, *5*(3), e20. doi:10.2196/jmir.5.3.e20 PMID:14517111

Cochand-Priollet, B., Koutroumbas, K., Megalopoulou, T. M., Pouliakis, A., Sivolapenko, G., & Karakitsos, P. (2006). Discriminating benign from malignant thyroid lesions using artificial intelligence and statistical selection of morphometric features. *Oncology Reports*, *15*, 1023–1026. PMID:16525694

Demichelis, F., Della Mea, V., Forti, S., Dalla Palma, P., & Beltrami, C. A. (2002). Digital storage of glass slides for quality assurance in histopathology and cytopathology. *Journal of Telemedicine and Telecare*, *8*(3), 138–142. doi:10.1177/1357633X0200800303 PMID:12097174

Dey, P., Logasundaram, R., & Joshi, K. (2013). Artificial neural network in diagnosis of lobular carcinoma of breast in fine-needle aspiration cytology. *Diagnostic Cytopathology*, *41*(2), 102–106. doi:10.1002/dc.21773 PMID:21987420

Drozdov, I., Ouzounis, C. A., Shah, A. M., & Tsoka, S. (2011). Functional Genomics Assistant (FUGA): A toolbox for the analysis of complex biological networks. *BMC Research Notes*, *4*(1), 462. doi:10.1186/1756-0500-4-462 PMID:22035155

Eugster, M. J., Schmid, M., Binder, H., & Schmidberger, M. (2013). Grid and cloud computing methods in biomedical research. *Methods of Information in Medicine*, *52*(1), 62–64. PMID:23318694

Fowsantear, W., Argo, E., Pattinson, C., & Cash, P. (2013). Comparative proteomics of Helicobacter species: The discrimination of gastric and enterohepatic Helicobacter species. *Journal of Proteomics*. doi:10.1016/j.jprot.2013.07.016 PMID:23899588

Fung, K. M., Hassell, L. A., Talbert, M. L., Wiechmann, A. F., Chaser, B. E., & Ramey, J. (2012). Whole slide images and digital media in pathology education, testing, and practice: The Oklahoma experience. *Analytical Cellular Pathology (Amsterdam)*, *35*(1), 37–40. doi:10.1155/2012/103857 PMID:21965282

Gagnon, M., Inhorn, S., Hancock, J., Keller, B., Carpenter, D., Merlin, T., ... Whalen, R. (2004). Comparison of cytology proficiency testing: Glass slides vs. virtual slides. *Acta Cytologica, 48*(6), 788–794. doi:10.1159/000326447 PMID:15581163

Garrison, J. A., Schardt, C., & Kochi, J. K. (2000). Web-based distance continuing education: A new way of thinking for students and instructors. *Bulletin of the Medical Library Association, 88*(3), 211–217. PMID:10928706

Georgiou, A., & Westbrook, J. I. (2006). Computerised Order Entry Systems and Pathology Services - A Synthesis of the Evidence. *The Clinical Biochemist. Reviews / Australian Association of Clinical Biochemists, 27*(2), 79–87. PMID:17077878

Ghaznavi, F., Evans, A., Madabhushi, A., & Feldman, M. (2013). Digital imaging in pathology: Whole-slide imaging and beyond. *Annual Review of Pathology, 8*(1), 331–359. doi:10.1146/annurev-pathol-011811-120902 PMID:23157334

Giovagnoli, M. R., Cenci, M., Olla, S. V., & Vecchione, A. (2002). Cervical false negative cases detected by neural network-based technology. Critical review of cytologic errors. *Acta Cytologica, 46*(6), 1105–1109. doi:10.1159/000327115 PMID:12462090

Glaser, J. (2011). Cloud computing can simplify HIT infrastructure management. *Healthcare Financial Management, 65*(8), 52–55. PMID:21866720

GlobalData. (2012). *Snapshot: The US cloud computing market for medical imaging*. Retrieved 22/08/2013, from http://www.medicaldevice-network.com/features/featuresnapshot-the-us-cloud-computing-market-for-medical-imaging

Greenbaum, D., & Gerstein, M. (2011). The role of cloud computing in managing the deluge of potentially private genetic data. *The American Journal of Bioethics, 11*(11), 39–41. doi:10.1080/15265161.2011.608242 PMID:22047125

Gutman, D. A., Cobb, J., Somanna, D., Park, Y., Wang, F., Kurc, T., ... Cooper, L. A. (2013). Cancer Digital Slide Archive: An informatics resource to support integrated in silico analysis of TCGA pathology data. *Journal of the American Medical Informatics Association, 20*(6), 1091–1098. doi:10.1136/amiajnl-2012-001469 PMID:23893318

Halligan, B. D., Geiger, J. F., Vallejos, A. K., Greene, A. S., & Twigger, S. N. (2009). Low cost, scalable proteomics data analysis using Amazon's cloud computing services and open source search algorithms. *Journal of Proteome Research, 8*(6), 3148–3153. doi:10.1021/pr800970z PMID:19358578

Haymart, M. R., Cayo, M., & Chen, H. (2009). Papillary thyroid microcarcinomas: Big decisions for a small tumor. *Annals of Surgical Oncology, 16*(11), 3132–3139. doi:10.124510434-009-0647-6 PMID:19653044

Hipp, J. D., Lucas, D. R., Emmert-Buck, M. R., Compton, C. C., & Balis, U. J. (2011). Digital slide repositories for publications: Lessons learned from the microarray community. *The American Journal of Surgical Pathology, 35*(6), 783–786. doi:10.1097/PAS.0b013e31821946b6 PMID:21552111

Izadi-Mood, N., Sarmadi, S., & Sanii, S. (2013). Quality control in cervicovaginal cytology by cytohistological correlation. *Cytopathology*, *24*(1), 33–38. doi:10.1111/j.1365-2303.2011.00926.x PMID:21929578

Jemal, A., Bray, F., Center, M. M., Ferlay, J., Ward, E., & Forman, D. (2011). Global cancer statistics. *CA: a Cancer Journal for Clinicians*, *61*(2), 69–90. doi:10.3322/caac.20107 PMID:21296855

Karakitsos, P., Cochand-Priollet, B., Pouliakis, A., Guillausseau, P. J., & Ioakim-Liossi, A. (1999). Learning vector quantizer in the investigation of thyroid lesions. *Analytical and Quantitative Cytology and Histology*, *21*(3), 201–208. PMID:10560492

Karakitsos, P., Megalopoulou, T. M., Pouliakis, A., Tzivras, M., Archimandritis, A., & Kyroudes, A. (2004). Application of discriminant analysis and quantitative cytologic examination to gastric lesions. *Analytical and Quantitative Cytology and Histology*, *26*(6), 314–322. PMID:15678613

Karakitsos, P., Stergiou, E. B., Pouliakis, A., Tzivras, M., Archimandritis, A., Liossi, A. I., & Kyrkou, K. (1996). Potential of the back propagation neural network in the discrimination of benign from malignant gastric cells. *Analytical and Quantitative Cytology and Histology*, *18*(3), 245–250. PMID:8790840

Khurana, K. K. (2012). Telecytology and its evolving role in cytopathology. *Diagnostic Cytopathology*, *40*(6), 498–502. doi:10.1002/dc.22822 PMID:22619124

Kondoh, H., Teramoto, K., Kawai, T., Mochida, M., & Nishimura, M. (2013). Development of the regional EPR and PACS sharing system on the infrastructure of cloud computing technology controlled by patient identifier cross reference manager. *Studies in Health Technology and Informatics*, *192*, 1073. PMID:23920847

Konganti, K., Wang, G., Yang, E., & Cai, J. J. (2013). SBEToolbox: A Matlab Toolbox for Biological Network Analysis. *Evolutionary Bioinformatics Online*, *9*, 355–362. doi:10.4137/EBO.S12012 PMID:24027418

Krishnamurthy, S., Mathews, K., McClure, S., Murray, M., Gilcrease, M., Albarracin, C., ... Liang, K. (2013). Multi-Institutional Comparison of Whole Slide Digital Imaging and Optical Microscopy for Interpretation of Hematoxylin-Eosin-Stained Breast Tissue Sections. *Archives of Pathology & Laboratory Medicine*, *137*(12), 1733–1739. doi:10.5858/arpa.2012-0437-OA PMID:23947655

Kubono, K. (2004). Quality management system in the medical laboratory--ISO15189 and laboratory accreditation. *Rinsho Byori*, *52*(3), 274–278. PMID:15137330

Kubono, K. (2007). Outline of the revision of ISO 15189 and accreditation of medical laboratory for specified health checkup. *Rinsho Byori*, *55*(11), 1029–1036. PMID:18154036

Kuo, A. M. (2011). Opportunities and challenges of cloud computing to improve health care services. *Journal of Medical Internet Research*, *13*(3), e67. doi:10.2196/jmir.1867 PMID:21937354

Landis, J. R., & Koch, G. G. (1977). The measurement of observer agreement for categorical data. *Biometrics*, *33*(1), 159–174. doi:10.2307/2529310 PMID:843571

Lee, J., Kim, S., Kim, P., Liu, X., Lee, T., Kim, K. M., ... Kang, W. K. (2013). A novel proteomics-based clinical diagnostics technology identifies heterogeneity in activated signaling pathways in gastric cancers. *PLoS One*, *8*(1), e54644. doi:10.1371/journal.pone.0054644 PMID:23372746

Leprevost, F. V., Lima, D. B., Crestani, J., Perez-Riverol, Y., Zanchin, N., Barbosa, V. C., & Carvalho, P. C. (2013). Pinpointing differentially expressed domains in complex protein mixtures with the cloud service of PatternLab for Proteomics. *Journal of Proteomics, 89*, 179–182. doi:10.1016/j.jprot.2013.06.013 PMID:23796493

Li, G., Zhao, F., & Cui, Y. (2013). Proteomics using mammospheres as a model system to identify proteins deregulated in breast cancer stem cells. *Current Molecular Medicine, 13*(3), 459–463. PMID:23331018

Lupse, O. S., Vida, M., & Stoicu-Tivadar, L. (2012). Cloud computing technology applied in healthcare for developing large scale flexible solutions. *Studies in Health Technology and Informatics, 174*, 94–99. PMID:22491119

Madden, K., Flowers, L., Salani, R., Horowitz, I., Logan, S., Kowalski, K., ... Mohammed, S. I. (2009). Proteomics-based approach to elucidate the mechanism of antitumor effect of curcumin in cervical cancer. *Prostaglandins, Leukotrienes, and Essential Fatty Acids, 80*(1), 9–18. doi:10.1016/j.plefa.2008.10.003 PMID:19058955

Marchevsky, A. M., Tsou, J. A., & Laird-Offringa, I. A. (2004). Classification of individual lung cancer cell lines based on DNA methylation markers: Use of linear discriminant analysis and artificial neural networks. *The Journal of Molecular Diagnostics, 6*(1), 28–36. doi:10.1016/S1525-1578(10)60488-6 PMID:14736824

Markin, R. S., & Whalen, S. A. (2000). Laboratory automation: Trajectory, technology, and tactics. *Clinical Chemistry, 46*(5), 764–771. PMID:10794775

Markopoulos, C., Karakitsos, P., Botsoli-Stergiou, E., Pouliakis, A., Gogas, J., Ioakim-Liossi, A., & Kyrkou, K. (1997). Application of back propagation to the diagnosis of breast lesions by fine needle aspiration. *The Breast, 6*(5), 293–298. doi:10.1016/S0960-9776(97)90008-4

Mirza, H., & El-Masri, S. (2013). National Electronic Medical Records integration on Cloud Computing System. *Studies in Health Technology and Informatics, 192*, 1219. PMID:23920993

Mohammed, Y., Mostovenko, E., Henneman, A. A., Marissen, R. J., Deelder, A. M., & Palmblad, M. (2012). Cloud parallel processing of tandem mass spectrometry based proteomics data. *Journal of Proteome Research, 11*(10), 5101–5108. doi:10.1021/pr300561q PMID:22916831

Mouli, K. C., & Seshadri, U. (2013). Single to Multi Clouds for Security in Cloud Computing by using Secret Key Sharing. *International Journal of Computers and Technology, 10*(4), 1539–1545. doi:10.24297/ijct.v10i4.3254

Mun, S. K., Elsayed, A. M., Tohme, W. G., & Wu, Y. C. (1995). Teleradiology/telepathology requirements and implementation. *Journal of Medical Systems, 19*(2), 153–164. doi:10.1007/BF02257066 PMID:7602247

Murai, T. (2002). Future outlook for LAS, LIS. *Rinsho Byori, 50*(7), 698–701. PMID:12187708

Muth, T., Peters, J., Blackburn, J., Rapp, E., & Martens, L. (2013). ProteoCloud: A full-featured open source proteomics cloud computing pipeline. *Journal of Proteomics, 88*, 104–108. doi:10.1016/j.jprot.2012.12.026 PMID:23305951

Nagy, G. K., & Newton, L. E. (2006). Cytopathology proficiency testing: Where do we go from here? *Diagnostic Cytopathology*, *34*(4), 257–264. doi:10.1002/dc.20361 PMID:16544329

O'Brien, M. J., Takahashi, M., Brugal, G., Christen, H., Gahm, T., Goodell, R. M., ... Winkler, C. (1998). Digital imagery/telecytology. International Academy of Cytology Task Force summary. Diagnostic Cytology Towards the 21st Century: An International Expert Conference and Tutorial. *Acta Cytologica*, *42*(1), 148–164. PMID:9479334

Okada, M. (2002). Future of laboratory informatics. *Rinsho Byori*, *50*(7), 691–693. PMID:12187706

Pantanowitz, L., Hornish, M., & Goulart, R. A. (2009). The impact of digital imaging in the field of cytopathology. *CytoJournal*, *6*(1), 6. doi:10.4103/1742-6413.48606 PMID:19495408

Pantazopoulos, D., Karakitsos, P., Iokim-Liossi, A., Pouliakis, A., Botsoli-Stergiou, E., & Dimopoulos, C. (1998). Back propagation neural network in the discrimination of benign from malignant lower urinary tract lesions. *J Urol, 159*(5), 1619-1623. doi:10.1097/00005392-199805000-00057

Patel, R. P. (2012). Cloud computing and virtualization technology in radiology. [Review]. *Clinical Radiology*, *67*(11), 1095–1100. doi:10.1016/j.crad.2012.03.010 PMID:22607956

Pearlman, E. S., Wolfert, M. S., Miele, R., Bilello, L., & Stauffer, J. (2001). Utilization management and information technology: Adapting to the new era. *Clinical Leadership & Management Review*, *15*(2), 85–88. PMID:11299910

Pinco, J., Goulart, R. A., Otis, C. N., Garb, J., & Pantanowitz, L. (2009). Impact of digital image manipulation in cytology. *Archives of Pathology & Laboratory Medicine*, *133*(1), 57–61. doi:10.1043/1543-2165-133.1.57 PMID:19123737

Pouliakis, A., Athanasiadi, E., Karakitsou, E., Archondakis, S., Mourtzikou, A., Stamouli, M., ... Karakitsos, P. (2014b). ISO 15189:2012 Management Requirements for Cytopathology Laboratory Information Systems. *International Journal of Reliable and Quality E-Healthcare*, *3*(3), 37–57. doi:10.4018/ijrqeh.2014070103

Pouliakis, A., Iliopoulou, D., & Karakitsou, E. (2012). Design and Implementation Issues of an Information System Supporting Cervical Cancer Screening Programs. *Journal of Applied Medical Sciences*, *1*(1), 61–91.

Pouliakis, A., & Karakitsos, P. (2011). *Concepts of software design for population based cervical cencer screening*. Paper presented at the 36th European Congress of Cytology, Istanbul, Turkey.

Pouliakis, A., Margari, N., Spathis, A., Kottaridi, C., Stamouli, M., Mourtzikou, A., ... Karakitsos, P. (2014a). ISO 15189:2012 Technical Requirements for Cytopathology Laboratory Information Systems. *International Journal of Reliable and Quality E-Healthcare*, *3*(3), 58–80. doi:10.4018/ijrqeh.2014070104

Raab, S. S., Zaleski, M. S., Thomas, P. A., Niemann, T. H., Isacson, C., & Jensen, C. S. (1996). Telecytology: Diagnostic accuracy in cervical-vaginal smears. *American Journal of Clinical Pathology*, *105*(5), 599–603. doi:10.1093/ajcp/105.5.599 PMID:8623769

Renshaw, A. A. (2011). Quality improvement in cytology: Where do we go from here? *Archives of Pathology & Laboratory Medicine*, *135*(11), 1387–1390. doi:10.5858/arpa.2010-0606-RA PMID:22032562

Rosenthal, A., Mork, P., Li, M. H., Stanford, J., Koester, D., & Reynolds, P. (2010). Cloud computing: A new business paradigm for biomedical information sharing. *Journal of Biomedical Informatics*, *43*(2), 342–353. doi:10.1016/j.jbi.2009.08.014 PMID:19715773

Rudnisky, C. J., Tennant, M. T., Weis, E., Ting, A., Hinz, B. J., & Greve, M. D. (2007). Web-based grading of compressed stereoscopic digital photography versus standard slide film photography for the diagnosis of diabetic retinopathy. *Ophthalmology*, *114*(9), 1748–1754. doi:10.1016/j.ophtha.2006.12.010 PMID:17368543

Schaffer, A. A., Simon, R., Desper, R., Richter, J., & Sauter, G. (2001). Tree models for dependent copy number changes in bladder cancer. *International Journal of Oncology*, *18*(2), 349–354. PMID:11172603

Sciacovelli, L., Secchiero, S., Zardo, L., D'Osualdo, A., & Plebani, M. (2007). Risk management in laboratory medicine: Quality assurance programs and professional competence. *Clinical Chemistry and Laboratory Medicine*, *45*(6), 756–765. doi:10.1515/CCLM.2007.165 PMID:17579529

Shannon, P., Markiel, A., Ozier, O., Baliga, N. S., Wang, J. T., Ramage, D., ... Ideker, T. (2003). Cytoscape: A software environment for integrated models of biomolecular interaction networks. *Genome Research*, *13*(11), 2498–2504. doi:10.1101/gr.1239303 PMID:14597658

Shen, Z., & Yang, Z. (2001). The problems and strategy relevant to the quality management of clinical laboratories. *Clinical Chemistry and Laboratory Medicine*, *39*(12), 1216–1218. doi:10.1515/CCLM.2001.194 PMID:11798079

Sherman, M. E., Dasgupta, A., Schiffman, M., Nayar, R., & Solomon, D. (2007). The Bethesda Interobserver Reproducibility Study (BIRST): A web-based assessment of the Bethesda 2001 System for classifying cervical cytology. *Cancer*, *111*(1), 15–25. doi:10.1002/cncr.22423 PMID:17186503

Sohn, J., Do, K. A., Liu, S., Chen, H., Mills, G. B., Hortobagyi, G. N., ... Gonzalez-Angulo, A. M. (2013). Functional proteomics characterization of residual triple-negative breast cancer after standard neoadjuvant chemotherapy. *Annals of Oncology: Official Journal of the European Society for Medical Oncology*, *24*(10), 2522–2526. doi:10.1093/annonc/mdt248 PMID:23925999

Solomon, D., Davey, D., Kurman, R., Moriarty, A., O'Connor, D., Prey, M., ... Young, N. (2002). The 2001 Bethesda System: Terminology for reporting results of cervical cytology. *Journal of the American Medical Association*, *287*(16), 2114–2119. doi:10.1001/jama.287.16.2114 PMID:11966386

Stamataki, M., Anninos, D., Brountzos, E., Georgoulakis, J., Panayiotides, J., Christoni, Z., ... Karakitsos, P. (2008). The role of liquid-based cytology in the investigation of thyroid lesions. *Cytopathology*, *19*(1), 11–18. doi:10.1111/j.1365-2303.2007.00512.x PMID:17986263

Stergiou, N., Georgoulakis, G., Margari, N., Aninos, D., Stamataki, M., Stergiou, E., ... Karakitsos, P. (2009). Using a web-based system for the continuous distance education in cytopathology. *International Journal of Medical Informatics*, *78*(12), 827–838. doi:10.1016/j.ijmedinf.2009.08.007 PMID:19775933

Taylor, C. R. (2011). From microscopy to whole slide digital images: A century and a half of image analysis. *Applied Immunohistochemistry & Molecular Morphology*, *19*(6), 491–493. doi:10.1097/PAI.0b013e318229ffd6 PMID:22089486

Thrall, M., Pantanowitz, L., & Khalbuss, W. (2011). Telecytology: Clinical applications, current challenges, and future benefits. *Journal of Pathology Informatics*, *2*(1), 51. doi:10.4103/2153-3539.91129 PMID:22276242

Torres-Cabala, C., Bibbo, M., Panizo-Santos, A., Barazi, H., Krutzsch, H., Roberts, D. D., & Merino, M. J. (2006). Proteomic identification of new biomarkers and application in thyroid cytology. *Acta Cytologica*, *50*(5), 518–528. doi:10.1159/000326006 PMID:17017437

Tsilalis, T., Archondakis, S., Meristoudis, C., Margari, N., Pouliakis, A., Skagias, L., ... Karakitsos, P. (2012). Assessment of static telecytological diagnoses' reproducibility in cervical smears prepared by means of liquid-based cytology. *Telemedicine Journal and e-Health*, *18*(7), 516–520. doi:10.1089/tmj.2011.0167 PMID:22856666

Uppal, D. S., & Powell, S. M. (2013). Genetics/genomics/proteomics of gastric adenocarcinoma. *Gastroenterology Clinics of North America*, *42*(2), 241–260. doi:10.1016/j.gtc.2013.01.005 PMID:23639639

Vacata, V., Jahns-Streubel, G., Baldus, M., & Wood, W. G. (2007). Practical solution for control of the pre-analytical phase in decentralized clinical laboratories for meeting the requirements of the medical laboratory accreditation standard DIN EN ISO 15189. *Clinical Laboratory*, *53*(3-4), 211–215. PMID:17447659

Varlatzidou, A., Pouliakis, A., Stamataki, M., Meristoudis, C., Margari, N., Peros, G., ... Karakitsos, P. (2011). Cascaded learning vector quantizer neural networks for the discrimination of thyroid lesions. *Analytical and Quantitative Cytology and Histology*, *33*(6), 323–334. PMID:22590810

Vriesema, J. L., van der Poel, H. G., Debruyne, F. M., Schalken, J. A., Kok, L. P., & Boon, M. E. (2000). Neural network-based digitized cell image diagnosis of bladder wash cytology. *Diagnostic Cytopathology*, *23*(3), 171–179. doi:10.1002/1097-0339(200009)23:3<171::AID-DC6>3.0.CO;2-F PMID:10945904

Wall, D. P., Kudtarkar, P., Fusaro, V. A., Pivovarov, R., Patil, P., & Tonellato, P. J. (2010). Cloud computing for comparative genomics. *BMC Bioinformatics*, *11*(1), 259. doi:10.1186/1471-2105-11-259 PMID:20482786

Waxer, N., Ninan, D., Ma, A., & Dominguez, N. (2013). How cloud computing and social media are changing the face of health care. *Physician Executive*, *39*(2), 58–60, 62. PMID:23621068

Webb, G. (2012). Making the cloud work for healthcare: Cloud computing offers incredible opportunities to improve healthcare, reduce costs and accelerate ability to adopt new IT services. *Health Management Technology*, *33*(2), 8–9. PMID:22397112

Westbrook, J. I., Georgiou, A., & Rob, M. I. (2008). Computerised order entry systems: Sustained impact on laboratory efficiency and mortality rates? *Studies in Health Technology and Informatics*, *136*, 345–350. PMID:18487755

Williams, B. H., Mullick, F. G., Butler, D. R., Herring, R. F., & O'Leary, T. J. (2001). Clinical evaluation of an international static image-based telepathology service. *Human Pathology*, *32*(12), 1309–1317. doi:10.1053/hupa.2001.29649 PMID:11774162

Wright, A. M., Smith, D., Dhurandhar, B., Fairley, T., Scheiber-Pacht, M., Chakraborty, S., ... Coffey, D. M. (2013). Digital slide imaging in cervicovaginal cytology: A pilot study. *Archives of Pathology & Laboratory Medicine*, *137*(5), 618–624. doi:10.5858/arpa.2012-0430-OA PMID:22970841

Yamamura, Y., Nakajima, T., Ohta, K., Nashimoto, A., Arai, K., Hiratsuka, M., ... Goto, M. (2002). Determining prognostic factors for gastric cancer using the regression tree method. *Gastric Cancer*, *5*(4), 201–207. doi:10.1007101200200035 PMID:12491077

Yamashiro, K., Kawamura, N., Matsubayashi, S., Dota, K., Suzuki, H., Mizushima, H., ... Azumi, N. (2004). Telecytology in Hokkaido Island, Japan: Results of primary telecytodiagnosis of routine cases. *Cytopathology*, *15*(4), 221–227. doi:10.1111/j.1365-2303.2004.00147.x PMID:15324451

Yim, E. K., & Park, J. S. (2006). Role of proteomics in translational research in cervical cancer. *Expert Review of Proteomics*, *3*(1), 21–36. doi:10.1586/14789450.3.1.21 PMID:16445348

KEY TERMS AND DEFINITIONS

Cloud Computing: An online data-storage platform where the users can access and process the uploaded records though an Internet connection without any limitations posed by the hardware and/or software they may use.

Laboratory Information System (LIS): A group of digital software and applications that consist a computing system with capability to provide better management, monitoring and automation for laboratory procedures and activities.

Mobile Health Applications: Computer programs and digital applications that used for the practice of medicine and provision of healthcare services through the utilization of mobile devices such as tablets and smartphones.

Proficiency Testing (PT): The inter-laboratory testing scheme though which the performance of an individual laboratory to carry out specific tests and measurements is evaluated in comparison with the performance of other similar laboratories.

Telecytology: A concept of diagnostic evaluation and assessment of cytological smear-slides that have been converted into digital images and uploaded online so as to be accessible remotely by cytopathologists.

Quality Assurance (QA): The entire system of planning procedures and systematic activities that a laboratory has implemented into its Quality Management System and carries out so as to assure that the determined quality requirements for its provided services will be fulfilled.

Quality Control (QC): The testing techniques, analytical measurements and observation methods that a laboratory uses in order to ensure that the services it provides will fulfill the quality requirements as defined through the earlier QA process.

Chapter 9
Mathematical Models for Computer Virus:
Computer Virus Epidemiology

Stelios Zimeras
University of the Aegean, Greece

ABSTRACT

Computer viruses have been studied for a long time both by the research and by the application communities. As computer networks and the internet became more popular from the late 1980s on, viruses quickly evolved to be able to spread through the internet by various means such as file downloading, email, exploiting security holes in software, etc. In general, epidemic models assume that individuals go through a series of states at a certain constant set of rates. Different epidemic models have been proposed based on the characteristics of the systems and the topology of the network. In this chapter, an analysis of various epidemic models will be analyzed under differential mathematical systems.

INTRODUCTION

The threats to network security can be classified as hacking, inside attack, computer virus, the leak of secret message and modification of key data in the network. All these attacks and invasions aim at wrecking information that is stored in a server in different ways.

The term "computer virus", coined by Adleman in the early 1980's, is suggestive of Btrong analogies between computer viruses and their biological namesakes. Both attach themselves to a small functional unit (cell or program) of the host individual (organism or computer) and co-opt the resources of that unit for the purpose of creating more copies of the virus. By using up materials (memory) and energy (CPU), viruses can cause a wide spectrum of malfunctions in their hosts. Even worse, viruses can be toxic. Computer viruses are self-replicating software entities that attach themselves parasitically to existing programs (Whitten et al., 2004; Bentley, et al., 2004).

When a user executes an infected program (an executable file or boot sector), the viral portion of the code typically executes first. The virus looks for one or more victim programs to which it has to write

DOI: 10.4018/978-1-5225-8021-8.ch009

Copyright © 2019, IGI Global. Copying or distributing in print or electronic forms without written permission of IGI Global is prohibited.

access (typically the same set of programs to which the user has access), and attaches a copy of itself (perhaps a deliberately modified copy) to each victim. Under some circumstances, it may then execute a payload, such as printing a weird message, playing music, destroying data, *etc.* Eventually, a typical virus returns control to the original program, which executes normally. Unless the virus executes an obvious payload, the user is unlikely to notice that anything is amiss, and will be completely unaware of having helped a virus to replicate (Mollison, 1995; Skoudis, 2004). Viruses often enhance their ability to spread by establishing themselves as resident processes in memory, persisting long after the infected host finishes its execution (terminating only when the machine is shut down). As resident processes, they can monitor system activity continually, and identify and infect executables and boot sectors as they become available. Over a period of time, this scenario is repeated, and the infection may spread to several programs on the user's system. Eventually, an infected program may be copied and transported to another system electronically or via diskette. If this program is executed on the new system, the cycle of infection will begin anew. In this manner, computer viruses spread from program to program, and (more slowly) from machine to machine (Burger, 1991; Newman, 2002; Beutel, 2012; Kephart and White, 1993)

Lately, computer worms have become a major problem for large computer networks, causing considerable amounts of resources and time to be spent recovering from large-scale attacks. It is believed that understanding the factors influencing worm propagation in technological networks (such as the Internet, the World Wide Web, phone networks, IP networks, etc.) will suggest useful ways to control them (Mollison, 1995; Skoudis, 2004). So far, a few studies have employed simple epidemiological models to understand the general characteristics of virus spreading (Stallings, 2011). However, they become one of the most important factors for the security of any system.

Epidemiological models have traditionally been used to understand and predict the outcome of virus outbreaks in human or animal populations. However, the same models were recently applied to the analysis of computer virus epidemics. For example, using a simple model it has been shown that networks that have a topology similar to the Internet are highly vulnerable to viral attacks (Burger, 1991; Newman, 2002; Beutel, 2012; Kephart and White, 1993).

In general, epidemic models assume that individuals go through a series of states at a certain constant set of rates (Zimeras, 2016). Therefore, the elaboration of a model requires the definition of a set of possible states and a set of transition rates. The simplest model is referred as the *SIS* model (for *Susceptible-Infected- Susceptible*). Other more complex models include the *Susceptible-Infected-Removed* (SIR) model and the *Susceptible-Exposed-Infected-Removed* (SEIR) model (Bailey, 1975; Zimeras, 2016).

The topology also plays a role in determining the outcome of an outbreak. Technological networks appear to be best approximated using scale-free graphs or homogeneous graphs network in some cases. Markov models may be introduced to analyse the network topology of the spreading into the systems. In this work, we analyse various computer virus spread models.

COMPUTER VIRUS DEFINITION AND MODELLING

A computer virus is a malicious software that infects other programs by attacking them and transforms them (or part of them) into an infected body. This technique includes infection of the basic host program, attacking a new uninfected program partially, making some copies of the infected program into the system, spreading the infection inside the system, destroying whole or parts (Stallings, 2004).

During its lifetime, a virus goes through four phases (Stallings, 2004):

- **Dormant Phase:** In this phase, a virus is waiting for attacking under a specific event (e.g. date, another program or file, disc capacity).
- **Propagation Phase:** The virus attacking the system by copying itself in whole or in parts and infects the system.
- **Triggering Phase**: The virus is activated by spreading the infection into the whole system
- **Execution Phase:** The infected program is executed and sometimes is harmless (e.g. message on the screen) and other times destructive (e.g. damage data files)

Continuous study of possible models of a virus attack in a population with different properties led to further study of epidemics. Modelling an epidemic has three main goals. The first is to understand the mechanisms of diffusion and how different parameters affect the epidemic. The second objective is to make it possible to predict the course of the epidemic in the future, which includes the final size the epidemic and convergence time at steady state. Finally, the third objective is to define the mechanisms to deal with the epidemic and to prevent it under spreading conditions. So, to create an epidemic model is essential to make a set of assumptions about the nature of the population and its mechanisms of spreading. Based on the transition between conditions to a disease, the most studied models are (Zimeras, 2016):

- **Susceptible Infectious (SI) Model:** In the SI model, people who are susceptible to infections, when infected, remain in this state forever.
- **Susceptible Infectious Recovered (SIS) Model:** In the SIS model, individuals go through three situations, from susceptible ones that turn into infected and then again susceptible.
- **Susceptible Infectious Recovered (SIR) Model:** In the case of a SIR model, after some time, a person dies or is recovered due to the immune system and cannot spread the infection further.
- **Susceptible-Exposed-Infected-Removed (SEIR) Model:** In the case of the SEIR model, after some time, a person is exposed to a virus before dying or recovering and cannot spread further infection.

For the study of the above models, simulation of the dynamic systems must be considered to investigate the effects of the attacks. In general, a model is a simplified representation of a system ignoring trivial or useless details, and emphasizes those of interest. Especially an attack's model analyses the specifications of the attack as well as abilities and intentions. This analysis can be done by introducing attack's graphs which are a special case of scenarios' graphs. Attack charts illustrate ways in which a virus can invade the system. The system administrators analyze attack charts to understand the weaknesses of the system and to propose defensive measures.

Figure 1 illustrates the modelling process. It includes the following stages: initialization of the defence system, creation of the model, variables and parameters, the modelling and control, and finally, evaluation (Dinesh Kumar Saini, 2012).

A scenario graph is a representation of all of executable paths through a system that violates some condition correctness (Sheyner, 2004). Scenario graphs represent anything that can work

incorrectly in a system, giving the system the ability to analyze appropriate problems. A graph attack is a graphical connection between system security and network topology combined with the hosts' connectivity *(*Michael Lyle Artz 2002*)*. Examples are given in Figure 2.

The Attack Chart involves a collection of possible scenarios penetration into a computer network. Each penetration scenario is a series of steps of the attacker, ending with a specific target - access

Figure 1. Mathematical modelling procedure (Dinesh Kumar Saini, 2012)

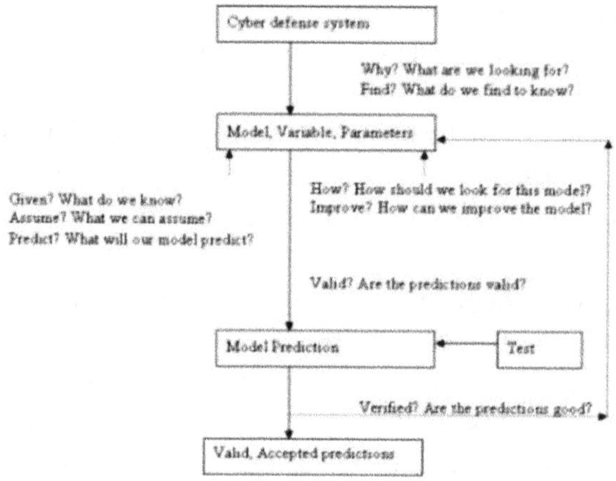

Figure 2. Examples of graph attack (Michael Lyle Artz 2002)

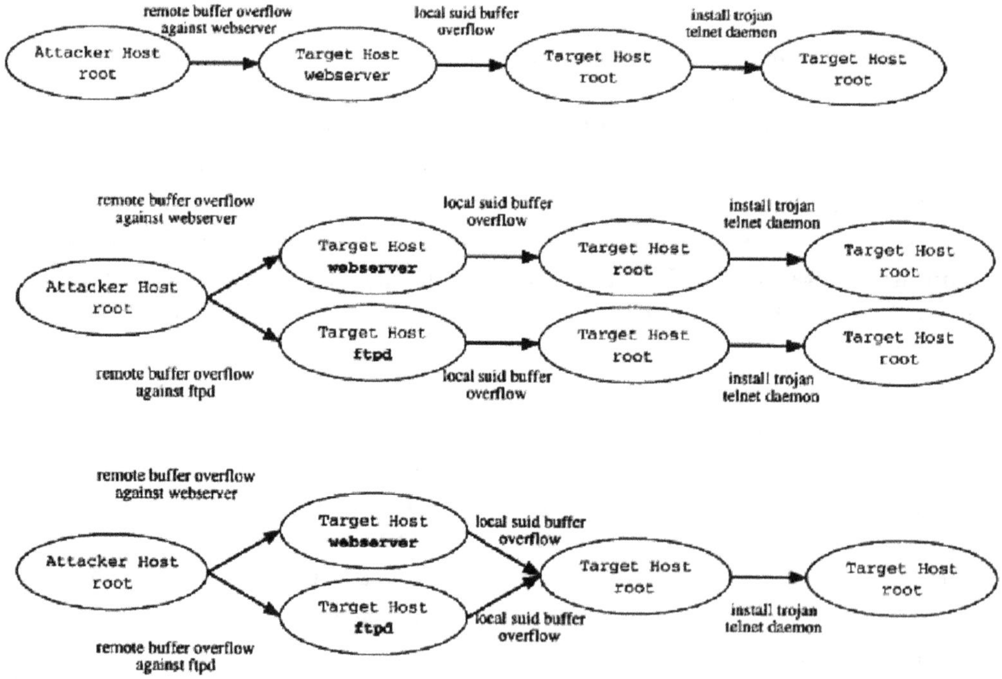

administrator on a particular host, access to a database, denial access to services. Summarizing, an attack graph is a collection of scenarios that show how a malicious virus can affect its target system (Sheyner, 2004).

A network is a group of computers that are interconnected by electronic circuits or wireless transmissions of various designs and technologies for the purpose of exchanging data or communicating information between them or their users. Different topology is given in Figure 3 (Zimeras, 2016).

Figure 3. Network topology

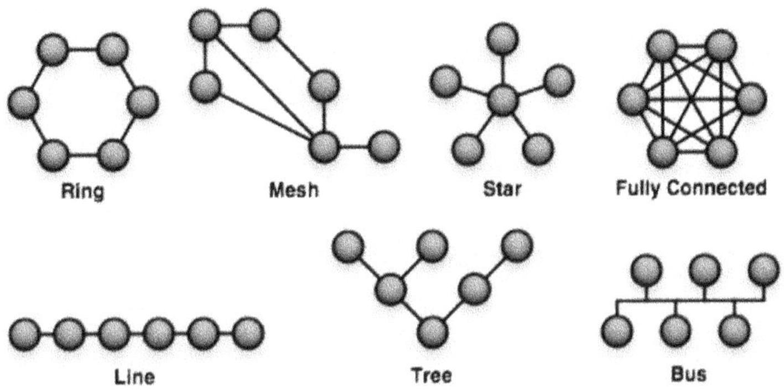

MATHEMATICAL MODELS OF COMPUTER VIRUS

The creation and spread of infectious diseases is a complex phenomenon with various factors such as the environment in which the population is exposed, and the dynamics of the studied population. The role of mathematics in epidemiology is to model the creation and spread of a virus.

SI and SIS Models

The SI (Susceptible Infectious Model) is the simplest epidemic model. In SI model, each host is susceptible to infection or already infected (Figure 4) (Hethcote, 2000; Diekmann et al., 2000; Kempe et al., 2000).

Susceptible hosts (S): These hosts do not currently have the virus and are capable of contracting the virus.

Infected computers (I): These hosts are currently infected with the virus and are capable of transmitting the virus to others.

The infectious rate, β, controls the rate of spread which represents the probability of transmitting disease between a susceptible and an infectious individual. The dynamics of I in a SI model are also known as logistic growth. The differential equitation for the SI model is given by (Anderson et al., 1992):

$$\frac{dS}{dt} = -\beta \frac{SI}{N}$$
$$\frac{dI}{dt} = \beta \frac{SI}{N} = \beta I \left(1 - \frac{I}{N}\right)$$

where N is the size of the population (N=S+I).

Figure 4. SI model

Susceptible Infectious Susceptible (SIS) Model

In the SIS model, individuals go through three situations, from susceptible ones that turn into infected and then again susceptible. The model is an extension of the SI model including one more stage, the susceptible (Figure 5) (Hethcote, 2000; Diekmann et al., 2000; Kempe et al., 2000)

Recovery rate, $\gamma = \frac{1}{D}$, is determined by the average duration, D, of infection. The differential equitation for the SIS model is given by (Anderson et al., 1992):

$$\frac{dS}{dt} = -\beta \frac{SI}{N} + \gamma I$$
$$\frac{dI}{dt} = \beta \frac{SI}{N} - \gamma I$$

The second equation is solved as follows.

$$\frac{dI}{dt} = \beta \frac{SI}{N} - \gamma I = \beta S \left(1 - \frac{I}{N}\right) - \gamma I = 0$$

There are two equilibrium solutions for the SIS model, the first is $I = 0$ (disease-free state), and the second is:

$$I = \frac{\left(\beta - \gamma\right) N}{\beta} = \left(1 - \frac{\gamma}{\beta}\right) N$$

For spreading disease, the condition is $\frac{dI}{dt} > 0$, and for $\frac{\beta}{\gamma} > 1$, the disease will spread and approach the second steady state; otherwise, it will eventually reach the disease-free state.

Also under the condition $S + I = N \Rightarrow \frac{dS}{dt} + \frac{dI}{dt} = 0$, the solution for $\frac{dI}{dt} > 0$ is

$$\frac{dI}{dt} = \left(\beta N - \gamma\right) I - \beta I^2$$

Figure 5. SIS model

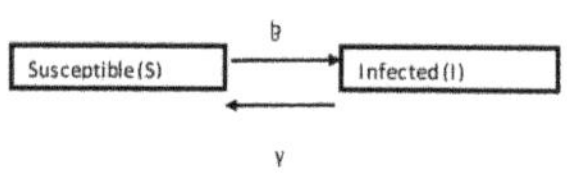

The solution of this equation using the transformation $I = \frac{1}{y}$ is given by

$$-\frac{y'}{y^2} = \left(\beta N - \gamma\right)\frac{1}{y} - \beta\frac{1}{y^2}$$

with general solution form $y\left(t\right) = Ce^{\left(y - N\beta\right)t} + \beta$. Thus

$$I\left(t\right) = \frac{1}{Ce^{\left(y - N\beta\right)t} + \beta}$$

Susceptible Infectious Recovered (SIR) Model

In the case of a SIR model, after some time, a person dies or is recovered due to the immune system and cannot spread further infection (Hethcote, 2000; Diekmann et al., 2000; Kempe et al., 2000)

In epidemiology, the SIR model is more commonly used as the most realistic model to transmit disease. The SIR model presents a behavior depending on the populations' characteristics. In other words, if the epidemic parameters have a critical value, the virus in a network dies before most of the population is infected. Kermack and McKendrick (1927) define a deterministic epidemic model with a stable N population and three states.

The infectious rate, β, controls the rate of spread which represents the probability of transmitting disease between a susceptible and an infectious individual. Recovery rate, γ, is determined by the average duration, D, of infection (Figure 6).

The R which represents the number of removed hosts. S, I and R represent the number of susceptible, infected, and recovered individuals, and N = S + I + R is the total population. The SIR model can be written as the following ordinary differential equation (ODE) (Anderson et al., 1992):

$$\frac{dS}{dt} = -\beta\frac{SI}{N}$$
$$\frac{dI}{dt} = \beta\frac{SI}{N} - \gamma I$$
$$\frac{dR}{dt} = \gamma I$$

Figure 6. SIR model

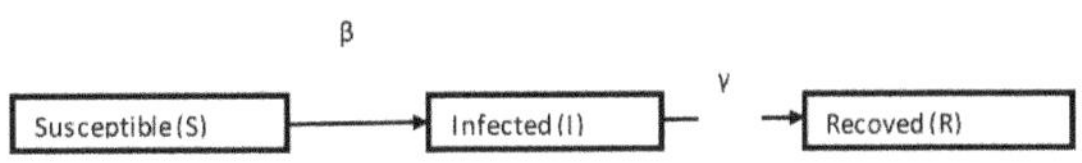

If a person is infected, then it can transmit the disease with infectious rate β at the same time depending on the contacts (healthy and not healthy people). This implies that the patient is capable of provoking

$$\frac{\beta}{N}NC = aC$$

the number of infections, at any time, with C the probability of contact.

Susceptible-Exposed-Infected-Removed (SEIR) Model

In the case of the SEIR model after some time, a person is exposed to a virus before dying or recovering and cannot spread infection further (Kermack and McKendrick, 1927). The infectious rate, β, controls the rate of spread which represents the probability of transmitting disease between a susceptible and an infectious individual. The incubation rate, σ, is the rate of latent individuals becoming infectious (average duration of incubation is 1/σ) (Keeling and Rohani, 2008). Recovery rate, γ= 1/D, is determined by the average duration, D, of infection (Figure 7). Many diseases have a latent phase during which the individual is infected but not yet infectious. This delay between the acquisition of infection and the infectious state can be incorporated into the SIR model by adding a latent/exposed population, E, and letting infected (but not yet infectious) individuals move from S to E and from E to I (Hethcote, 2000; Diekmann et. al., 2000; Kempe et. al., 2000).

The SEIR model can be written as the following ordinary differential equation (ODE) (Anderson et al., 1992):

$$\frac{dS}{dt} = -\beta\frac{SI}{N}$$
$$\frac{dE}{dt} = \beta\frac{SI}{N} - \sigma E$$
$$\frac{dI}{dt} = \sigma E - \gamma I$$
$$\frac{dR}{dt} = \gamma I$$

where N is the size of the population (N=S+E+I+R).

Figure 7. SEIR model

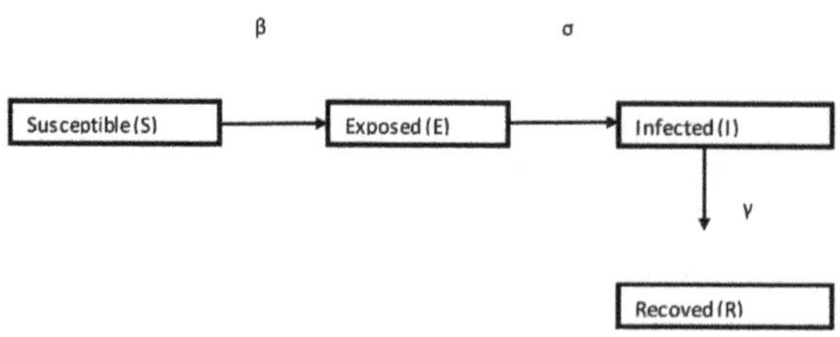

CONCLUSION

In this work, the analysis of computer virus modelling is introduced, and the description of the characteristics for the epidemiological model is illustrated. Based on that model, the dynamic equations system is explained considering the rate of infection for the computer network system and the final mathematical solutions are presented.

REFERENCES

Anderson, R. M., May, R. M., & Anderson, B. (1992). *Infectious Diseases of Humans Dynamics and Control*. New York: Oxford UP.

Artz. (2002). *NetSPA: A Network Security Planning Architecture*. MIT.

Bailey, N. T. J. (1975). *The Mathematical Theory of Infectious Diseases* (2nd ed.). London: Griffin.

Bentley, L., Dittman, K., & Whitten, J. (2004). *System analysis and design methods*. McGraw-Hill Higher Education.

Beutel, A., Prakash, B. A., Rosenfeld, R., & Faloutsos, C. (2012). Interacting viruses in networks: Can both survive? *KDD: Proceedings / International Conference on Knowledge Discovery & Data Mining. International Conference on Knowledge Discovery & Data Mining*, *12*, 426–434. doi:10.1145/2339530.2339601

Burger, R. (1991). Computer Viruses and Data Protection. *Abacus*.

Diekmann, O., & Heesterbeek, J. A. (2000). *Mathematical Epidemiology of Infectious Diseases: Model Building, Analysis and Interpretation*. New York: John Wiley & Sons, Incorporated.

Hethcote, H. W. (2000). The mathematics of infectious diseases. *SIAM Review*, *42*(4), 599–653. doi:10.1137/S0036144500371907

Keeling, M. J., & Rohani, P. (2008). *Modeling Infectious Diseases in Humans and Animals*. Princeton University Press.

Kempe, D., Kleinberg, J. M., & Tardos, É. (2003). *Maximizing the spread of influence through a social network*. SIGKDD.

Kephart, J. O., & White, S. R. (1993). Measuring and modeling computer virus prevalence. *IEEE Computer Society Symposium on Research in Security and Privacy*, 2-15. 10.1109/RISP.1993.287647

Kermack, W. O., & McKendrick, A. G. (1927). A contribution to the Mathematical Theory of Epidemics. *Proceedings of the Royal Society of London. Series A, Containing Papers of a Mathematical and Physical Character*, *115*(772), 700–711. doi:10.1098/rspa.1927.0118

Mollison, D. (1995). *The structure of Epidemic Models*. Cambridge University Press.

Newman, M. (2002). Spread of epidemic disease on networks. *Physical Review Letters*, *66*, 1–11. PMID:12241447

Saini, D. K. (2012). Cyber Defense: Mathematical Modeling and Simulation. *International Journal of Applied Physics and Mathematics*, *2*(5), 312–315. doi:10.7763/IJAPM.2012.V2.121

Sheyner, O. M. (2004). *Scenario Graphs and Attack Graphs*. Pittsburgh, PA: Carnegie Mellon University.

Skoudis, E. (2004). *Malware Fighting malicious code. Computer Networking and Distribution Systems*. Prentice Hall.

Stallings, W. (2011). *Cryptography and network Security*. Pearson Education Inc.

Whitten, J., Bentley, L., & Dittman, K. (2004). *Fundamentals of system analysis and design methods*. Academic Press.

Zimeras, S. (2016). Computer Virus Models and Analysis in M-Health IT Systems: Computer Virus Models. In. A. Moumtzoglou (Ed.), Health Innovations for Patient-Centered Care (pp. 284-297). IGI Global.

KEY TERMS AND DEFINITIONS

Downloaders: Malicious software that installs a set of harmful tools on a target machine.

Keyloggers: Captures keystrokes on a compromised system and collecting sensitive information (e.g., names, passwords) for the attacker.

Trojan Horse: A destructive program that masquerades as a benign application.

Virus: Malicious software that infects other programs by modifying them.

Worm: Program that can replicate itself and send copies from computer to computer across network connections.

Zombie Programs: Program that secretly activated on an infected machine for launching attacks on other machines.

Chapter 10
The Science of Individuality and Tailored M-Health Communication

Anastasius S. Moumtzoglou
P&A Kyriakou Children's Hospital, Greece

ABSTRACT

The era of the science of individuality promises to fully recognize the uniqueness of the individual who needs to be seen and treated with utter respect for his or her individuality. It will not be long until digitizing a person unlocks the cause for what is wrong, creating valuable knowledge that can save a life or markedly improve the quality of life. On the other hand, emerging m-health technologies provide fundamentally different ways of looking at tailored communication technology. As a result, tailored communications research is poised at a crossroads. It needs to both build on and break away from existing frameworks into new territory, realizing the necessary commitment to theory-driven research at basic, methodological, clinical, and applied levels. The chapter envisions tailored m-health communication in the context of the science of individuality, emphasizing the variability, stability, and centrality of the individual.

INTRODUCTION

The health care environment is currently changing to meet technology and societal trends which converge to bring into being new communication patterns that connect and coordinate the roles of healthcare stakeholders. At the same time, the healthcare industry is steering inexorably toward a distributed service design in which essential decision-making occurs at the point of care. One of the central engines of this shift towards decentralization and reorientation of health care services is mobile healthcare (M-Health). M-Health describes the use of a broad range of telecommunication and multimedia technologies within the wireless care delivery design and can be broadly defined as the delivery of healthcare services via mobile communication devices. M-Health establishes healthcare communities in which every stake-holder can participate. However, it disrupts the traditional service model where healthcare information,

DOI: 10.4018/978-1-5225-8021-8.ch010

Copyright © 2019, IGI Global. Copying or distributing in print or electronic forms without written permission of IGI Global is prohibited.

security and access is centrally managed, maintained and limited, transforming the healthcare sector and destroying components that are slow to adapt.

M-Health interventions range from simple to complex applications and systems that remotely coordinate and actively manage patient care. In this context, it offers an elegant solution to the problem of accessing the right information within highly fluid, distributed organizations. Moreover, it removes geography and time as barriers to care by establishing connectivity with remote locations and remote workers, creates new points of contact with patients, and changes the frequency and intensity of health care delivery. It also establishes effective new treatment modalities like telehealth, remote patient monitoring, self-care, and home health while it blurs the boundaries between professional medical advice and self-care. Overall, M-Health blends three bodies of knowledge: high technology, life sciences, and human factors.

Additionally, four prevailing theories are explaining the formation of health attitudes, intentions, or behaviors (Weinstein, 1993):

- The protection motivation theory.
- The health belief model.
- The theory of reasoned action.
- The subjective expected utility.

These theories share an underlying premise. Health intentions arise to avoid potential adverse outcomes through cognitive assessment and include a cost-benefit component. However, existing studies have largely ignored the role of various message tactics and individual characteristics, contrary to the protection motivation model (Rogers, 1985). Overall, health messages accommodate risk information in different formats (Keller, 2006):

- To increase perceptions of vulnerability.
- To include action steps.
- To provide comparative information to increase intentions.

By the same token, tailoring is a multi-dimensional communication strategy that involves the development of individualized messages that are based on the pre-assessment of critical variables or characteristics that are linked to the underlying model of behavior change. Several studies have found that tailored health messages demand greater attention for the following reasons:

- They are processed more intently.
- They contain less redundant information.
- They are perceived more positively by health consumers.

Specifically, the Elaboration Likelihood Model suggests that personal information enhances the strength of motivation and sensitivity to the argument, forcing the individual to expound on the message. Moreover, if the argument is forceful to senses, personal pertinence increases the probability for persuasion. Thus, tailoring creates an ideal environment for persuasion and health behavior change. Studies of tailored communication are exploding in an array of disciplines. In health education, studies have shown that tailored print materials are generally more effective than non-tailored ones (Prochaska et al., 1993;

Campbell et al., 1994; Skinner et al., 1994; Strecher et al., 1994; Kreuter and Strecher, 1996; Brug et al., 1996, 1998; Brennan et al., 1998; Bull & Jamrozik, 1998; Dijkstra et al., 1998a,b; Marcus et al., 1998).

Computing technologies have considerably contributed to the sophistication of tailoring as they can facilitate theory-based assessment of tailoring. Web-based tailored interventions have multiple advantages over single-mode, static interventions:

- Abounding access probability to expert care and feedback.
- Capability to switch between modalities and formats of different learning styles and literacy levels.
- Asynchronous and synchronous communication.
- A vast array of interactive components to strengthen user experiences and support skills development, behavior/goal monitoring, and progress tracking.

The objective of the chapter is to envision tailored M-Health communication in the context of the science of individuality, emphasizing the variability, stability and centrality of the individual.

BACKGROUND

Internet Health Coalition (2000) defines health information as 'the information for staying well, preventing and managing disease and making other decisions related to health and health care.' Bates (2009) states 'information behavior is the currently preferred term used to describe the many ways in which human beings interact with information.' It is also the concept used in information studies to refer to a sub-discipline that engages in research conducted to understand the human relationship to information. Wilson (2000) defines information behavior as 'the totality of human behavior relating to sources and channels of information, including both active and passive information seeking and information use. Thus, information behavior involves face-to-face communication with others, as well as the passive reception of information. Pettigrew et al. (2001) point out that information behavior phenomena are part of the human communicative process. Furthermore, Savolainen (2008) has introduced information practice as a co-ordinate concept for the information behavior. He considers that both concepts refer to how individuals deal with information, but from somewhat different perspectives.

Derr (1983) states that information may be needed without being desired while Chatman and Pendleton (1995) separate information need and information want. The concept of 'desire for information' is also used to describe the amount (and frequency) an individual would like to have information (Fourie, 2008). In other words, information could be important in an individual´s life, but yet that person may have no interest in gaining it. According to Fidel (2012), information needs can be unconscious, but information wants (or desire for information) can usually be put into words by the individual.

Information seeking is assumed to be an essential element in decision-making and health outcomes (Johnson, Andrews & Allard, 2001; Rimer et al., 2004). Human information behavior research has recognized information seeking as the central form of interaction that individuals employ to get information (Fidel, 2012). It can be active or passive. Active information seeking has been defined as 'the purposive seeking for information as a consequence of a need to satisfy some goal' (Wilson, 2000).

Information searching is seen as a narrower and more focused concept while information use is a poorly defined concept linked to the information need (Wilson, 1999). According to Cole and Leide

(2006) information use is a process in which an environmental stimulus, which includes stimuli obtained from reading, viewing, and listening activities, modifies the user´s knowledge structure. Wilson (2000) states that information use behavior 'consists of the physical and mental acts involved in incorporating the information found in the person's existing knowledge base.' Information is interpreted and internalized by the individual in order to construct knowledge, and this knowledge may result in further action (Savolainen, 2008).

The concept of 'information reception' has been used to define the first stages of the information use process. The stages include noticing, filtering, evaluating, and comparing the content of the obtained information (Nahl & Bilal, 2007). In information studies, in addition to the cognitive viewpoint, information use has been considered from the constructivist and socio-constructivist viewpoints (Talja et al., 2005). These viewpoints have a lot in common as they all present information use as processes occurring within the human mind. They share the assumptions that a human being is an information processor. Moreover, comparing and interpreting qualities of things is fundamental to the information use process and that the reception of information is mediated by an individual´s existing state of knowledge. (Savolainen, 2009; Talja et al., 2005).

Health behavior has been studied by several social cognition theories and models that are widely used in health promotion. Many of these theories or models can be defined as statements about causal relationships between individual-level factors (such as knowledge, attitudes, motivation, sociodemographic factors, personality) and health behavior change. For health providers, they provide conceptual frameworks for developing effective health promotion programs, campaigns, and interventions (Campbell & Quintiliani, 2006; Schwarzer, 2008). Their theoretical constructs help in analyzing behavioral health problems and are also used as a basis to tailor health information and messages (Kreuter et al., 1999). However, no single theory or model can account for all complexities of behavior change, and therefore theories and models should be seen as complementary rather than competing.

Social cognition models have been divided into:

- Motivational models.
- Behavioral enaction models.
- Multistage models of behavior change.
- Health Action Process Approach (HAPA) by Schwarzer (2008).

Motivational models imply that motivation is sufficient for successful behavioral enaction. Behavioral enaction models focus on bridging the 'gap' between motivation, intention and behavior. Stage-based health behavior change models propose that behavior change is a non-continuous process occurring through stages. Each stage refers to differing individual barriers. In this context, the transtheoretical model of behavior change (TTM) argues that individuals move through a series of five stages of change. According to this model, when adopting a particular health behavior, an individual can be at one of five stages:

- Precontemplation.
- Contemplation.
- Preparation.
- Action or maintenance.

People in action or maintenance stages may also relapse and then recycle between stages. It has been stated that different kinds of information, messages and support are needed for people in different stages of change (Rimer & Kreuter, 2006).

The TTM also includes other theoretical constructs. They can be used to explain what motivates an individual to progress through the stages of change toward a healthy change in behavior. Self-efficacy is one of the significant incentives of whether a person will progress through the stages. Self-efficacy originates from the Social Cognitive Theory and is defined as the confidence in individual abilities to overcome barriers and adopt a particular behavior (Toscos & Connelly, 2010). It can be seen as situation specific, but it has also been conceptualized as a stable, trait-like disposition (Contrada & Goyal, 2004). According to Bandura (2006), it is not a global trait but a differentiated set of self-beliefs.

Increasing awareness and enhancing intentions are significant predictors of health behavior and included in many behavioral change theories and models. Individuals are often unaware of their risk behavior, making it unlikely that they would consider a behavioral change. Awareness of the relationship between behavior and outcome may also be significant, especially in earlier stages of behavioral change (Brug et al., 1994).

Behavioral intentions are defined as 'plans individuals have about whether or not they intend to perform the recommended behavior' (Murray-Johnson & Witte, 2003). However, a definite intention may not be enough for behavioral change (Sheeran, 2005; Webb & Sheeran, 2006), especially for complex, habitual behaviors. Such behaviors depend very much on personal abilities and environmental opportunities (Brug, Oenema & Ferreira, 2005).

Likewise, health communication can be partly responsible for all aspects of disease prevention and health promotion. It has been defined as 'the crafting and delivery of messages and strategies, based on consumer research, to promote the health of individuals and communities' (Roper, 1993). In health communication, health information or messages can be delivered to a general audience or segmented, targeted audiences (Evans, 2006). Traditionally, health promotion materials have been generic (Kreuter et al., 1999; Johnson & Case, 2012). In generic mass media, communication materials are intended to appeal to a large group of people (Brug, Oenema & Campbell, 2003). A relatively large undifferentiated audience receives identical information content (Kreuter & Wray, 2003). In many cases, as much information as possible is provided, and individuals need to find the relevant information on their own. However, it is likely that only individuals, who are already motivated, are willing to search through lengthy brochures for information that applies to their situation (Brug et al., 2003).

Although health information is widely available, appropriate information suited to particular individual needs cannot often be found (Williamson, 2005). However, people do not always access or obtain information that could be beneficial to them (Chatman & Pendleton, 1995). One reason for this could be that the individual´s information needs can be unconscious, and thus they are not aware of them (Fourie, 2008; Case, 2012). In addition, individuals do not always know how to express their information needs (Fourie, 2008). Moreover, other psychological and cognitive barriers can inhibit the recognition of information need (Johnson, Andrews & Allard, 2001).

Overall, it has been concluded that general health communication is not sufficient to meet the information needs of individuals (Docherty et al., 2008). In this context, progress in technology has led to a tailored approach to health communication. It involves soliciting information from individuals or querying information about individuals from existing records. It is consequential because it combines the potential for delivering cost-effective health communications to reach an enormous audience combined with the benefits of interpersonal communication. The reason is that communications that are tailored to be responsive to the solicited information can be used to imitate the transactional and response-dependent qualities of interpersonal communication. An interactive cycle of tailored feedback and response can be repeated to assist in motivating health behavior change. Along the way, both source and message factors can be dynamically modified to realize the advantages inherent in interpersonal channels, advantages proven essential for persuading individuals to change their health behavior.

This approach, known as tailoring, has been defined as any combination of information or change strategies intended to reach one specific person. This definition highlights the two features of a tailored approach that distinguishes it from other approaches:

- The collection of messages is intended for a particular person.
- The messages are based on individual-level factors.

The rationale for a tailored approach is grounded in the theory that explains how people process information. Petty and Cacioppo's (1986) Elaboration Likelihood Model (ELM) provides a method of understanding this process. They have proposed the central and peripheral routes to attitude formation and change. The central route involves a cognitive component and necessitates effort on the part of the individual. Studies have shown that messages processed via the central route lead to more firmly held beliefs and attitudes and result in lasting attitude change. It is, therefore, considered to be more effective in changing attitudes than general information. Subsequently, the theory suggests the following rationale for a tailored approach:

- By tailoring materials, superfluous information is eliminated.
- The remaining information is more personally relevant to the message recipient.
- The message recipient will pay more attention to the information if it is personally relevant.
- The unshared needs of a person will be useful in enacting and sustaining the desired behavior change

Tailoring enhances cognitive conditions for information processing and acceptance. A common aim of tailoring merely is to increase attention and comprehension. Apparently, attention to information is a prerequisite for the information to have any impact. Attention is gained by communicating to the information receiver that the information addresses his or her preferences and needs (Hawkins et al., 2008). Rimer and Kreuter (2006) argue that at least four approaches to tailoring can be used to enhance health communication. The approaches are as follows:

- Matching content to information needs and interests.
- Providing information in a meaningful context.
- Using design, production and channel elements to capture attention and enhance message processing.
- Presenting the requested information.

In conclusion, tailoring of health information is a means to overcome the problems related to the provision of general health information. It attempts to provide carefully selected information suitable for an individual and consequently may lower or remove psychological or cognitive barriers to information use and decision-making. It makes easier for the receiver to interpret, understand and trust information (Te´eni, 2001) while increasing the perceived personal relevance of health information. Consequently, it helps engage individuals and create ideal conditions for persuasion and attitude or behavior change to occur (Lustria et al., 2009).

Furthermore, tailoring and targeting are not discrete categories of communication, but overlapping segments of the continua (Hawkins et al., 2008). They combine the benefits of interpersonal communication and mass media (Evans, 2006). Tailoring imitates and automates the process of person-to-person counselling by providing more customized information than the mass media. Similarly, targeted communication is intended to reach some population subgroup based on characteristics presumed to be shared by the group's members

Despite these fundamental differences between tailoring and targeting, the rationale for both approaches is quite similar. The more one knows about the intended recipients of communication; the better able one will be to make the message relevant to them. There are, however, situations in which each approach would seem to have an advantage over the other. Tailored health messages should have an advantage over targeted messages when there is significant variability within the target audience.

Finally, because tailoring is a form of data-based communication, it should only be considered as a message strategy when a mechanism exists for gathering or accessing information from the target population on the critical determinants of change. That is one reason that tailoring has been applied so often in health care settings. Individual-level data are already routinely gathered there; tailoring assessments can be integrated or added to existing structures without disrupting practice norms or patient expectations.

THE SCIENCE OF INDIVIDUALITY AND TAILORED M-HEALTH COMMUNICATION

Unquestionably, m-health communication requires extensive data, which currently flows from the beneficiaries towards data centers. Such data include a multitude of health and well-being information collected manually or automatically. Moreover, algorithms are required to process such information and alert when health-related actions should be taken. On the other hand, nowadays, there are technologies which provide both the data storage and processing capacity while the mobile device (especially the mobile phone), as well as inter-connectable devices (health gadgets), may serve as data acquisition points on the individual level.

However, there is a significant deficiency of contemporary medicine which is reflected by the use of experts to make recommendations or guidelines for a significant proportion of decisions for which no or minimal data exists. These guidelines are published in major specialty journals which have a pronounced impact, as they are believed to represent the standard of care. Overall, there is too much literature which is evidenced by the statistic that only 0.5 per cent of the 38 million published papers are cited more than two hundred times, and half were never cited. Moreover, when pooled analyses of prior studies are published, many relevant papers are excluded (Topol, 2012).

In fact, this should be considered 'eminence-based medicine.' (Topol, 2012).

Better studies might be part of the solution. However, as we can accrue more meaningful data and information for individuals, the hope is that we can override our dependence on such recommendations. We need evidence which is built not on populations but individuals.

Fortunately, our capacity to get just that information is rapidly arising. An era which is characterized by the right drug and dose, at the right cost and timing has begun (Topol, 2012). Medicine for the common good is not sufficient. A rebooted life science, instead of a mass-population-directed strategy, would leverage the science of individuality, getting the relevant digital readout from an individual to shape a therapy. We now, for the first time, have the devices to promote a level of prescription precision we have never seen before (Topol, 2012).

The era of individualized medicine ultimately promises to do away with terms like 'cryptogenic' and 'essential,' fully recognizing the uniqueness of the individual who needs to be seen and treated with utter respect for his or her individuality. It will not be long until digitizing a person unlocks the cause for what is wrong, creating valuable knowledge that can save a life or markedly improve the quality of life. That is a major outgrowth of the science of individuality.

In this context, the entire classification system of medical conditions and diagnoses is about to be rewritten. Instead of our current reductionist model for which individuals are unwisely assigned to such categories as one of two types of diabetes or cancer of a particular organ, the science of individuality will promote a new molecular taxonomy that invokes the main biologic basis, regarding genes or pathways.

On the other hand, communication has always been a fundamental component of effective health care and health promotion. In this context, throughout the last decade, tailoring systems have been developed for an extensive variety of applications providing information for:

- Patients at significant risk of developing chronic conditions.
- Patients who already have chronic conditions such as migraines, asthma, and diabetes that require long-term continuing treatment.
- Patients undergoing more short-term intensive treatment such as for cancer.

The goal of these systems has also been diverse, supporting the patient's role, health promotion advice, and behavior change interventions.

However, improvement of ICT and mobile health has increased the potential for tailored communication (Rimer & Kreuter 2006). Computer automation allows for the rapid processing of individual responses and matches individuals´ answers to individually tailored messages (Kreuter et al., 1999; Noar et al., 2011). In this kind of computer-generated tailored communication (also called computer-tailoring), the combined expertise of health promoters is translated into a computer expert system (Dijkstra & De Vries, 1999). Content knowledge is needed both to determine the correct information for different kinds of individuals and to devise the decision rules on which the computer program is based (Brug, Campbell &Assema, 1999). Moreover, tailoring can be static or dynamic. In static tailoring, one baseline assessment is provided on which all tailored information is based. In dynamic tailoring, the assessment is repeated before providing pieces of tailored information or feedback (Krebs, Prochaska & Rossi, 2010).

Computer-generated tailored information can be delivered via various channels. Channel selection can be guided by audience preferences and campaign goals.

Tailored information can be delivered via:

- Print.
- Telephone call.
- Face to face.
- Mobile phone text message.

- CD-ROM.
- Computer kiosk.
- The Internet.

Computer-tailored but print-delivered interventions are deemed the 'first generation'; interventions using interactive media are deemed the 'second generation' of tailored health communication (Oenema, Brug & Lechner, 2001). The 'third generation' interventions refer to interventions delivered via mobile and remote devices such as mobile phones and handheld computers (Norman et al., 2007).

Information and communication technologies (ICT) such as the Internet and mobile phones provide new opportunities for the delivery of innovative interventions (Pratt et al., 2012). Health behavior change programs and campaigns delivered via the Internet have become increasingly popular for the promotion of lifestyle-related health behaviors (Kroeze, Werkman & Brug, 2006). Availability, transferability, relatively small cost, and customization are some of the benefits of selecting web-based programs and campaigns as well as a perception of anonymity, which may be appealing to reluctant or self-conscious participants. In addition, Web-based health behavior programs and campaigns appear to be cost-effective (Norman et al., 2007; Tate et al., 2009; Webb et al., 2010). The Internet is increasingly used by private and public healthcare organizations in their communications and information transfer (Eng, 2002). The concept of eHealth involves the use of ICT to improve health in general and the healthcare system in particular (Eysenbach, 2001; Chau & Hu, 2004). Furthermore, mobile health (mHealth) is thought to be the next step in computerized health interventions (Riley et al., 2011).

The research on health behavior change has also led to the development of technologies supporting behavior changes (Consolvo et al., 2006; Nawyn et al., 2006). These so-called persuasive technologies (Fogg, 2003) embed motivational strategies into everyday electronic devices to encourage and sustain long-term health behavior changes. They attempt to shape, reinforce or change behaviors, attitudes, feelings or thoughts about an issue, object or action (Berkovsky et al., 2012). According to Oinas-Kukkonen (2013) behavior change support systems are the primary focus of research in the area of persuasive technologies (Lehto, 2013). A fundamental challenge in persuasion is that the target audiences are large and heterogeneous including users with wide-ranging goals, needs and preferences (Berkovsky et al., 2012). The solutions for this can be the targeting and tailoring of health communication. (Noar et al., 2009).

In addition, tailored health behavior change programs usually refer to computer-tailored programs commonly delivered by a computer or the Internet (Suggs et al., 2006). In a tailored program, for instance, tools for building self-regulatory skills can be combined with tailored health feedback messages (Lustria et al., 2009). Goal setting and action planning (Brug et al., 2005) or observational learning, providing role models, supporting emotional coping and allowing reinforcement by virtual rewards (Toscos & Connolly, 2010), can help to bridge the information behavior gap.

Other projects around the world are using natural language generation techniques that allow more interactivity. Interactivity is defined as the capability of new communication systems to 'talk back' to the user as do individuals participating in a conversation (Rogers, 1986). Although there is interest in producing tailoring systems that enable enhanced interactivity, few studies have been able to demonstrate the effectiveness of health behavior. Cawsey, Grasso & Jones (1999) developed a nutritional tailoring system based on a dialog with the user. The users receive suggestions for improving the meal after making some meal choices. They can answer back to each tip in various ways, asserting objections or rejecting it outright. Another example is the Patient Education and Activation System (PEAS) project, which was designed to prepare individuals to take an active role in health care decisions (McRoy & Liu-Perez, 1998).The project investigated strategies for helping people to identify their health care concerns.

These strategies combine a multimodal computer interface with intelligent tutoring and intelligent discourse processing. As PEAS interacts with a patient, it varies the content and pace of the interaction and suggests relevant learning activities.

Because of the restraints of existing tools and techniques, several of the most experimental projects attempt to use more sophisticated techniques, taking ideas from information technology and using Natural Language Generation (NLG) methods (Reiter & Sripanda, 2003). The basic idea behind most of these systems is to:

- Represent explicit information about the patient.
- Represent general rules about communication.
- Generate text from a database of health-related information.

Achieving this, with only limited knowledge of how humans tailor their communications has proven to be very difficult. In practice, however, even these systems have lacked access to a knowledge base that contains fundamental determinants of the selected behavior. As a result, NLG approaches that incorporate tailoring on health behavior determinants have been limited.

More frequently the tailoring systems are developed using NLG. Consequently, they embrace the understanding that the same semantic information can be conveyed through text and sentence structures. A multi-argument formation, which is critical to expanding communications in health behavior change, embodies two types of knowledge acquisition (KA) techniques:

- Working with experts in a structured fashion, think-aloud protocols, sorting and laddered grids.
- Learning from data sets of correct solutions.

In this light, a new conceptual framework is needed to broaden the scope and boundaries of tailored communications research in the era of the science of individuality. The traditional communications model consists of a source, a message, a channel of delivery, a receiver, and an effect on the receiver. Anything that impedes message transfer through the channel is considered 'noise'. This basic model, developed before the science of individuality, could not anticipate the new tools that are now available. Ideally, both sender and receiver continually adapt their presentations until both are satisfied that knowledge has been appropriately transferred. As computers become faster, multimedia, interactive communications are now also possible, using sophisticated expert systems and inference engines to reduce 'noise'. Virtual reality can help individuals 'pre-live' the future consequences of their decisions and explore the effect of their lifestyle choices on their biology and social and emotional well-being. Palmtop computers and personal organizers make it possible to provide 'on demand' information in 'real time'. The concept of a computer 'coach' that is available on demand is rapidly becoming a reality.

ISSUES, CONTROVERSIES, PROBLEMS

The most significant barriers to information use and information reception are psychological and cognitive. For instance, an individual may feel bombarded with too much information. This kind of situation is called information overload, and it may lead to information avoidance (Case, 2012). Information overload is directly related to information use because the experience of information overload affects the way in which information sources are selected or rejected. According to Savolainen (2008), there is no consensus among researchers about the definition of information overload and whether the phenomenon exists. Eysenbach (2003) states 'individuals who are exposed to excessive information may make poor health decisions that can potentially have harmful effects on outcomes.'

Additionally, the terminology used in health information may be complicated and presented in a way that the information receiver does not understand (Docherty et al., 2008; Fourie, 2008). Coping with differences between 'lay language' and professional terminology can be a barrier to information use and decision-making (McKenzie, 2002; Brennan & Safran, 2005; Eriksson-Backa, 2008). Thus, one way to avoid the experience of information overload or avoidance is to become information literate.

The Medical Library Association (2003) defines health information literacy as a 'set of abilities needed to: recognize a health information need; identify information sources and use them to retrieve relevant information; assess the quality of the information and its applicability to a particular situation; and analyze, understand, and use the information to make good health decisions'.

On the other hand, no studies to date have directly compared tailored and targeted approaches to health communication. One particular area of inquiry would be to test the variability of the principal determinants of the intended outcome. More variability on the key determinants of some expected outcome is associated with the tailored messages being superior to targeted messages. Such studies would provide valuable information contributing to greater evidence-based practice in health communication.

However, analysis elucidated that well-suited non-tailored materials can function as well or better than tailored materials. At the same time, moderate and poor-fitting non-tailored materials were usually subordinate to both approaches. These findings suggest two critical points. First, there is considerable variation in the effectiveness of any single communication approach. Second, current tailored print communications may be no more effective than generic materials that are well matched to a particular person.

Nevertheless, the art of creating tailored health communication is still evolving. The tailored print materials tested to date probably lie in the middle of a continuum from entirely generic to perfectly tailored health communication. However, enhanced tailored communication addresses not only behavioral constructs from a few selected theories of health behavior change but also factors such as:

- Learning style.
- Preferred media.
- Cultural norms and values.
- Need for cognition.
- Use of emotional versus cognitive appeals.

As a result, research on tailored health communication should identify and test new types of tailoring variables that could improve behavior change and health messages.

Moreover, studies of tailored content matching have compared a group of targeted communication with the experimental group. In effect, the designs tested if tailoring is more efficient than little or no segmentation and customization. In this context, research questions should focus on the attributes of tailoring:

- The cognitive and behavioral determinant goals.
- The strategies to achieve them.

One obvious way to approach such designs is the presence versus absence of specific attributes, but many creative alternatives are also possible. Beyond this, research should also address the circumstances different tailoring tactics elicit different results. It is also necessary to compare specific tailoring strategies and tactics. One method is a dismantling design. Another approach, the parametric or 'dosing' model, examines the effects of the same tailoring strategy but various intensities. Third, individual tailoring strategies may be added to those with some degree of tailoring.

Finally, because segmentation and customization rely on information about individuals, individual-based assessments are considered to be indispensable to tailored interventions. However, such assessments can have an independent impact on behavior.

SOLUTIONS AND RECOMMENDATIONS

Tailored communications can come in an unlimited number of forms, including tailored telephone counselling and voice response systems. As the information superhighway evolves, the World Wide Web will bring accessibility to interactive multimedia intervention technologies.

Given such rapid technological advances, tailored communications may now reduce 'noise' by gathering detailed personal information for input at the source and then presenting appropriate messages through the channel. Computer-based delivery options can simulate a conversation by tailoring information, in real time, based on user responses. The potential for rapid feedback in real time provides the capability to modify subsequent messages and/or deliver repeated communications.

Such factors offer qualitative advances in the communication model of the 1960s. As a result, the theoretical models of the future must continuously evolve to keep pace with new technologies.

Theories of behavior change must also guide tailored message algorithms. In the last 30 years, Social Cognitive Theory has served as an overarching theoretical framework; one that has identified specific mediating mechanisms that lead to behavior change. Related models emphasize different potential mediating mechanisms that are thought to be most relevant to creating tailored communications (Glanz et al., 1997). They range from the Health Belief Model, the Theory of Reasoned Action, and the Transtheoretical Stages of Change Model to more recent theories of risk perception such as the Precaution Adoption Model (Weinstein, 1993).

Research can help identify what specific mediating mechanisms and processes are best targeted to enhance tailored message effects. Such variables include:

- Intrinsic versus extrinsic motivation.
- Emotional blunting versus monitoring.

- Availability and type of coping responses.
- Self-efficacy expectations.
- Variety of proximal and distal outcome expectations.
- Appraisal of the decisional balance between the advantages and disadvantages of changing behavior.

Neural nets and intelligence technologies blur the boundaries between computer learning algorithms and the human brain. Intelligence research can inform tailored communications research and vice versa. Current advanced tailoring technology uses deductive and inductive inferencing systems to generate new data points based on an individual's profile information. Artificial intelligence applications, such as heuristics and neural networks hold much promise for generating tailored content from generic content and for modifying intervention curricula and presentation based on individual case observations.

Moreover, the particular neurobiological substrate determines the parameters and limits of the tailored communications. Basic mechanisms might include individual differences in speed of information processing and preferences regarding modes of message delivery. Research on risk perception and optimistic versus pessimistic bias can further contribute to improving understanding of how to present information to patients and what questions to ask.

In the final analysis, the impact of computer and provider delivered tailored messages may also hinge on the receiver's perceptions of self-efficacy, outcome expectations, and feelings of empowerment. Depending upon how messages are framed, receivers may feel more or less empowered and more or less self-confident. As a result, we need to understand more about how computer versus human experts influence the receiver's perceptions of empowerment and self-efficacy.

Within Anderson's (1998) interdisciplinary biopsychosocial framework, the interface between biobehavioral and biosocial disciplines is particularly relevant for advancing theory and guiding research on the mediating mechanisms underlying tailored communications. Models of self-control or self- regulation, derived from Social Cognitive Theory, are at the heart of understanding behavior change for tailored communications. However, different biological, psychological, or social mechanisms underlie change for different target behaviors and populations.

Prior research offers little specific guidance about how to bridge the gap between theory and application. The gap between theory and practice raises fundamental questions about how to define the boundaries and limits of tailoring in actual practice. That raises the issue of whether the principles of stepped care should be considered when designing future tailored interventions. A stepped-care model would first disseminate a relatively brief inexpensive and less sophisticated tailored intervention. Only the subset who failed to respond would then be stepped up. This type of model that combines stepped care with tailoring has been proposed to improve the cost-effectiveness. It provides a rational means of allocating finite resources to achieve the most significant population impact by reserving the more complicated and expensive interventions for a smaller group who have failed at all previous steps.

Despite the intuitive appeal of stepped-care models to tailoring, it is also possible that a very inexpensive intervention produce little change. Very little research to date has addressed these issues. Ultimately, future research should provide information relevant to the costs of tailoring per incremental increase in the outcome and population impact. It should also shed light on linking such gains to measures of quality-adjusted life years saved. Cost-effectiveness and cost-benefit information are critical for informing health policy and convincing payers to consider investing in tailored message technologies over other ideas within their budget allocations.

In summary, traditional communication theories need to be expanded, or new ones developed. Bridges must be built between communication and behavior change theory. Standardization of language, models, mechanisms, and measures is needed to advance the field, producing unique additions to outcome variance. More research must focus on how to define and identify the mediators that optimize the impact of tailored communications. Variables that cut across biopsychosocial domains should be incorporated into a single model or theory of tailored communications. Future research on theory and mechanisms should conduct a more prospective process to outcome evaluations of causal pathways and examine the predictive and incremental value of new variables and mechanisms over and above existing ones. A broader theoretical model must also incorporate other disciplines and bodies of knowledge beyond those listed above. Some of the significant factors in developing a credible and trusting relationship among humans is the consistency of responses over time. Finally, a fundamental issue that deserves more attention is who should receive tailored messages.

FUTURE RESEARCH DIRECTIONS

It is complicated to employ persuasive argumentation theories to behavioral change communication. Moreover, research in argumentation has been concerned only with the structure of single arguments. Likewise, NLG systems do not explore the planning mechanisms that would account for the generation of text. One also needs a theory that would describe (Ajzen, 1991):

- How arguments could be put together.
- Why particular multi-argument structures are more persuasive.

Some of the computational tailoring systems have attempted to combine theories of argumentation with behavioral theories. They realized that if an intervention aims to induce people to modify their behavior, particular theories of the advising process are necessary. These interventions have used Stages of Change and the Health Belief Model (Grasso, 1998). However, all of these systems have been difficult to move into real-world environments primarily because of the entanglement of using NLG techniques to generate multi-argument structures in domains as complex as health behavior.

In addition, little is known in the reusable NLG resources while the nonlinguistic tailoring approach has other limitations. It is possible that the integration of both the nonlinguistic tailoring approach and computer science methods is essential for the development of tailored messages. To design a system whose ultimate aim is to try influencing the user's behavior, very diverse sources of knowledge have to be integrated.

Theories of argumentation and persuasive structure are perhaps what is needed to build on and extend current tailoring research. In addition, additional types of tailoring variables should be tested. Theory must adopt the most parsimonious strategies without omitting essential mechanisms. That will require the adoption of a common language and standard measures for the underlying mechanism and processes. For the unification of the more sophisticated technologies, theory, and real-world applications, joint research is needed. As such, it remains to be seen whether the advances of the tailoring process will deliver the tailored health communication approaches sufficient to engineer an impact on:

- Improved decision-making.
- Patient health behavior.
- Chronic disease management.

CONCLUSION

Robinson et al. (1998) cautioned that health communications applications hold great promise but can cause harm. They encouraged health care providers to speed the advancement of knowledge and evaluate its safety, quality, and utility. They also proposed a standardized reporting template to:

- Guide developers and evaluators.
- Conduct evaluations.
- Help clinicians, purchasers, and consumers judge their quality, efficacy, and efficiency of disclosed results.

Of critical importance is the need for research on implementation to elucidate the mechanisms for cost-effective diffusion of tailored interventions to populations. Safeguards must also ensure confidentiality and ethical standards to protect consumers. Finally, theory and applications are lagging behind the rapid pace of technological advances. Standardization of language, research designs, methods, and measures are crucial along with developing broader interdisciplinary conceptual models. The gap between technology, theory, and application can be closed by:

- Providing opportunities for basic research into the fundamental mechanisms of tailored communications.
- Broadening theories of behavior change for tailored communications research.
- Enhancing message effectiveness and practical impact on outcomes.

It remains to be seen whether the revolution in the science of individuality and m-health will provide the tools to engineer sufficient impact on tailored communication.

REFERENCES

Ajzen, I. (1991). The theory of planned behavior. *Organizational Behavior and Human Decision Processes*, *50*(2), 179–211. doi:10.1016/0749-5978(91)90020-T

Anderson, N. B. (1998). Levels of analysis in health science: A framework for integrating sociobehavioral and biomedical research. *Annals of the New York Academy of Sciences*, *840*(1), 563–576. doi:10.1111/j.1749-6632.1998.tb09595.x PMID:9629283

Bandura, A. (2006). Guide for constructing self-efficacy scales. In T. Urban & F. Pajares (Eds.), *Self-efficacy Beliefs of Adolescents*. Charlotte, NC: Information Age Publishing.

Barton, A. J. (2010). Using mobile health technology to enhance patient-centered care. *Clinical Nurse Specialist CNS, 24*(5), 233–234. PMID:20716974

Bates, M. J. (2009). Information Behavior. In M. J. Bates & M. N. Maack (Eds.), *Encyclopedia of Library and Information Sciences* (3rd ed.). New York, NY: CRC Press. doi:10.1081/E-ELIS3-120043263

Berkovsky, S., Freyne, J., & Oinas-Kukkonen, H. (2012). Influencing individually: Fusing personalization and persuasion. *ACM Transactions on Interactive Intelligent Systems, 2*(2), 1–8. doi:10.1145/2209310.2209312

Brennan, L. K., Kreuter, M. W., Caburnay, C. A., & Wilshire, B. L. (1998). *Linking smokers to smoking cessation programs: does perceived importance of specific program characteristics predict cessation?* Paper presented at the Society of Behavioral Medicine Conference, New Orleans, LA.

Brennan, P. F., & Safran, C. (2005). Empowered consumers. In D. Lewis, G. Eysenbach, R. Kukafka, P. Z. Stavri, & H. Jimison (Eds.), *Consumer Health Informatics: informing consumers and improving health care*. New York, NY: Springer. doi:10.1007/0-387-27652-1_2

Brug, J., Campbell, M., & van Assema, P. (1999). The application and impact of computer-generated personalized nutrition education: A review of the literature. *Patient Education and Counseling, 36*(2), 145–156. doi:10.1016/S0738-3991(98)00131-1 PMID:10223019

Brug, J., Oenema, A., & Campbell, M. (2003). Past, present, and future of computer-tailored nutrition education. *The American Journal of Clinical Nutrition, 77*(4), 1028S–1034S. doi:10.1093/ajcn/77.4.1028S PMID:12663313

Brug, J., Oenema, A., & Ferreira, I. (2005). Theory, evidence and Intervention Mapping to improve behavior nutrition and physical activity interventions. *The International Journal of Behavioral Nutrition and Physical Activity, 2*(2). PMID:15807898

Brug, J., Steenhaus, I., van Assema, P., & de Vries, H. (1996). The impact of computer-tailored nutrition intervention. *Preventive Medicine, 25*(3), 236–242. doi:10.1006/pmed.1996.0052 PMID:8781000

Brug, J., van Assema, P., Kok, G., Lenderink, T., & Glanz, K. (1994). Self-rated dietary fat intake: Association with objective assessment of fat, psychosocial factors, and intention to change. *Journal of Nutrition Education, 26*(5), 218–223. doi:10.1016/S0022-3182(12)80890-9

Bull, F. C., & Jamrozik, K. (1998). Advice on exercise from a family physician can help sedentary patients to become active. *American Journal of Preventive Medicine, 15*(2), 85–94. doi:10.1016/S0749-3797(98)00040-3 PMID:9713663

Campbell, M. K., DeVellis, B. M., Strecher, V. J., Ammerman, A. S., DeVellis, R. F., & Sandler, R. S. (1994). Improving dietary behavior: The effectiveness of tailored messages in primary care settings. *American Journal of Public Health, 84*(5), 783–787. doi:10.2105/AJPH.84.5.783 PMID:8179049

Campbell, M. K., & Quintiliani, L. M. (2006). Tailored interventions in public health. Where does tailoring fit in interventions to reduce health disparities? *The American Behavioral Scientist, 49*(6), 775–793. doi:10.1177/0002764205283807

Case, D. O. (2012). *Looking for Information. A Survey of Research on Information Seeking, Needs, and Behavior*. Bingley, UK: Emerald.

Cawsey, A., Grasso, F., & Jones, R. B. (1999). A conversational model for health promotion on the World Wide Web. Artificial intelligence in medicine. *Proceedings of the Joint European Conference on Artificial Intelligence in Medicine and Medical Decision Making*.

Chatman, E. A., & Pendleton, V. E. M. (1995). Knowledge gap, information-seeking and the poor. *The Reference Librarian*, *23*(49/50), 135–145. doi:10.1300/J120v23n49_10

Chau, P. Y. K., & Hu, P. J. (2004). Technology Implementation for Telemedicine Programs. *Communications of the ACM*, *47*(2), 87–92. doi:10.1145/966389.966396

Cole, C., & Leide, J. E. (2006). A cognitive framework for human information behavior: The place of metaphor in human information organizing behavior. In A. Spink & C. Cole (Eds.), *New Directions in Human Information Behavior* (pp. 171–202). Dordrecht, Germany: Springer. doi:10.1007/1-4020-3670-1_10

Consolvo, S., Everitt, K. M., Smith, I., & Landay, J. A. (2006). Design requirements for technologies that encourage physical activity. In *Proceedings of CHI 2006*. Montréal, Canada. ACM Press.

Contrada, R. J., & Goyal, T. M. (2004). Individual differences, health and illness: the role of emotional traits and generalized expectancies. In The SAGE Handbook of Health Psychology (pp. 143–169). London, UK: SAGE Publications Ltd.

Derr, R. L. (1983). A conceptual analysis of information need. *Information Processing & Management*, *19*(5), 273–278. doi:10.1016/0306-4573(83)90001-8

Dijkstra, A., De Vries, H., & Roijackers, J. (1998a). Computerized tailored feedback to change cognitive determinants of smoking: A Dutch field experiment. *Health Education Research*, *13*(2), 197–206. doi:10.1093/her/13.2.197 PMID:10181018

Dijkstra, A., De Vries, H., & Roijackers, J. (1998b). Longterm effectiveness of computer-generated tailored feedback in smoking cessation. *Health Education Research*, *13*(2), 207–214. doi:10.1093/her/13.2.207 PMID:10181019

Dijkstra, A., & Vries, H. (1999). The development of computer-generated tailored interventions. *Patient Education and Counseling*, *36*(1), 193–203. doi:10.1016/S0738-3991(98)00135-9 PMID:10223023

Docherty, A., Owens, A., Asadi-Lari, M., Petchey, R., Williams, J., & Carter, Y. H. (2008). Knowledge and information needs of informal caregivers in palliative care: A qualitative systematic review. *Palliative Medicine*, *22*(2), 153–171. doi:10.1177/0269216307085343 PMID:18372380

Eng, T. R. (2002). E-health research and evaluation: Challenges and opportunities. *Journal of Health Communication*, *7*(4), 267–272. doi:10.1080/10810730290001747 PMID:12356287

Eriksson-Backa, K. (2008). Access to health information: perceptions of barriers among elderly in a language minority. *Information Research*, *13*(4).

Evans, W. D. (2006). How social marketing works in health care. *British Medical Journal*, *332*(7551), 1207–1210. PMID:16710002

Eysenbach, G. (2001). What is e-health? *Journal of Medical Internet Research, 3*(2), e20. doi:10.2196/jmir.3.2.e20 PMID:11720962

Eysenbach, G. (2003). The impact of the Internet on cancer outcomes. *CA: a Cancer Journal for Clinicians, 53*(6), 356–370. doi:10.3322/canjclin.53.6.356 PMID:15224975

Fidel, R. (2012). *Human Information Interaction: An Ecological Approach to Information Behavior.* Cambridge, MA: MIT Press. doi:10.7551/mitpress/9780262017008.001.0001

Fogg, B. J. (2003). *Persuasive Technology: Using Computers to Change What We Think and Do.* New York, NY: Morgan Kaufmann. doi:10.1016/B978-155860643-2/50011-1

Fourie, I. (2008). Information needs and information behaviour of patients and their family members in a cancer palliative care setting: an exploratory study of an existential context from different perspectives. *Information Research, 13*(4).

Glanz, K., Lewis, F. M., & Rimer, B. K. (Eds.). (1997). *Health Behavior and Health Education.* San Francisco, CA: Jossey-Bass Publishers.

Grasso, F. (1998). Exciting avocados and dull pears: combining behavioral and argumentative theory for producing effective advice. In *Proceedings of the 20th Annual Meeting of the Cognitive Science Society* (pp. 436-41). Hillsdale, NJ: Erlbaum Associates.

Hawkins, R. P., Kreuter, M., Resnicow, K., Fishbein, M., & Dijkstra, A. (2008). Understanding tailoring in communicating about health. *Health Education Research, 23*(3), 454–466. doi:10.1093/her/cyn004 PMID:18349033

Johnson, J. D., Andrews, J. E., & Allard, S. (2001). A model for understanding and affecting cancer genetics information seeking. *Library & Information Science Research, 23*(4), 335–349. doi:10.1016/S0740-8188(01)00094-9

Johnson, J. D., & Case, D. O. (2012). *Health Information Seeking.* New York, NY: Peter Lang Publishing.

Keller, P. (2006). Regulatory Focus and Efficacy of Health Messages. *The Journal of Consumer Research, 33*(June), 109–114. doi:10.1086/504141

Krebs, P., Prochaska, J. O., & Rossi, J. S. (2010). Defining what works in tailoring: A meta-analysis of computer-tailored interventions for health behavior change. *Preventive Medicine, 51*(3–4), 214–221. doi:10.1016/j.ypmed.2010.06.004 PMID:20558196

Kreuter, M. W., Farrell, D., Olevich, L., & Brennan, L. (1999). *Tailoring health messages: Customizing communication with computer technology.* Mahwah, NJ: Erlbaum.

Kreuter, M. W., & Strecher, V. J. (1996). Do tailored behavior change messages enhance the effectiveness of health risk appraisals? Results from a randomized trial. *Health Education Research, 11*(1), 97–105. doi:10.1093/her/11.1.97 PMID:10160231

Kreuter, M. W., & Wray, R. J. (2003). Tailored and targeted health communication: Strategies for enhancing information relevance. *American Journal of Health Behavior, 27*(1Suppl 3), S227–S232. doi:10.5993/AJHB.27.1.s3.6 PMID:14672383

Kroeze, W., Werkman, A., & Brug, J. (2006). A systematic review of randomized trials on the effectiveness of computer-tailored education on physical activity and dietary behaviors. *Annals of Behavioral Medicine, 31*(3), 205–223. doi:10.120715324796abm3103_2 PMID:16700634

Lehto, T. (2013). *The Importance of Persuasive Systems Design in Enhancing Consumers´ Perceptions and Adoption of Health Behavior Change Support Systems* (Doctoral dissertation). University of Oulu, Department of Information Processing Science.

Lustria, M. L., Cortese, J., Noar, S. M., & Glueckauf, R. L. (2009). Computer-tailored health interventions delivered over the Web: Review and analysis of key components. *Patient Education and Counseling, 74*(2), 156–173. doi:10.1016/j.pec.2008.08.023 PMID:18947966

Marcus, B. H., Emmons, K. M., Simkin-Silverman, L. R., Linnan, L. A., Taylor, E. R., Bock, B. C., ... Abrams, D. B. (1998). Evaluation of motivationally tailored versus standard self-help physical activity interventions at the workplace. *American Journal of Health Promotion, 12*(4), 246–253. doi:10.4278/0890-1171-12.4.246 PMID:10178617

McKenzie, P. J. (2002). Communcation barriers and information-seeking counterstrategies in accounts of practitioner-patient encounters. *Library & Information Science Research, 24*(1), 31–47. doi:10.1016/S0740-8188(01)00103-7

McRoy, S. W., Liu-Perez, A., & Ali, S. S. (1998). Interactive computerized health care education. *Journal of the American Medical Informatics Association, 5*(4), 347–356. doi:10.1136/jamia.1998.0050347 PMID:9670132

Medical Library Association. (2003). *Health Information Literacy: Definitions*. Retrieved April 20, 2015, from https://www.mlanet.org/resources/healthlit/define.html

Murray-Johnson, L., & Witte, K. (2003). Looking toward the future: health message design strategies. In T. L. Thompson, A. M. Dorsey, K. I. Miller, & R. Parrott (Eds.), *Handbook of Health Communication*. Mahwah, NJ: Lawrence Erlbaum Associates Inc.

Nahl, D., & Bilal, D. (2007). *Information and Emotion: The Emergent Affective Paradigm in Information Behavior Research and Theory*. Medford, NJ: Information Today.

Nawyn, J., Intille, S. S., & Larson, K. (2006). Embedding behavior modification strategies intoa consumer electronic device: a case study. In *Proceedings of UbiComp 2006, Ubiquitous Computing: 8th International Conference*. Berlin: Springer. 10.1007/11853565_18

Noar, S. M., Harrington, N. G., & Aldrich, R. S. (2009). The role of message tailoring in the development of persuasive health communication messages. In C. S. Beck (Ed.), *Communication Yearbook 33* (pp. 73–133). New York, NY: Routledge.

Noar, S. M., Harrington, N. G., Van Stee, S. K., & Aldrich, R. S. (2011). Tailored Health Communication to Change Lifestyle Behaviors. *American Journal of Lifestyle Medicine, 5*(2), 112–122. doi:10.1177/1559827610387255

Norman, G. J., Zabinski, M. F., Adams, M. A., Rosenberg, D. E., Yaroch, A. L., & Atienza, A. A. (2007). A review of eHealth interventions for physical activity and dietary behavior change. *American Journal of Preventive Medicine*, *33*(4), 336–345. doi:10.1016/j.amepre.2007.05.007 PMID:17888860

Oenema, A., Brug, J., & Lechner, L. (2001). Web-based tailored nutrition education: Results of a randomized controlled trial. *Health Education Research*, *16*(6), 647–660. doi:10.1093/her/16.6.647 PMID:11780705

Oinas-Kukkonen, H. (2013). A foundation for the study of Behavior Change Support Systems. *Personal and Ubiquitous Computing*, *17*(6), 1223–1235. doi:10.100700779-012-0591-5

Pettigrew, K. E., Fidel, R., & Bruce, H. (2001). Conceptual frameworks in information behavior. *Annual Review of Information Science & Technology*, *35*, 43–78.

Petty, R. E., & Cacioppo, J. T. (1986). The elaboration likelihood model of persuasion. *Advances in Experimental Psychology*, *19*, 123–205. doi:10.1016/S0065-2601(08)60214-2

Pratt, M., Sarmiento, O. L., Montes, F., Ogilvie, D., Marcus, B. H., Perez, L. G., & Brownson, R. C. (2012). The implications of megatrends in information and communication technology and transportation for changes in global physical activity. *Lancet*, *380*(9838), 282–293. doi:10.1016/S0140-6736(12)60736-3 PMID:22818940

Prochaska, J. O., DiClemente, C. C., Velicer, W. F., & Rossi, J. S. (1993). Standardized, individualized, interactive and personalized self-help programs for smoking cessation. *Health Psychology*, *12*(5), 399–405. doi:10.1037/0278-6133.12.5.399 PMID:8223364

Reiter, E., & Sripanda, S. (2003). Acquiring correct knowledge from natural language generation. *Journal of Artificial Intelligence Research*, *18*, 491–516. doi:10.1613/jair.1176

Riley, W. T., Rivera, D. E., Atienza, A. A., Nilsen, W., Allison, S. M., & Mermelstein, R. (2011). Health behavior models in the age of mobile interventions: Are our theories up to the task? *Translational Behavioral Medicine*, *1*(1), 53–71. doi:10.100713142-011-0021-7 PMID:21796270

Rimer, B. K., Briss, P. A., Zeller, P. K., Chan, E. C., & Woolf, S. H. (2004). Informed decision making: What is its role in cancer screening? *Cancer*, *101*(5Suppl), 1214–1228. doi:10.1002/cncr.20512 PMID:15316908

Rimer, B. K., & Kreuter, M. W. (2006). Advancing tailored health communication: A persuasion and message effects perspective. *Journal of Communication*, *56*(s1), S184–S201. doi:10.1111/j.1460-2466.2006.00289.x

Rippen, H., & Risk, A. (2000). eHealth Code of Ethics. *Journal of Medical Internet Research*, *2*(2), e9. doi:10.2196/jmir.2.2.e9

Robinson, T. N., Patrick, K., Eng, T. R., & Gustafson, D. (1998). An evidence-based approach to interactive health communication. *Journal of the American Medical Association*, *280*(14), 1264–1269. doi:10.1001/jama.280.14.1264 PMID:9786378

Rogers, E. M. (1986). *Communication Technology: The New Media in Society*. New York: The Free Press.

Rogers, R. W. (1985). Attitude Change and Information on Integration in Fear Appeals. *Psychological Reports*, *56*(1), 179–182. doi:10.2466/pr0.1985.56.1.179

Roper, W. L. (1993). Health communication takes on new dimensions at CDC. *Public Health Reports*, *108*(2), 179–183. PMID:8385358

Savolainen, R. (2008). *Everyday Information Practices. A Social Phenomenological Perspective*. Lanham, MD: Scarecrow.

Savolainen, R. (2009). Information use and information processing: Comparison of conceptualizations. *The Journal of Documentation*, *65*(2), 187–207. doi:10.1108/00220410910937570

Schwarzer, R. (2008). Modeling health behavior change: How to predict and modify the adoption and maintenance of health behaviors. *Applied Psychology*, *57*, 1–29.

Sheeran, P. (2005). Intention–Behavior Relations: A Conceptual and Empirical Review. In W. Stroebe & M. Hewstone (Eds.), *European Review of Social Psychology*. Chichester, UK: John Wiley & Sons. doi:10.1002/0470013478.ch1

Skinner, C. S., Strecher, V. J., & Hospers, H. (1994). Physician recommendations for mammography: Do tailored messages make a difference? *American Journal of Public Health*, *84*(1), 43–49. doi:10.2105/AJPH.84.1.43 PMID:8279610

Strecher, V. J., Kreuter, M. W., Den Boer, D.-J., Kobrin, S., Hospers, H. J., & Skinner, C. S. (1994). The effects of computer-tailored smoking cessation messages in family practice settings. *The Journal of Family Practice*, *39*, 262–270. PMID:8077905

Suggs, L. S., Cowdery, J. E., & Carroll, J. B. (2006). Tailored program evaluation: Past, present, future. *Evaluation and Program Planning*, *29*(4), 426–432. doi:10.1016/j.evalprogplan.2006.08.003 PMID:17950872

Talja, S., Tuominen, K., & Savolainen, R. (2005). Isms in information science: Constructivism, collectivism and constructionism. *The Journal of Documentation*, *61*(1), 70–101. doi:10.1108/00220410510578023

Tate, D. F., Finkelstein, E. A., Khavjou, O., & Gustafson, A. (2009). Cost effectiveness of Internet interventions: Review and recommendations. *Annals of Behavioral Medicine*, *38*(1), 40–45. doi:10.100712160-009-9131-6 PMID:19834778

Te'eni, D. (2001). Review: A cognitive-affective model of organizational communication for designing IT. *MIS Quaterly*, *25*(2), 251–312. doi:10.2307/3250931

Topol, E. J. (2012). *The creative destruction of medicine: how the digital revolution will create better health care*. New York: Basic Books.

Toscos, T., & Connelly, K. (2010). Using behavior change theory to understand and guide technological interventions. In B. M. Hayes & A. William (Eds.), *Health Informatics: A patient-centered approach to diabetes* (pp. 295–326). Cambridge, MA: MIT Press. doi:10.7551/mitpress/9780262014328.003.0011

Webb, T. L., Joseph, J., Yardley, L., & Michie, S. (2010). Using the Internet to promote health behavior change: A systematic review and meta-analysis of the impact of theoretical basis, use of behavior change techniques, and mode of delivery on efficacy. *Journal of Medical Internet Research*, *12*(1), e4. doi:10.2196/jmir.1376 PMID:20164043

Webb, T. L., & Sheeran, P. (2006). Does change behavioral intentions engender behavior change? A meta-analysis of the experimental evidence. *Psychological Bulletin*, *132*(2), 249–268. doi:10.1037/0033-2909.132.2.249 PMID:16536643

Weinstein, N. D. (1993). Testing four competing theories of health-protective behavior. *Health Psychology*, *12*(4), 324–333. doi:10.1037/0278-6133.12.4.324 PMID:8404807

Williamson, K. (2005). Where one size does not fit all: Understanding the needs of potential users of a portal to breast cancer knowledge online. *Journal of Health Communication: International Perspectives*, *10*(6), 567–580. doi:10.1080/10810730500228961 PMID:16203634

Wilson, T. D. (1999). Models in information behaviour research. *The Journal of Documentation*, *55*(3), 249–270. doi:10.1108/EUM0000000007145

Wilson, T. D. (2000). Human information behavior. *Information Science Research*, *3*(2), 49–55.

KEY TERMS AND DEFINITIONS

Health Behavior: Behavior directed at promoting, protecting and maintaining health.

Health Communication: Informing, influencing, and motivating about important health issues.

Health Information: Information for staying well, preventing and managing disease, and making other decisions related to health and healthcare.

M-Health: It describes the use of a broad range of telecommunication and multimedia technologies within wireless care delivery design and can be broadly defined as the delivery of healthcare services via mobile communication devices.

Science of Individuality: The science which acknowledges that each human needs to be seen and treated with utter respect for his or her individuality.

Tailored Health Communication: Any combination of information strategies intended to reach an individual.

Targeted Health Communication: It corresponds to a process appealing to a defined population subgroup.

Chapter 11
The Nexus of M-Health and Self-Care

Anastasius S. Moumtzoglou
P&A Kyriakou Children's Hospital, Greece

ABSTRACT

Self-care emerged from the concept of health promotion in the 1970s while from 2000 onwards the term self-management gained popularity, with a greater focus on long-term conditions and the trend towards more holistic models of care. Although self-management and self-care are often used interchangeably, a distinction between the two concepts can be made. Both can be considered in terms of a continuum, with self-care at one end as "normal activity" and self-management an extension of this. Self-management support is the assistance given to patients in order to encourage daily decisions that improve health-related behaviors and clinical outcomes. The chapter envisions these concepts on a continuum with one pole representing mobile health and the other self-care. It concludes that self-management support is the nexus of mobile health and self-care.

INTRODUCTION

The health care environment is currently changing to meet technology and societal trends which converge to bring into being new communication patterns that connect and coordinate the roles of healthcare stakeholders. At the same time, the healthcare industry is steering inexorably toward a distributed service design in which essential decision-making occurs at the point of care. One of the central engines of this shift towards decentralization and reorientation of health care services is mobile healthcare (M-Health). M-Health describes the use of a broad range of telecommunication and multimedia technologies within wireless care delivery design and can be broadly defined as the delivery of healthcare services via mobile communication devices. M-Health establishes healthcare communities in which every stakeholder can participate. However, it disrupts the traditional service model where healthcare information, security and access is centrally managed, maintained and limited, transforming the healthcare sector and destroying components that are slow to adapt.

DOI: 10.4018/978-1-5225-8021-8.ch011

Copyright © 2019, IGI Global. Copying or distributing in print or electronic forms without written permission of IGI Global is prohibited.

M-Health interventions range from simple to complex applications and systems that remotely coordinate and actively manage patient care. In this context, it offers an elegant solution to the problem of accessing the right information where and when it is needed within highly fluid, distributed organizations. Moreover, it removes geography and time as barriers to care by establishing connectivity with remote locations and remote workers, creates new points of contact with patients, and changes the frequency and intensity of health care delivery. It also establishes effective new treatment modalities like telehealth, remote patient monitoring, self-care, and home health while it blurs the boundaries between professional medical advice and self-care. Overall, M-Health blends three bodies of knowledge: high technology, life sciences, and human factors.

Self-care emerged from the concept of health promotion in the 1970s. The 1980s there was increasing recognition of 'partnership' with health care professionals, and the 1990s saw more emphasis on the continuity of self-care and so-called 'growth' models. From 2000 onwards the term 'self-management' gained popularity, with a greater focus on long-term conditions and the trend towards more holistic models of care.

Although 'self-management' and 'self-care' are often used interchangeably, a distinction between the two concepts can be made. Both can be considered in terms of a continuum, with self-care at one end as 'normal activity' and self-management an extension of this.

Self-management is principally justified in two different but interlinked ways. The first is that long-term conditions are most effectively managed when patients and professionals work in partnership, combining their different skills and expertise. Secondly, reference is made to the growing older population and incidence of long-term conditions and the increasing demands on health services that result from these trends. In this context, supporting people to become more efficient self-managers of their conditions is presented as an essential strategy for managing health care demand and ensuring the long-term sustainability of health services.

Attempts to encourage and enable people to self-manage have focused on two primary strategies:

- Educational, training and peer-support programs that are provided separately from clinical health care consultations and tend to have little connection to the patients' usual clinical care.
- Approaches to health care meetings in which clinicians put a strong emphasis on supporting people to manage their conditions rather than rely on the clinician.

On the other hand, self-management support is the assistance given to patients in order to encourage daily decisions. It may be viewed in two ways:

- As a portfolio of techniques and tools that help patients choose healthy behaviors.
- As a fundamental transformation of the patient-caregiver relationship into a collaborative partnership.

The purpose of the self-management support is to aid patients take an active role in their treatment.

Education is a feature of self-management support. In self-management support interventions, this is often in the form of patients teaching more about their health condition, the circumstances that trigger and potential options for managing symptom exacerbation.

Thus, the objective of the chapter is to argue that the different concepts of mobile health, self-management support, and self-eare are interconnected and reflect a continuum with one pole representing mobile health and the other self-care. Analysis and interpretation goes beyond summarizing and synthesizing concepts and evidence. It takes concepts apart and puts them back together in a new perspective.

Specifically, the premise that mobile health, self-management support, and self-care reflect a continuum with one pole representing mobile health and the other self-care will come into existence by exploring historical and conceptual information in the background. In this context, the concepts of self-care, self -management, self-management support, and M-Health will be defined and examined. The rationale of the presentation is to show the evolution and conceptual relationship of the concepts of self-care, self -management and self-management support and provide relevant information about the distinct concept of M-Health. The main section of the chapter explicates the nexus of M-Health and self-care by reframing self-management support within patient-centeredness. The rationale and the sequence for developing the arguments is that patient-centeredness involves patients in decisions as well as in their health and health care. Involving patients in decisions relates to the concept of shared decision making while involving patients in their health and health care implies the concepts of self-management support and care and support planning. The presentation, at this point, emphasizes the presentation of existing self-management support tools that embrace the dimensions of information, patient empowerment, and behavior change. Finally, the chapter concludes by providing a discussion of relevant issues, controversies, problems, and emerging trends relating to the conceptualization of the main argument.

BACKGROUND

The term self-care is often associated with a lack of theoretical clarity and confusion because its scope and boundaries are difficult to define (Soderhamn, 2000; Barlow et al., 2002; Clark, 2003). It is frequently viewed as a spectrum starting from the individual responsibility people take in managing the daily choices that they make in relation to their lifestyle, maintaining their health and preventing illness (Chambers, 2006).

Several definitions of self-care have been proposed over the past few decades that highlight the broad spectrum of activities that self-care seems to encompass. Levin et al. (1977), state that self-care is 'the process whereby patients deliberately act on their behalf in health, promotion, prevention of illness, and the detection and treatment of health deviations'. Orem (1995), states that self-care is 'the practice of activities that individuals initiate and perform on their behalf in maintaining life, health, and well-being' and that self-care is 'an adult's continuous contribution to his or her continued existence, health, and well-being'. These definitions clearly acknowledge that the nature of self-care encourages individuals to adopt responsibility for undertaking their self-care but also highlight the spectrum of activities considered to fall within the sphere of self-care.

In reflecting the earlier discussion on the medical and social ideologies associated with self-care, the Department of Health (2005) defines self-care as 'the actions individuals and carers take for themselves, their children, their families, and others to stay fit and maintain good physical and mental health, meet social and psychological needs, prevent illness or accidents, care for minor ailments and long-term conditions, and maintain health and well-being after an acute illness or discharge from hospital.'

Although, these definitions view self-care as occurring without professional assistance, Levin and Idler (1983) have acknowledged that in carrying out self-care 'individuals are informed by technical knowledge and skills derived from the pool of both professional and lay experience.' Hickey et al. (1986) also proposed that self-care be interactive with healthcare professionals, rather than being independent of professional care. Moreover, Orem (1995) stated that a large part of self-care includes knowing when to seek medical advice and participating in interactions with health professionals.

Although the previous discussion has highlighted the different focus of each of the definitions presented above, all of the definitions highlight several key themes that can be considered central to the concept of self-care. The prominent idea is that of the patient being encouraged to take a more active role in, and a greater level of control over, its self-care. As Rodgers et al. (1999) acknowledged self-care transcends the idea of patients as dependent, customary recipients of health services to one where patients become a provider of a large part of their care. Ultimately, the choices for self-care are within the control of the patient, rather than, for example, the health professional (Rodgers and Hay, 1998). Recently, studies supported the potential of a caritative caring culture and compassionate community to form the basis for the reawakening of the natural self-care ability (Arman & Hok, 2016) and the influence of empowerment of habitual health behavior (Eyuboglu & Schulz, 2016).

As a result, the second theme is the idea of self-care, occurring not in isolation from health professionals' provision of care, but in collaboration with health professionals. Self-care is often seen as the antithesis of formal care delivered by health professionals (Dill et al., 1995). However, it should be seen as an approach that requires and promotes a greater level of collaboration between patients and health professionals (Paterson and Sloan, 1994; Rodgers and Hay, 1998; Kolbe, 2002; Redman, 2005; Chambers, 2006). It is an approach that should acknowledge the importance of actively listening to patients about why, when and how they self-care (Ryan et al., 2007). It should also appropriately guide and support patients in their self-care practices (Richardson and Ream, 1997; Rodgers and Hay, 1998; Koch et al., 2004).

A number of theories and conceptual models, rooted in different disciplines, seem relevant to the concept of self-care. However, there are few which have been explicitly posited as a model designed to underpin self-care research and self-care in clinical practice and few which have been empirically tested for their utility. Fu et al. (2004) identified five theoretical or conceptual models central to the idea of self-care and symptom management. These included:

- The Self Care Model (Orem, 1991; 1995).
- The Conceptual Model for Symptom Management (Larson et al., 1994; Dodd et al., 2001).
- The Common Sense Model (Leventhal et al., 1984, 1997, 2001).
- The Symptom Interpretation Model (Teel et al., 1997).
- The Theory of Unpleasant Symptoms (Lenz et al., 1995; 1997).

The Self Care Model (Orem, 1991; 1995) focuses on determining the extent of one's ability to carry out self-care. The Conceptual Symptom Management Model focuses on the subjective symptom experiences of individuals, the influence factors, the symptom management strategies and symptom outcomes. The Common Sense Model or Leventhal's Self-Regulation Model (Leventhal et al, 1984, 1997, 2001) theorizes that the perception of fear and threat resulting from the experience of a symptom are determining factors in the initiation of one's self-care (Fu et al., 2004). The Symptom Interpretation Model (Teel et al, 1997) postulates that an individual receives and recognizes a stimulus from a symptom and makes a decision about how to manage that symptom (Fu et al., 2004). Finally, the Theory of Unpleasant Symptoms (Lenz et al, 1995; 1997) argues that the same factors that influence symptom experience lead to similar alleviating interventions for more than one symptom (Fu et al., 2004).

Policy support for self-care has been firmly established in a number of published reports such as:

- 'The NHS Plan' (Department of Health, 2000).
- 'The Expert Patient' (Department of Health, 2001).
- 'Supporting People with Long Term Conditions' (Department of Health, 2005a).
- 'Self-Care – a real choice' (Department of Health, 2005b).
- 'Our Health, Our Care, Our Say' (Department of Health, 2006a).

Additionally, a focus on self-care has also been encouraged by the Scottish healthcare system with the publication of:

- The 'Partnership for Care' (Scottish Executive, 2003).
- The 'National Framework for Service Change in Scotland' (Scottish Executive, 2005a).
- The 'Delivering for Health' (Scottish Executive, 2005b).

These reports appear to have acknowledged the changing focus of chronic disease management and service provision within the NHS. More, political support for self-care may also have been influenced by:

- The recent moves towards the greater patient and public involvement in healthcare (Hubbard et al., 2005).
- The growing evidence base on involving patients in decision-making related to their care (Degner et al., 1997; Beaver et al., 1999; Davison et al., 1999, 2004).

Such calls reinforce support for a move away from the existing top-down model of care to a culture where patients' subjective experiences are considered an essential contribution to understanding the experience of illness.

Overall, definitions of self-care are wide-ranging as they refer to individual responsibilities for healthy lifestyle behaviors required for human development, functioning and coping with health conditions. Self-care suggests that individuals use their attributes to improve poor health (Akinsola, 2001) and includes the actions individuals and carers take to maintain their health and meet social and psychological needs. Positive self-care behaviors include:

- Lifestyle
- Symptoms
- Therapy

Self-management refers to strategies, skills and methods by which individuals effectively direct their activities toward the achievement of their objectives. In computer science, it refers to the process by which pre-programmed computer systems will manage their operation without human intervention. It is understood both as an educative process and an outcome. As an educative process, self-management programs include the participation in education, and the preparation of individuals to manage their health conditions.

In health care, self-management refers to the individual's ability to manage:

- Symptoms
- Treatment

- Physical and psychosocial consequences
- Lifestyle changes

It is also linked with models of coping with adversity through self-help, self-reliance, and family and community reliance (Newbould et al., 2006). The emergence and development of self-management programs can be attributed to:

- The interest of policy-makers.
- The increasing numbers of people seeking to control their approaches to living with illness.
- The increase in awareness of the need to address chronic illnesses.
- The belief that promoting self-management has the potential to help individuals enhance their quality of life.
- The process of demographic and epidemiological transition.
- The emergence of new attitudes towards healthcare delivery.

From a technology standpoint, self-management tools can be categorized into four pillars regarding their use (Sutton & Vatavuk, 2014):

- Subordinate (they do not include much involvement from the patient).
- Structured (allow for self-management in a defined way).
- Collaborative (enable better collaboration between the patient and provider).
- Autonomous (do not require the regular involvement of a healthcare provider).

Although 'self-management' and 'self-care' are often used interchangeably, a distinction between the two concepts can be made. Both can be considered in terms of a continuum, with self-care at one end as 'normal activity', and self-management an extension of this. It is defined as managing 'ailments' either with or without the assistance of a health care professional. Likewise, self-management support is the help health care professionals give to patients with chronic disease in order to stimulate everyday decisions that ameliorate health-related behaviors and clinical outcomes. Self-management support, an important component of person-centered care (de Iongh et al., 2015), may be thought in two ways:

- A portfolio of techniques and tools that assist patients choose healthy behaviors.
- A radical change of the patient-caregiver interrelationship into a synergetic partnership.

The intention of self-management support is to assist patients to become informed about their conditions and take an active role in their treatment. The concept of self-management support has evolved to encompass a wide variety of interventions with different intentions. It is largely a result of various disciplines having contributed to its evolution. There is an important distinction to make between 'self-management' and 'self-management support'. The former takes account of the fact that individuals are self-managing (to a greater or lesser extent) all the time in their daily lives. Self-management, therefore, refers to the behaviors that individuals engage in outside of the health care framework. Self-management support refers to individuals' support for their self-management goals and activities by health care professionals.

Self-management support emanated from a social model of health and disability. The voluntary sector and service user groups were influential in the development of lay-led programs of support. Early models of self-management support were grounded in educational approaches. However, psychological influences became more prominent, especially from the late 1990s onwards, with the realization that behavioral change is not predicted by improvements in knowledge alone.

Mobile health became functional in biomedical engineering and started with looking at wireless and sensor technologies that could be incorporated to monitor people's health at a distance. M-Health implementation came out in developing countries out of access necessity. Mobile phones have been around for years, but it was not until 1976 that mobile phones first appeared in Japan. However, much work happened predominantly in the early millennium when M-Health started to develop mobile health applications for cell phones. The early days there were things like remote cardiac monitors that evolved to look at diabetes monitoring and other types of sensor technologies. The early programs provided support tools for supply chain management while mobile communications gave access to areas that people never had using fixed line telephones. More recent, M-Health evolvement provided access to emergency medical transportation services, facilitated patient-doctor encounter, and there was a movement to personal digital assistants use.

There is no standardized definition of M-Health. In most cases, mobile health or M-Health is defined as 'medical and public health practice supported by mobile devices, such as mobile phones, patient monitoring devices, personal digital assistants (PDAs), and other wireless devices'. It involves:

- The use and capitalization on a mobile phone's core utility of voice and short messaging service.
- More complex functionalities and applications including general packet radio service (GPRS), third and fourth-generation mobile telecommunications (3G and 4G systems), global positioning system (GPS), and Bluetooth technology.

M-Health is increasingly being used in the healthcare field since its use is becoming a cost-effective method of identifying and monitoring health issues. It also provides health professionals with:

- Access to patient data.
- Access to various information sources.

Individuals can use M-Health to obtain resource materials on health issues, and patients can self-monitor and transmit information to their health care provider.

While the timely emergence of M-Health will not resolve the myriad problems, it offers unique opportunities to increase efficiency and improve the quality and access to care. Moreover, with rapid consumer adoption of smartphones, physicians can now perform two-way video conferencing. Patients and physicians have access to medical records and vital signs. Wireless technology will also allow physicians to serve more patients despite geographical limitations.

On current trends, M-Health embraces medical and public health practice sustained by mobile phones, patient monitoring devices, personal digital assistants (PDAs), and tablet PCs. The spread of 3G and 4G networks has boosted the use of mobile applications offering healthcare services. 4G is a mobile network, IP-based, providing connection via the best network using seamless roaming and independent radio access technologies. In 4G mobile systems, different access technologies are combined in the best possible way for different communication environments and service requirements. They promise much larger data rates supporting full mobility while enabling wireless connection and access to multimedia services with high-quality voice and high-definition video. In addition, the availability of satellite navigation technologies in mobile devices supports safety and autonomy of patients. Through sensors and mobile applications, M-Health permits the accumulation of extensive medical, physiological, lifestyle, daily activity and environmental data.

Consequently, M-Health serves evidence-driven care practice and research activities while expediting patients' access to health information and accommodating lifestyle and wellbeing applications, counseling systems, health information and medication reminders. However, beyond clinical connectivity, M-Health is a field that came to light holding the promise of quality improvement, cost reduction, wholesale gains in population health, access to care and better allocation of health-delivery resources. With M-Health, healthcare professionals can continuously monitor and manage health conditions. As a result, M-Health becomes embedded into a number of care delivery strategies, including the medical home, a health information exchange, the care team and patient-centric healthcare.

In its fullest flowering, M-Health it is expected to address the most intractable problems of healthcare quality and cost, chronic disease management, public health, wellness, and prevention. However, the impact of M-Health is just beginning to be felt as it results in more personalized medication and treatment and contributes to the empowerment of patients.

THE NEXUS OF M-HEALTH AND SELF-CARE

Patient-centered care is more than a method of communication. It focuses on patients' preferences, experienced needs and values in decisions about care and treatment. It has a broadened perspective of illness, in which patients' experiences and control are prominent. It also focuses on interactions, striving for an alliance between patients and professionals working together and having common grounds and goals (Epstein et al., 2005; Glasgow et al., 2008; Mead et al., 2000; Michie et al., 2003; Stewart et al., 2000; Swedish Agency for Health and Care Services Analysis, 2012). Howie et al. (2004) reported that patient-centeredness is based on the patients' concerns, putting emphasis on giving the patients time to express these concerns.

Patient-centeredness pertains to patient empowerment which is grounded in equality and respect. As a result, It features self-determining agents with some control over their health and health care and conceptualizes personal control and self-efficacy. For patient empowerment, it is important that patients have knowledge and skills to define and achieve their goals (Funnell et al., 2003; Nyatanga et al., 2002). It is furthermore important that care be planned and performed from this perspective (Ekman et al. 2011; Funnell & Anderson, 2003). In this context, the features of patient empowerment are mapped into agenda, goal setting and its follow up regarding self-management support.

Ovearll, patient-centeredness involves patients in decisions as well as in their health and health care. Involving patients in decisions relates to the concept of shared decision making while involving patients in their health and health care implies the concepts of self-management support and care and support planning.

Concurrently, the concept of self-management support has evolved to encompass a wide variety of interventions with different intentions that is the result of various disciplines having contributed to its evolution. Moreover, a multitude of approaches have been tested to support self-management. These range from more passive information sharing approaches at one end of the spectrum to more active behavioral change interventions at the other. Another way to conceptualize self-management support is to divide interventions into those that focus on building knowledge and technical skills versus those that aim to develop self-efficacy.

The most promising way of supporting self-management involves a person empowerment and activation. There is also strong evidence suggesting that improved self-efficacy is associated with better clinical outcomes (Hibbard & Mahoney, 2010; Remmers et al., 2009; Cunningham, Lockwood & Cunningham, 1991). These approaches include:

- Motivational interviewing by telephone or in person.
- Group or individual education programs with an active component.
- Coaching with proactive goal setting and follow up.
- Programs based on psychological and emotional support that acknowledge people's stage of change.

Individual and group education sessions are the most commonly evaluated interventions of this type though there is also an increasing focus on telephone coaching by nurses.

In this context, the Patient Activation Measure (PAM), a tool for measuring the level of patient engagement, was designed to assess an individual's knowledge, skill and confidence for self-management. It was developed as a 22 item scale, resulting in a 13 item short form, which asks people about their beliefs, knowledge and confidence for engaging in a broad range of health behaviors. It suggested four stages of activation that patients go through on their way to becoming fully activated in managing their health:

- Knowledge.
- Skills.
- Confidence.
- Behavior.

However, it is difficult to categorize approaches in self-management support because there is a wide variation. Historically, approaches built on patient compliance have been frequently used in health care. The approach emphasizes that health care professionals define the problems and give advice about solutions (Funnell et al., 2000). On the other hand, the patients are expected to follow the advice and instructions (Lutfey et al., 1999). Patients that do not follow the advice have frequently been labeled as non-compliant (Lutfey et al., 1999). Non-compliance, though, is invalid and not useful construct for understanding the behavior of patients. The patient is viewed as the source of the problem when adapting to a compliance approach. In addition, the solution is that the patient must change and follow the recommendations for lifestyle changes (Anderson & Funnell, 2000). Because of the criticism of the concept of compliance, alternative terms have been developed. The term adherence has a larger focus on the provider–patient relationship and the patient's involvement in care. Therefore, adherence has been seen as a more patient-centered concept than compliance (Vlasnik et al., 2005). Differently, other researchers state that adherence represents a broader interpretation and understanding of factors that affect a person's ability to follow treatment recommendations.

Anyhow, providing information about people's condition and how to manage it is an important component of supporting self-management and patient-centered care. Information can be provided using leaflets, websites, email, text messages, electronic forums, by telephone and in person individually or in groups. A great deal has been written about different ways to provide information to people with health conditions. There is some evidence that written motivational leaflets or letters can help people feel more confident to raise their concerns and discuss their symptoms (Glasgow et al., 2003). There is sparse evidence that such methods improve self-management behavior or clinical outcomes. Other reviews suggest that printed materials can enhance knowledge (Dally et al., 2002: van Boeijen et al., 2005; Roberts et al., 2010) but may not impact behavior when used alone (Morisson, 2001: Gibson et al., 2004).

On the other hand, findings are mixed. Some trials suggest that postal educational materials are as effective for improving symptoms and self-efficacy as group education sessions (Lorig et al., 2004). There is also evidence that combining written information with lectures or other educational activities can be more effective than written information alone (Forster et al., 2004; Seals & Keith, 1997).

It is worth considering the characteristics of the most effective written information tools. There is some evidence that targeting and personalizing written information is more effective than standardized printed materials (Kennedy et al., 2003; Lafata et al., 2002; Sethares & Elliott, 2004; Enwald & Huotari, 2010).

Self-management support can also be delivered using audiovisual technology, computers and the mass media (Oermann, Webb & Ashare, 2003; Grilli, Ramsay & Minozzi, 2004; Buchbinder, 2008; Williams et al., 2010). Moreover, there is evidence that providing structured education programs by video/DVD, audio or computer may be as effective as in person education groups (Cordina, McElnay & Hughes, 2001; Samoocha et al., 2010).

Other novel approaches have also been tried. A number of computer-based peer to peer communities and electronic groups have been set up to support self-management. Some descriptive studies suggest that computer chat rooms, coaching, and other online forums can provide a good motivator for self-care (Hoffman-Goetz & Donelle, 2007; Barrera et al., 2002; Stinson et al., 2010). However, the effect on clinical outcomes is uncertain. Another novel approach is using text messages or pager messages as reminders and support mechanisms (Simoni et al., 2009; Faridi et al., 2008).

Systematic reviews and randomized trials have found that when used alone, information provision can improve some health behaviors. However, when used as part of a broader support initiative, information provision has been found to be useful. Especially if it is targeted or personalized to account for people's individual needs (Kennedy et al., 2003).

Decision support tools support self-management and encourage service users and carers to (Maly et al., 1996; Laffel et al., 2003):

- Take more responsibility for their care.
- Assist self-control in the long term conditions.
- Encourage adoption of care protocols.
- Have an impact on quality of life.

However, reviews about written decision aids suggest that such aids affect attitudes and knowledge rather than behavior.

A number of strategies have been experimented to increase people's involvement in healthcare processes and decision making as a way of facilitating self-management. Sometimes people are given their medical records to keep and bring to each consultation, which is known as patient held records. However, a number of reviews and trials suggest that patient held records have limited effects on self-management.

There is also interest in making records available electronically for service users (Ball, Smith & Bakalar, 2007; Winkelman, Leonard & Rossos, 2005; Currell & Urquhart, 2004). A randomized trial in the US provided patient records online to people with heart failure. After one year, those who had access to their records online were more likely to adhere to treatment, but there were no differences in self-efficacy or satisfaction with care (Ross et al., 2004). That implies that the patient held records might have some impact on self-management strategies, but it is unequivocal. The evidence is excessively diversified to suggest that the patient held records were a useful enabler for self-management.

Studies have also attempted to explore why action plans and agenda setting seem to work well, but few firm conclusions are possible. Plans and agenda setting appear to be better when care plans are provided and supported in primary care compared to secondary care. This approach may be better as a 'preventive' measure rather for those with the most severe disease, or for those who are hospitalized for the first time (Osman et al., 2002).

Self-monitoring involves service users monitoring their symptoms in order to track their progress, modify their behavior and judge when to seek help (Bradley & Blenkinsopp, 1996). Self-monitoring is often linked with electronic monitoring devices, but this term can also refer to written management plans and systems to help patient's self-refer to health services (Coster et al., 2000). Randomized trials suggest that electronic self-monitoring may have some clinical benefits (Mailloux et al., 1996; Siebenhofer et al., 2008; Menendez-Jandula et al., 2005). However, there are some conflicting findings (Coster et al., 2000).

Finally, schemes that use telecommunications systems such as the internet or telephone lines to transfer or record monitoring information are often referred to as 'telemonitoring'. Telemonitoring is not always strictly 'self-monitoring' as it may involve interaction between service users and health professionals (Biermann, Dietrich & Standl, 2000; Kruger et al., 2003). However, it is another way to support self-management although there is mixed evidence about the value of telemonitoring (de Lusignan et al., 2001). Notwithstanding, it is well received by patients and providers (De Clercq, Hasman & Wolffenbuttel, 2003; Cho et al., 2006).

To summarize, the evidence suggests that not all mechanisms to support self-management have equal outcomes. While information provision and building technical skills are necessary, this is just one aspect of self-management support. Approaches have been found to have more sustainable impact on behavior, clinical outcomes and healthcare resource use when:

- People's motivations and needs are recognized.
- The stage of change is taken into account.
- People are emotionally and psychologically supported.

Conclusively, the concepts of mobile health, self-management support, and self-care could be apparently thought on a continuum with one pole representing mobile health and the other representing self-care. In this context, self-management support is the nexus of mobile health and self-care.

ISSUES, CONTROVERSIES, PROBLEMS

While self-care and self-management concepts have been discussed in detail in the literature, the differences between and relationships among the concepts are not apparent. Richard and Shea (2011), argue that self-care involves 'the ability to care for oneself and the performance of activities necessary to achieve, maintain, or promote optimal health'. It may also be viewed as a continuum ranging from complete independence to complete reliance on medical care (Wilkinson and Whitehead, 2009).

Self-management is the ability of the individual to manage symptoms, treatments, lifestyle changes and psychosocial, cultural, and spiritual consequences of chronic diseases in conjunction with family, community and healthcare professionals (Wilkinson and Whitehead, 2009), an ability and process that individuals use in conscious attempts to gain control of his or her disease, rather than being controlled by it (Thorne et al., 2003).

On the other hand, there is a consensus among scholars that the term self-management, which is different from disease-management, can apply to health promotion activities as well as to those related to acute or chronic illness (Wagner et al., 2002; Lorig and Holman, 2003; Jerant et al., 2005; Wilde and Garvin, 2007).

Moreover, there are a number of barriers to self-management, and self-management support. The Macmillan self-management study (Fenlon & Foster, 2009) identified the following number of obstacles to self-management:

- Lack of, or limited, support and help from health care professionals.
- Lack of information.
- Conflicting advice.
- Lack of financial information.
- Limited access to others' experiences.
- Emotional barriers.
- Lacking focus.

It also identified specific factors that affect the engagement in self-management support. Specifically, self-management programs are more available to those who are well educated. Finally, information sources are also better utilized by those who are better educated.

SOLUTIONS AND RECOMMENDATIONS

The results from previous studies show that three strategies are used to achieve self-care objectives (Burney, Nadeem, Zain, 2010). The first strategy is the maintenance of health which is intended to avoid numerous afflictions such as early death, accident-related handicaps, psychological illnesses, behavioral problems and heart discomforts. The second important mobile-related, self-care strategy deals with chronic illnesses which form the primary challenge of the health system. The third strategy for self-care achievement is the application of mobile health for acute illnesses. Moreover, mobile health services for self-care have to be performed based on the following factors:

- The provision of quick replies to medical care users.
- The provision of medical consultations and communications.
- The development of a robust infrastructure.
- The applications of health services in three different areas of self-care.

The use of mobile technology has the potential to improve self-management. Providing access to health information refers to a patient, caregiver, or provider being able to obtain patient-specific health information through a mobile device. This sharing of information may take place with:

- A personal health record.
- A social network.

Alternatively, in the form of sending/collecting physiological and other health data.

Personal Health Records refer to a group of technologies that help patients track their health care services, access health records and manage their health information. The patient controls the Personal Health Record and chooses whether to share the health information with family members, caregivers, and providers. Personal Health Records enable patients to store and share historical information about their diagnoses, medications, and hospitalizations.

Current applications of Personal Health Records tend to target essential functions such as:

- Storage of a patient's medical history.
- Access to vital health records.
- Support for diet changes and wellness activities.
- Assistance with medication management.
- Secure forum for patient-clinician communication.

Social networking and care coordination technologies support seniors and their care providers. These social networks utilize a variety of means to facilitate communication between patients including discussion groups, chat, messaging, email, video, and file-sharing. While currently more often web-based, these social networking and care coordination programs are becoming ever more accessible on mobile devices.

Online social networking emerged as a way to connect peers independent of geography. Currently available M-Health social networking and care coordination technologies include Kaiser Permanente Texting using MobileStorm, mPro Appointment Reminders and Patient Diary Cards, Smile Reminder, Tyze, and Kinnexxus.

Moreover, a high percentage of older adults are challenged by:

- Chronic illnesses.
- Improper medication use.
- Falls and injuries.
- Frailty.
- Limited access to their personal health information.

Chronic disease and medication management, safety monitoring, and improved access to personal health information provide significant opportunities for the application of M-Health technologies. The primary goals of fall detection technologies distinguish falls from daily activities and then contact authorities who can quickly assist the individual. In this context, fall detection M-Health systems can be active, passive or a combination. Active systems are devices that users must activate to obtain assistance, most commonly by pushing a button. Passive systems contain the use of sensors to monitor movement continuously and utilize specific algorithms and alert systems to inform of potential falls. Some passive systems provide a backup system where users can activate the device for assistance. A range of passive fall detection devices are based around an M-Health platform and make use of a variety of sensors, including:

- Motion and pressure sensors.
- Accelerometers.
- Gyroscopes.

Finally, algorithms are utilized to set thresholds for alert notification tailored to each older adult by monitoring patterns of movement and behavior.

Location tracking technologies enable locating older adults. The majority of these techniques involve the older adult carrying the location tracking device or mobile enabled tracking device, like a cell phone. These technologies vary in range and accuracy of location due to selected tracking techniques, signal activation methods, and technology support systems.

Currently, there are different types of tracking methods. GPS technology location systems utilize satellites to locate individuals, but they are limited in their coverage, as signals are often lost in areas of high-density. Some location tracking technologies require remote activation while others provide an automatic stream of the user's location. Location information can also be available to providers and family caregivers or third party vendors and/or the authorities. Some location tracking devices require activation through the supplier, who then provides law enforcement personnel with location information of the older adult. Other tools provide algorithms with set alerts to notify providers, neighbors, family, and friends when the older adults leave a particular area. Finally, integration of multiple tracking techniques with mobile phones and other devices is becoming commonplace. As tracking techniques have resolution or accessibility limitations in particular fields, hardware platforms and network infrastructures that utilize multiple methods may make attractive options for location tracking.

The availability of such M-Health technology interventions for wellness is rapidly growing. Currently, available mobile health wellness technology interventions are categorized according to three primary wellness functions, fitness, nutrition, and quality of life. Furthermore, the number of M-Health interventions for medication adherence has been rapidly expanding in both variety and sophistication. These technologies can assist:

- Proper medication information.
- Patient education.
- Medication organization.
- Dispensing, dose reminders.
- Notification when doses are missed.

The primary functions that M-Health technologies can provide in the medication administration continuum are fill, remind, dispense, and report. M-Health technology interventions for these features can include:

- SMS medication reminders.

- SMS, email, and phone calls to healthcare professionals when a dose is missed.
- Mobile pill dispensers as a connector to cell phones or standalone devices.
- A smartphone application providing medication instructions.

The pill phone, which was developed by Verizon in 2008, is a cell phone software system that has fill, remind, and report functionality. The software can be used on particular cell phones and operates on basic cell phone models or smartphones. Reminders can be created around what drugs to take at what times. Older adults can reply to the alert saying they took the medication, skipped it, or may 'snooze' the alert to receive it at a later time.

In the same context, a number of diagnostic/monitoring devices can provide alert notifications to patients and caregivers via email, text, or a phone call. The systems will lock away the dispensed medication and alert up to four caregivers that a dose was missed. Dispensing and alert history is daily uploaded to a web support system allowing caregiver and clinician review.

FUTURE RESEARCH DIRECTIONS

The contemporary culture perceives healthcare as an entitlement while the goal of self-management technologies is to have patients collaborate with the healthcare providers. As a result, quality care becomes synonymous with convenient care, and education for self-management will begin as early as school age. Healthcare will not be aimed at certain illnesses, but at the care plan of the patient. In this context, the contemporary way of managing patients will quickly be obsolete as intelligent software steps in. Paper documentation will become uncommon, and mobile technology will become ubiquitous. Medical records will become profoundly detailed and personalized, as the acquisition of data becomes streamlined. Moreover, as medical records increase in number and reliability, datasets and analytics will start to play a role in diagnoses. Moreover, sensors will display their potential through mobile devices. They will be embedded in ubiquitous items and transform data collection and real-time analysis feedback into the new, normal industry standards. The integration of mobile devices into the lives of ordinary people through wearable technology will be a useful platform through which maximum impact can be achieved. Progressive methods of disease management will be continuously updated with the information provided by cloud data. It is obvious that mobile devices will operate on touchscreen platforms while innovations in human-computer interaction will drive the usefulness of M-Health.

Overall, M-Health has the potential:

- To improve the quality of care through self-management support.
- To reduce the strain on resources and healthcare workers.
- To redefine the roles of physicians, nurses, pharmacies, clinical research.
- To shift the point of care.

However, the continuum of mobile health, self-management support, and self-care as well as the self-management support as the nexus of mobile health and self-care should be thoroughly examined.

CONCLUSION

Despite the abundance of health apps, empirical evidence for their contribution to health management is limited (Anderson & Emmerton, 2016). However, the concepts of mobile health, self-management support, and self-care could be theoretically thought on a continuum with one pole representing mobile health and the other self-care. In this framework, self-management support is the nexus of mobile health and self-care.

In light of this, the increasing recognition of consumers' role in self-care, the engagement with technology and investment in mobile health apps will lead to the development, endorsement and appropriate use of quality, evidence-based health apps. The result will be a holistic, integrated approach which will cater for stakeholders with different literacy and demographic characteristics (Anderson & Emmerton, 2016).

REFERENCES

Akinsola, H. (2001). Fostering hope in people living with AIDS in Africa: The role of primary health-care workers. *The Australian Journal of Rural Health*, *9*(4), 158–165. doi:10.1046/j.1038-5282.2001.00358.x PMID:11488699

Anderson, K., & Emmerton, L. (2016). Contribution of mobile health applications to self-management by consumers: Review of published evidence. *Australian Health Review*, *40*(5), 591–597. doi:10.1071/AH15162 PMID:26681206

Anderson, R. M., & Funnell, M. M. (2000). Compliance and adherence are dysfunctional concepts in diabetes care. *The Diabetes Educator*, *26*(4), 597–604. doi:10.1177/014572170002600405 PMID:11140071

Arman, M., & Hok, J. (2016). Self-care follows from compassionate care - chronic pain patients' experience of integrative rehabilitation. *Scandinavian Journal of Caring Sciences*, *30*(2), 374–381. doi:10.1111cs.12258 PMID:26395196

Ball, M. J., Smith, C., & Bakalar, R. S. (2007). Personal health records: Empowering consumers. *Journal of Healthcare Information Management*, *21*(1), 76–86. PMID:17299929

Barlow, J., Wright, C., Sheasby, J., Turner, A., & Hainsworth, J. (2002). Self management approaches for people with chronic conditions: A review. *Patient Education and Counseling*, *48*(2), 177–187. doi:10.1016/S0738-3991(02)00032-0 PMID:12401421

Barrera, M. Jr, Glasgow, R. E., McKay, H. G., Boles, S. M., & Feil, E. G. (2002). Do internet-based support interventions change perceptions of social support?: An experimental trial of approaches for supporting diabetes self management. *American Journal of Community Psychology*, *30*(5), 637–654. doi:10.1023/A:1016369114780 PMID:12188054

Beaver, K., Bogg, J., & Luker, K. (1999). Decision making role preferences and information needs: A comparison of colorectal and breast cancer. *Health Expectations*, *2*(4), 266–276. doi:10.1046/j.1369-6513.1999.00066.x PMID:11281903

Biermann, E., Dietrich, W., & Standl, E. (2000). Telecare of diabetic patients with intensified insulin therapy. A randomized clinical trial. *Studies in Health Technology and Informatics*, *77*, 327–332. PMID:11187566

Bradley, C., & Blenkinsopp, A. (1996). Over the counter drugs: The future for self medication. *BMJ (Clinical Research Ed.)*, *312*(7034), 835–837. doi:10.1136/bmj.312.7034.835 PMID:8608296

Buchbinder, R. (2008). Self-management education en masse: effectiveness of the Back Pain: Don't Take It Lying Down mass media campaign. *The Medical Journal of Australia*, *189*(10Suppl), S29–S32. PMID:19143582

Burney, S. M. A., Nadeem, M., & Zain, A. (2010). Information and Communication Technology in Healthcare Management Systems: Prospects for Developing countries. *International Journal of Computers and Applications*, *4*, 1.

Chambers, R. (2006). Guest editorial: The role of the health professional in supporting self care. *Quality in Primary Care*, *14*, 129–131.

Cho, J. H., Chang, S. A., Kwon, H. S., Choi, Y.-H., Ko, S.-H., Moon, S.-D., ... Yoon, K.-H. (2006). Long-term effect of the internet-based glucose monitoring system on HbA1c reduction and glucose stability: A 30-month follow up study for diabetes management with a ubiquitous medical care system. *Diabetes Care*, *29*(12), 2625–2631. doi:10.2337/dc05-2371 PMID:17130195

Clark, N. M. (2003). Management of chronic disease by patients. *Annual Review of Public Health*, *24*(1), 289–313. doi:10.1146/annurev.publhealth.24.100901.141021 PMID:12415147

Cordina, M., McElnay, J. C., & Hughes, C. M. (2001). Assessment of a community pharmacy-based program for patients with asthma. *Pharmacotherapy*, *21*(10), 1196–1203. doi:10.1592/phco.21.15.1196.33894 PMID:11601666

Coster, S. (2000). Monitoring blood glucose control in diabetes mellitus: A systematic review. *Health Technology Assessment*, *4*(12). PMID:10944740

Cunningham, A. J., Lockwood, G. A., & Cunningham, J. A. (1991). A relationship between perceived self-efficacy and quality of life in cancer patients. *Patient Education and Counseling*, *17*(1), 71–78. doi:10.1016/0738-3991(91)90052-7 PMID:1997998

Currell, R., & Urquhart, C. (2004). Nursing record systems: effects on nursing practice and health care outcomes. *Cochrane Review, 2*.

Dally, D. L., Dahar, W., Scott, A., Roblin, D., & Khoury, A. T. (2002). The impact of a health education program targeting patients with high visit rates in a managed care organization. *American Journal of Health Promotion*, *17*(2), 101–111. doi:10.4278/0890-1171-17.2.101 PMID:12471862

Davison, B. J., Kirk, P., Degner, L. F., & Hassard, T. H. (1999). Information and patient participation in screening for prostate cancer. *Patient Education and Counseling*, *37*(3), 255–263. doi:10.1016/S0738-3991(98)00123-2 PMID:14528551

Davison, B. J., Parker, P. A., & Goldenberg, S. L. (2004). Patients' preferences for communicating a prostate cancer diagnosis and participating in medical decision making. *BJU International*, *93*(1), 47–51. doi:10.1111/j.1464-410X.2004.04553.x PMID:14678366

De Clercq, P. A., Hasman, A., & Wolffenbuttel, B. H. (2003). A consumer health record for supporting the patient-centered management of chronic diseases. *Medical Informatics and the Internet in Medicine*, *28*(2), 117–127. doi:10.1080/14639230310001600506 PMID:14692588

de Iongh, A., Fagan, P., Fenner, J., & Kidd, L. (2015). *A practical guide to self-management support: Key components for successful implementation*. London: The Health Foundation.

de Lusignan, S., Wells, S., Johnson, P., Meredith, K., & Leatham, E. (2001). Compliance and effectiveness of 1 year's home telemonitoring. The report of a pilot study of patients with chronic heart failure. *European Journal of Heart Failure*, *3*(6), 723–730. doi:10.1016/S1388-9842(01)00190-8 PMID:11738225

Degner, L., Krisjanson, L. J., Bowman, D., Sloan, J. A., Carriere, K. C., O'Neil, J., ... Mueller, B. (1997). Informational needs and decisional preferences in women with breast cancer. *Journal of the American Medical Association*, *277*(18), 1485–1492. doi:10.1001/jama.1997.03540420081039 PMID:9145723

Department of Health. (2000). *The NHS Plan. A plan for investment. A plan for reform*. London: Department of Health.

Department of Health. (2005a). *Supporting People with Long Term Conditions: an NHS and Social Care Model to support local innovation and integration*. London: Department of Health.

Department of Health. (2005b). *Self Care: A real choice*. London: Department of Health.

Department of Health. (2006a). *Our Health, Our Say*. London: Department of Health.

Department of Health Department of Health. (2001). *The Expert Patient: a new approach to chronic disease management for the 21st century*. London: Department of Health.

Dill, A., Brown, P., Ciambrone, D., & Rakowski, W. (1995). The meaning and practice of self care by older adults: A qualitative assessment. *Research on Aging*, *17*(1), 8–41. doi:10.1177/0164027595171002

Dodd, M. J., Janson, S., Facione, N., Faucett, J., Froelicher, E. S., Humphreys, J., ... Taylor, D. (2001). Advancing the science of symptom management. *Journal of Advanced Nursing*, *335*(5), 668–676. doi:10.1046/j.1365-2648.2001.01697.x PMID:11298204

Eastman, C., & Marzillier, J. S. (1984). Theoretical and Methodological Difficulties in Bandura's Self-Efficacy Theory. *Cognitive Therapy and Therapy*, *8*(3), 213–229. doi:10.1007/BF01172994

Ekman, I., Swedberg, K., Taft, C., Lindseth, A., Norberg, A., Brink, E., ... Sunnerhagen, K. S. (2011). Person-centered care—Ready for prime time. *European Journal of Cardiovascular Nursing*, *10*(4), 248–251. doi:10.1016/j.ejcnurse.2011.06.008 PMID:21764386

Enwald, H. P., & Huotari, M. L. (2010). Preventing the obesity epidemic by second generation tailored health communication: An interdisciplinary review. *Journal of Medical Internet Research*, *12*(2), e24. doi:10.2196/jmir.1409 PMID:20584698

Epstein, R. M., Franks, P., Fiscella, K., Shields, C. G., Meldrum, S. C., Kravitz, R. L., & Duberstein, P. R. (2005). Measuring patient-centered communication in patient physician consultations: Theoretical and practical issues. *Social Science & Medicine*, *61*(7), 1516–1528. doi:10.1016/j.socscimed.2005.02.001 PMID:16005784

Eyuboglu, E., & Schulz, P. J. (2016). Do health literacy and patient empowerment affect self-care behaviour? A survey study among Turkish patients with diabetes. *BMJ Open*, *6*(3), e010186. doi:10.1136/bmjopen-2015-010186 PMID:26975936

Faridi, Z., Liberti, L., Shuval, K., Northrup, V., Ali, A., & Katz, D. L. (2008). 'Evaluating the impact of mobile telephone technology on type 2 diabetic patients' self management: The NICHE pilot study.'. *Journal of Evaluation in Clinical Practice*, *14*(3), 465–469. doi:10.1111/j.1365-2753.2007.00881.x PMID:18373577

Fenlon, D., & Foster, C. (2009). Self management support: a review of the evidence. Southampton, Macmillan Research Unit, University of Southampton.

Forster, A., Smith, J., & Young, J. (2004). *Information provision for stroke patients and their caregivers (Cochrane Review)*. Chichester, UK: John Wiley & Sons.

Fu, M. R., LeMone, P., & McDaniel, R. (2004). An integrated approach to an analysis of symptom management in patients with cancer. *Oncology Nursing Forum*, *31*(1), 65–70. doi:10.1188/04.ONF.65-70 PMID:14722589

Funnell, M. M., & Anderson, R. M. (2000). The problem with compliance in diabetes. *Journal of the American Medical Association*, *284*(13), 1709. doi:10.1001/jama.284.13.1709-JMS1004-6-1 PMID:11015809

Funnell, M. M., & Anderson, R. M. (2003). Patient empowerment: A look back, a look ahead. *The Diabetes Educator*, *29*(3), 454–464. doi:10.1177/014572170302900310 PMID:12854337

Gibson, P. G., Powell, H., & Coughlan, J. (2004). *Limited (information only) patient education programs for adults with asthma (Cochrane Review)*. Chichester, UK: John Wiley & Sons.

Glasgow, N. J., Ponsonby, A. L., & Yates, R. (2003). Proactive asthma care in childhood: General practice based randomised controlled trial. *BMJ (Clinical Research Ed.)*, *327*(7416), 659. doi:10.1136/bmj.327.7416.659 PMID:14500440

Glasgow, R. E., Peeples, M., & Skovlund, S. E. (2008). Where is the patient in diabetes performance measures? *Diabetes Care*, *31*(5), 1046–1050. doi:10.2337/dc07-1845 PMID:18445728

Grilli, R., Ramsay, C., & Minozzi, S. (2004). *Mass media interventions: effects on health services utilisation (Cochrane Review)*. Chichester, UK: John Wiley & Sons.

Hibbard, J. H., & Mahoney, E. (2010). Toward a theory of patient and consumer activation. *Patient Education and Counseling*, *78*(3), 377–381. doi:10.1016/j.pec.2009.12.015 PMID:20188505

Hickey, T., Dean, K., & Holstein, B. (1986). Emerging trends in gerontology and geriatrics: Implications for the self-care of the elderly. *Social Science & Medicine*, *23*(12), 1363–1369. doi:10.1016/0277-9536(86)90299-6 PMID:3823991

Hoffman-Goetz, L., & Donelle, L. (2007). Chat room computer-mediated support on health issues for aboriginal women. *Health Care for Women International*, *28*(4), 397–418. doi:10.1080/07399330601180057 PMID:17454185

Howie, J. G. R., Heaney, D., & Maxwell, M. (2004). Quality, core values and the general practice consultation: Issues of definition, measurement and delivery. *Family Practice*, *21*(4), 458–468. doi:10.1093/fampra/cmh419 PMID:15249538

Hubbard, G., Kidd, L., Donaghy, E., MacDonald, C., Simpson, M., Haig, A., & Walker, S. (2005). *Phase 1 Report: Literature Review: Involvement of people affected by cancer in research, policy and planning and practice*. University of Stirling.

Jerant, A., von Frederichs-Fitzwater, M., & Moore, M. (2005). Patient's perceived barriers to active self-management of chronic conditions. *Patient Education and Counseling*, *57*(3), 300–307. doi:10.1016/j.pec.2004.08.004 PMID:15893212

Kennedy, A., Robinson, A., Hann, M., Thompson, D., & Wilkin, D. (2003). A cluster-randomised controlled trial of a patient-centred guidebook for patients with ulcerative colitis: Effect on knowledge, anxiety and quality of life. *Health & Social Care in the Community*, *11*(1), 64–72. doi:10.1046/j.1365-2524.2003.00399.x PMID:14629234

Koch, T., Jenkin, P., & Kralik, D. (2004). Chronic illness self management: Locating the 'self'. *Journal of Advanced Nursing*, *48*(5), 484–492. doi:10.1111/j.1365-2648.2004.03237.x PMID:15533086

Kolbe, J. (2002). The influence of socioeconomic and psychological factors on patient adherence to self management strategies: Lessons learned in asthma. *Disease Management & Health Outcomes*, *10*(9), 551–570. doi:10.2165/00115677-200210090-00004

Kruger, D. F., White, K., Galpern, A., Mann, K., Massirio, A., McLellan, M., & Stevenson, J. (2003). Effect of modem transmission of blood glucose data on telephone consultation time, clinic work flow, and patient satisfaction for patients with gestational diabetes mellitus. *Journal of the American Academy of Nurse Practitioners*, *15*(8), 371–375. doi:10.1111/j.1745-7599.2003.tb00410.x PMID:14509102

Lafata, J. E., Baker, A. M., Divine, G. W., McCarthy, B. D., & Xi, H. (2002). The use of computerized birthday greeting reminders in the management of diabetes. *Journal of General Internal Medicine*, *17*(7), 521–530. doi:10.1046/j.1525-1497.2002.10901.x PMID:12133142

Laffel, L. M., Vangsness, L., Connell, A., Goebel-Fabbri, A., Butler, D., & Anderson, B. J. (2003). Impact of ambulatory, family-focused teamwork intervention on glycemic control in youth with type 1 diabetes. *The Journal of Pediatrics*, *142*(4), 409–416. doi:10.1067/mpd.2003.138 PMID:12712059

Larson, P. J., Carrieri-Kohlman, V., Dodd, M. J., Douglas, M., Faucett, J., Froelicher, E. S., ... Underwood, P. (1994). A model for symptom management. *Image--the Journal of Nursing Scholarship*, *26*, 154–164. PMID:7829111

Lenz, E., Pugh, L., Milligan, R., Gift, A., & Suppe, E. (1997). The middle range theory of unpleasant symptoms: An update. *Advances in Nursing Science*, *19*(3), 14–27. doi:10.1097/00012272-199703000-00003 PMID:9055027

Lenz, E., Suppe, E., Pugh, L., & Milligan, R. (1995). Collaborative development of middle range nursing theories: Toward a theory of unpleasant symptoms. *Advances in Nursing Science*, *17*(3), 1–13. doi:10.1097/00012272-199503000-00003 PMID:7778887

Leventhal, H., Benyamini, Y., Brownlee, S., Diefenbach, M., Leventhal, E. A., Patrick-Miller, L., & Robitaille, C. (1997). Illness representations: theoretical foundations. In K. J. Petrie & J. A. Weinman (Eds.), *Perceptions of Health and Illness: Current Research and Applications* (pp. 19–45). Harwood Academic Publishers.

Leventhal, H., Leventhal, E. A., & Cameron, L. (2001). Representations, procedures and affect in illness self regulation: a perceptual-cognitive model. In A. Baum, T. Revenson, & J. Singer (Eds.), *Handbook of Health Psychology* (pp. 19–47). New York: Earlbaum.

Leventhal, H., Nerenz, D. R., & Steel, D. J. (1984). Illness representations and coping with health threats. In A. Baum, S. E. Taylor, & J. E. Singer (Eds.), Handbook of Psychology and Health (Vol. 4, pp. 219–252). Hillsdale, NJ: Erlbaum.

Levin, L. S., & Idler, E. L. (1983). Self-care in health. *Annual Review of Public Health*, *4*(1), 181–201. doi:10.1146/annurev.pu.04.050183.001145 PMID:6860437

Levin, L. S., Katz, A., & Holst, E. (1977). *Self-Care: Lay Initiatives in Health*. New York Prodist.

Lorig, K., & Holman, H. (2003). Self-Management Education: History, Definition, Outcomes, and Mechanisms. *Annals of Behavioral Medicine*, *26*(1), 1–7. doi:10.1207/S15324796ABM2601_01 PMID:12867348

Lorig, K. R., Ritter, P. L., Laurent, D. D., & Fries, J. F. (2004). Long-term randomized controlled trials of tailored-print and small-group arthritis self management interventions. *Medical Care*, *42*(4), 346–354. doi:10.1097/01.mlr.0000118709.74348.65 PMID:15076811

Lutfey, K. E., & Wishner, W. J. (1999). Beyond "compliance" is "adherence". Improving the prospect of diabetes care. *Diabetes Care*, *22*(4), 635–639. doi:10.2337/diacare.22.4.635 PMID:10189544

Mailloux, L. U., Kapikian, N., Napolitano, B., Mossey, R. T., Bellucci, A. G., Wilkes, B. M., ... Miller, I. J. (1996). Home hemodialysis: Patient outcomes during a 24-year period of time from 1970 through 1993. *Advances in Renal Replacement Therapy*, *3*(2), 112–119. doi:10.1016/S1073-4449(96)80050-1 PMID:8814916

Maly, R. C., Abrahamse, A. F., Hirsch, S. H., & … . (1996). What influences physician practice behavior? An interview study of physicians who received consultative geriatric assessment recommendations. *Archives of Family Medicine*, *5*(8), 448–454. doi:10.1001/archfami.5.8.448 PMID:8797548

Mead, N., & Bower, P. (2000). Patient-centredness: A conceptual framework and review of the empirical literature. *Social Science & Medicine*, *51*(7), 1087–1110. doi:10.1016/S0277-9536(00)00098-8 PMID:11005395

Menendez-Jandula, B., Souto, J. C., Oliver, A., Montserrat, I., Quintana, M., Gich, I., ... Fontcuberta, J. (2005). Comparing self management of oral anticoagulant therapy with clinic management: A randomized trial. *Annals of Internal Medicine*, *142*(1), 1–10. doi:10.7326/0003-4819-142-1-200501040-00006 PMID:15630104

Michie, S., Miles, J., & Weinman, J. (2003). Patient-centredness in chronic illness: What is it and does it matter? *Patient Education and Counseling*, *51*(3), 197–206. doi:10.1016/S0738-3991(02)00194-5 PMID:14630376

Morrison, A. (2001). Effectiveness of printed patient educational materials in chronic illness: A systematic review of controlled trials. *J Manag Pharm Care*, *1*(1), 51–62. doi:10.1300/J234v01n01_07

Newbould, J., Taylor, D., & Bury, M. (2006). Lay-led self-management in chronic illness: A review of the evidence. *Chronic Illness*, *2*(4), 249–261. doi:10.1177/17423953060020040401 PMID:17212872

Nyatanga, L., & Dann, K. L. (2002). Empowerment in nursing: The role of philosophical and psychological factors. *Nursing Philosophy*, *3*(3), 134–139. doi:10.1046/j.1466-769X.2002.00107.x

Oermann, M. H., Webb, S. A., & Ashare, J. A. (2003). Outcomes of videotape instruction in clinic waiting area. *Orthopedic Nursing*, *22*(2), 102–105. doi:10.1097/00006416-200303000-00006 PMID:12703393

Orem, D. E. (1991). *Nursing: Concepts of Practice* (4th ed.). St Louis, MO: Mosby.

Orem, D. E. (1995). *Nursing: Concepts of Practice* (5th ed.). St Louis, MO: Mosby.

Osman, L. M., Calder, C., Godden, D. J., Friend, J. A., McKenzie, L., Legge, J. S., & Douglas, J. G. (2002). A randomised trial of self management planning for adult patients admitted to hospital with acute asthma. *Thorax*, *57*(10), 869–874. doi:10.1136/thorax.57.10.869 PMID:12324673

Paterson, B. L., & Sloan, J. (1994). A phenomenological study of the decision making experience of individuals with long standing diabetes. *Canadian Journal of Diabetes Care*, *18*(4), 10–19.

Redman, B. K. (2005). The ethics of self management preparation for chronic illness. *Nursing Ethics*, *12*(4), 360–369. doi:10.1191/0969733005ne801oa PMID:16045244

Remmers, C., Hibbard, J., Mosen, D. M., Wagenfield, M., Hoye, R. E., & Jones, C. (2009). Is patient activation associated with future health outcomes and healthcare utilization among patients with diabetes? *The Journal of Ambulatory Care Management*, *32*(4), 320–327. doi:10.1097/JAC.0b013e3181ba6e77 PMID:19888008

Richard, A., & Shea, K. (2011). Delineation of Self-care and AssociatedConcepts. *Journal of Nursing Scholarship*, *43*, 255–264. PMID:21884371

Richardson, A., & Ream, E. K. (1997). Self care behaviours initiated by chemotherapy patients in response to fatigue. *International Journal of Nursing Studies*, *34*(1), 35–43. doi:10.1016/S0020-7489(96)00031-4 PMID:9055119

Roberts, L., Little, P., Chapman, J., Cantrell, T., Pickering, R., & Langridge, J. (2010). The back home trial: General practitioner-supported leaflets may change back pain behavior. *Spine*, *27*(17), 1821–1828. doi:10.1097/00007632-200209010-00002 PMID:12221342

Rodgers, A., Flowers, J., & Pencheon, D. (1999). Improving access needs a whole systems approach. *British Medical Journal*, *319*(7214), 866–867. doi:10.1136/bmj.319.7214.866 PMID:10506023

Rogers, A., & Hay, S. (1998). Self-care and access to health care. In A. Rodgers & S. Hay (Eds.), *Opportunities for Improving Access to Care*. NHSE Anglia and Oxford Region Milton Keynes.

Ross, S. E., Moore, L. A., Earnest, M. A., Wittevrongel, L., & Lin, C.-T. (2004). Providing a web-based online medical record with electronic communication capabilities to patients with congestive heart failure: Randomized trial. *Journal of Medical Internet Research*, *6*(2), e12. doi:10.2196/jmir.6.2.e12 PMID:15249261

Samoocha, D., Bruinvels, D. J., Elbers, N. A., Anema, J. R., & van der Beek, A. J. (2010). Effectiveness of web-based interventions on patient empowerment: A systematic review and meta-analysis. *Journal of Medical Internet Research*, *12*(2), e23. doi:10.2196/jmir.1286 PMID:20581001

Scottish Executive. (2003). *Partnership for Care: Scotland's Health White Paper.* Scottish Executive.

Scottish Executive. (2005a). *A National Service Framework for Service Change in the NHS in Scotland: Building a Health Service Fit for the Future*. Edinburgh, UK: Scottish Executive.

Scottish Executive. (2005b). *Delivering for Health*. Edinburgh, UK: Scottish Executive.

Seals, T. D., & Keith, M. R. (1997). Influence of patient information leaflets on anticonvulsant drug compliance in prison. *American Journal of Health-System Pharmacy*, *54*(22), 2585–2587. PMID:9397219

Greenfield, McManus, & Wilson. (2007). Self care – has DIY gone too far? *The British Journal of General Practice*, *57*, 907–908. PMID:17132376

Sethares, K. A., & Elliott, K. (2004). The effect of a tailored message intervention on heart failure readmission rates, quality of life, and benefit and barrier beliefs in persons with heart failure. *Heart & Lung*, *33*(4), 249–260. doi:10.1016/j.hrtlng.2004.03.005 PMID:15252415

Siebenhofer, A., Rakovac, I., Kleespies, C., Piso, B., & Didjurgeit, U. (2008). Self-management of oral anticoagulation reduces major outcomes in the elderly. A randomized controlled trial. *Thrombosis and Haemostasis*, *100*(6), 1089–1098. PMID:19132235

Simoni, J. M., Huh, D., Frick, P. A., Pearson, C. R., Andrasik, M. P., Dunbar, P. J., & Hooton, T. M. (2009). Peer support and pager messaging to promote antiretroviral modifying therapy in Seattle: A randomized controlled trial. *JAIDS Journal of Acquired Immune Deficiency Syndromes*, *52*(4), 465–473. doi:10.1097/QAI.0b013e3181b9300c PMID:19911481

Soderhamn, O. (2000). Self care activity as a structure: A phenomenological approach. *Scandinavian Journal of Occupational Therapy*, *7*(4), 183–189. doi:10.1080/110381200300008724

Stewart, M., Brown, J. B., Donner, A., McWhinney, I. R., Oates, J., Weston, W. W., & ... . (2000). The impact of patient-centered care on outcomes. *The Journal of Family Practice*, *49*(9), 796–804. PMID:11032203

Stinson, J. N., McGrath, P. J., Hodnett, E. D., Feldman, B. M., Duffy, C. M., Huber, A. M., ... White, M. E. (2010). An internet-based self-management program with telephone support for adolescents with arthritis: A pilot randomized controlled trial. *The Journal of Rheumatology*, *37*(9), 1944–1952. doi:10.3899/jrheum.091327 PMID:20595280

Sutton, C., & Vatavuk, J. (2014). *The journey from self-care management to virtual care for all*. Retrieved July 20, 2018, from https://www.telushealth.co/item/the-journey-from-self-care-management-to-virtual-care-for-all/

Swedish Agency for Health and Care Services Analysis (2012). *Patient centeredness in Sweden's health system- an external assessment and six steps for progress*. Author.

Teel, S., Meek, P., McNamura, A., & Watson, V. (1997). Perspectives unifying symptom interpretations. *Image Journal of Scholarly Inquiry*, *29*, 175–181. PMID:9212516

Thorne, S., Paterson, B., & Russell, C. (2003). The structure of everyday self-care decision making in chronic illness. *Qualitative Health Research*, *13*(10), 1337–1352. doi:10.1177/1049732303258039 PMID:14658350

van Boeijen, C. A., & ... . (2005). Efficacy of self-help manuals for anxiety disorders in primary care: A systematic review. *Family Practice*, *22*(2), 192–196. doi:10.1093/fampra/cmh708 PMID:15710643

Vlasnik, J. J., Aliotta, S. L., & DeLor, B. (2005). Medication adherence: Factors influencing compliance with prescribed medication plans. *The Case Manager*, *16*(2), 47–51. doi:10.1016/j.casemgr.2005.01.009 PMID:15818344

Wagner, E., Davis, C., Shaefer, J., Von Korff, M., & Austin, B. (2002). A survey of leading chronic disease management programs: Are they consistent with literature? *Journal of Nursing Care Quality*, *16*(2), 67–80. doi:10.1097/00001786-200201000-00008

Wilde, M. H., & Garvin, S. (2007). A concept analysis of self-monitoring. *Journal of Advanced Nursing*, *57*(3), 339–350. doi:10.1111/j.1365-2648.2006.04089.x PMID:17233653

Wilkinson, A., & Whitehead, L. (2009). Evolution of the concept of self-care and implications for nurses: A literature review. *International Journal of Nursing Studies*, *46*(8), 1143–1147. doi:10.1016/j.ijnurstu.2008.12.011 PMID:19200992

Williams, A., Hagerty, B. M., Brasington, S. J., Clem, J. B., & Williams, D. A. (2010). Stress Gym: Feasibility of deploying a web-enhanced behavioral self-management program for stress in a military setting. *Military Medicine*, *175*(7), 487–493. doi:10.7205/MILMED-D-09-00216 PMID:20684452

Winkelman, W. J., Leonard, K. J., & Rossos, P. G. (2005). Patient-perceived usefulness of online electronic medical records: Employing grounded theory in the development of information and communication technologies for use by patients living with chronic illness. *Journal of the American Medical Informatics Association*, *12*(3), 306–314. doi:10.1197/jamia.M1712 PMID:15684128

KEY TERMS AND DEFINITIONS

M-Health: It describes the use of a broad range of telecommunication and multimedia technologies within wireless care delivery design and can be broadly defined as the delivery of healthcare services via mobile communication devices.

Patient Activation: It is the individual's knowledge, skill, and confidence for managing his health and healthcare.

Patient Empowerment: It features self-determining agents with some control over their health and health care and conceptualizes personal control and self-efficacy.

Patient-Centered Care: It is more than a method of communication which focuses on patients' preferences, experienced needs and values in decisions about care and treatment.

Self-Care: It emerged from the concept of health promotion in the 1970s and describes what people do for themselves to establish and maintain their health and prevent and deal with illness.

Self-Management: The taking of responsibility for one's behavior and wellbeing.

Self-Management Support: It is the assistance given to patients in order to encourage daily decisions that improve health-related behaviors and clinical outcomes.

Compilation of References

Adams, K., & Corrigan, J. M. (2003). *Priority Areas for National Action: Transforming Health Care Quality*. Washington, DC: National Academies Press.

Adibi, S. (2015). Mobile Health A Technology Road Map. Academic Press.

Ajzen, I. (1991). The theory of planned behavior. *Organizational Behavior and Human Decision Processes*, *50*(2), 179–211. doi:10.1016/0749-5978(91)90020-T

Akinsola, H. (2001). Fostering hope in people living with AIDS in Africa: The role of primary health-care workers. *The Australian Journal of Rural Health*, *9*(4), 158–165. doi:10.1046/j.1038-5282.2001.00358.x PMID:11488699

Albouy, B., Treuillet, S., Lucas, Y., Barre, H., & Pichaud, J. C. (2005). Depth and color analysis of wounds using digital camera. *ITBM-RBM*, *26*(4), 240–242. doi:10.1016/j.rbmret.2005.06.001

Al-Falahy, N., & Alani, O. Y. (2017). Technologies for 5G Networks: Challenges and Opportunities. *IEEE IT Professional*, *19*(1), 12–20. doi:10.1109/MITP.2017.9

Al-Janabi, S., Huisman, A., Willems, S. M., & Van Diest, P. J. (2012). Digital slide images for primary diagnostics in breast pathology: A feasibility study. *Human Pathology*, *43*(12), 2318–2325. doi:10.1016/j.humpath.2012.03.027 PMID:22901465

Allen, J. K., Stephens, J., Dennison Himmelfarb, C. R., Stewart, K. J., & Hauck, S. (2013). Randomized Controlled Pilot Study Testing Use of Smartphone Technology for Obesity Treatment. *Journal of Obesity*, *7*. doi:10.1155/2013/151597 PMID:24392223

Al-Shaqsi, S. (2010). Models of International Emergency Medical Service (EMS) Systems. *Oman Medical Journal*, *25*(4), 320–323. doi:10.5001/omj.2010.92 PMID:22043368

Amadi-Obi, A., Gilligan, P., Owens, N., & O'Donnell, C. (2014). Telemedicine in pre-hospital care: A review of telemedicine applications in the pre-hospital environment. *International Journal of Emergency Medicine*, *7*(1), 29. doi:10.118612245-014-0029-0 PMID:25635190

American Medical Association. (2018), *CPT® (Current Procedural Terminology)*. Retrieved from https://www.ama-assn.org/practice-management/cpt-current-procedural-terminology

Anderson, K., & Emmerton, L. (2016). Contribution of mobile health applications to self-management by consumers: Review of published evidence. *Australian Health Review*, *40*(5), 591–597. doi:10.1071/AH15162 PMID:26681206

Anderson, N. B. (1998). Levels of analysis in health science: A framework for integrating sociobehavioral and biomedical research. *Annals of the New York Academy of Sciences*, *840*(1), 563–576. doi:10.1111/j.1749-6632.1998.tb09595.x PMID:9629283

Anderson, R. M., & Funnell, M. M. (2000). Compliance and adherence are dysfunctional concepts in diabetes care. *The Diabetes Educator*, *26*(4), 597–604. doi:10.1177/014572170002600405 PMID:11140071

Anderson, R. M., May, R. M., & Anderson, B. (1992). *Infectious Diseases of Humans Dynamics and Control.* New York: Oxford UP.

Anliker, U., Ward, J. A., Lukowicz, P., Tröster, G., Dolveck, F., Baer, M., ... Vuskovic, M. (2004). AMON: A wearable multi parameter medical monitoring and alert systems. *IEEE Transactions on Information Technology in Biomedicine*, *8*(4), 415–427. doi:10.1109/TITB.2004.837888 PMID:15615032

Aqueveque, P., Gutierrez, C., Saavedra, F., & Pino, E. J. (2017). Monitoring Physiological Variables of Mining Workers at High Altitude. *IEEE Transactions on Industry Applications*, *53*(3), 2628–2634. doi:10.1109/TIA.2017.2675360

Arbabi, S., Jurkovich, G. J., Wahl, W. L., Franklin, G. A., Hemmila, M. R., Taheri, P. A., & Maier, R. V. (2004). A comparison of prehospital and hospital data in trauma patients. *The Journal of Trauma*, *56*(5), 1029–1032. doi:10.1097/01.TA.0000123036.20919.4B PMID:15179242

Archondakis, S. (2014). Static Telecytological Applications for Proficiency Testing. In A. Information Resources Management (Ed.), Nanotechnology: Concepts, Methodologies, Tools, and Applications (pp. 556-568). Hershey, PA: IGI Global. doi:10.4018/978-1-4666-5125-8.ch023

Archondakis, S. (2013). The Use of Static Telemedical Applications of Cytopathology for Proficiency Testing. *International Journal of Reliable and Quality E-Healthcare*, *2*(2), 47–53. doi:10.4018/ijrqeh.2013040104

Archondakis, S. (2015). The Use of Information Systems in a Modern Cytopathology Laboratory. In A. Moumtzoglou, A. Kastania, & S. Archondakis (Eds.), *Laboratory Management Information Systems: Current Requirements and Future Perspectives* (pp. 208–236). Hershey, PA: Medical Information Science Reference. doi:10.4018/978-1-4666-6320-6.ch011

Archondakis, S., Georgoulakis, J., Stamataki, M., Anninos, D., Skagias, L., Panayiotides, I., ... Karakitsos, P. (2009). Telecytology: A tool for quality assessment and improvement in the evaluation of thyroid fine-needle aspiration specimens. *Telemedicine Journal and e-Health*, *15*(7), 713–717. doi:10.1089/tmj.2009.0037 PMID:19694595

Archondakis, S., Stathopoulou, A., & Sitaras, I. (2011). ISO 15189:2007: Implementation in a Laboratory Information System. In A. Moumtzoglou & A. Kastania (Eds.), *E-Health Systems Quality and Reliability: Models and Standards* (pp. 64–72). Hershey, PA: Medical Information Science Reference. doi:10.4018/978-1-61692-843-8.ch006

Archondakis, S., Vavoulidis, E., & Nasioutziki, M. (2016). The Use of Mobile Health Applications for Quality Control and Accreditational Purposes in a Cytopathology Laboratory. In M. Anastasius (Ed.), *M-Health Innovations for Patient-Centered Care* (pp. 262–283). Hershey, PA: IGI Global.

ArduinoI. D. E. (2018). Retrieved from https://www.arduino.cc/

Arman, M., & Hok, J. (2016). Self-care follows from compassionate care - chronic pain patients' experience of integrative rehabilitation. *Scandinavian Journal of Caring Sciences*, *30*(2), 374–381. doi:10.1111cs.12258 PMID:26395196

Arthur, G. (2010). *Wound care: Innovation and chronic care drives market growth.* Retrieved from http://www.trilogy-capital.com/sci/sci_woundcare.pdf

Artz. (2002). *NetSPA: A Network Security Planning Architecture*. MIT.

Astion, M. L., & Wilding, P. (1992). Application of neural networks to the interpretation of laboratory data in cancer diagnosis. *Clinical Chemistry*, *38*(1), 34–38. PMID:1733603

Atalay, O., Kennon, W. R., & Demirok, E. (2015). Weft- Knitted Strain Sensor for Monitoring Respiratory Rate and Its Electro-Mechanical Modelling. *IEEE Sensors Journal*, *15*(1), 110–122. doi:10.1109/JSEN.2014.2339739

Athanasiadi, E., Pouliakis, A., Bilirakis, E., Fragoulakis, V., Bilirakis, C., & Karakitsos, P. (2014). Quality Indicators for Cervical Cancer Screening Programs: The Role of Computerized Systems. *International Journal of Reliable and Quality E-Healthcare*, *3*(4), 19–37. doi:10.4018/ijrqeh.2014100102

Auguste, L., & Palsana, D. (2015). Mobile Whole Slide Imaging (mWSI): A low resource acquisition and transport technique for microscopic pathological specimens. *BMJ Innovations*, *1*(3), 137–143. doi:10.1136/bmjinnov-2015-000040

Aujoulat, I., D' Hoore, W., & Deccache, A. (2007). Patient empowerment in theory and practice: Polysemy or cacophony? *Patient Education and Counseling*, *66*(1), 13–20. doi:10.1016/j.pec.2006.09.008 PMID:17084059

Bachmann, D. J., Jamison, N. K., Martin, A., Delgado, J., & Kman, N. E. (2015). Emergency Preparedness and Disaster Response: There's An App for That. *Prehospital and Disaster Medicine*, *30*(5), 486–490. doi:10.1017/S1049023X15005099 PMID:26369629

Bailey, N. T. J. (1975). *The Mathematical Theory of Infectious Diseases* (2nd ed.). London: Griffin.

Baker, S., Wei Xiang and Atkinson, I. (2017). Internet Of things for smart Healthcare: Technologies, Challenges and Opportunities. *Journal of IEEE ACCESS*.

Ball, M. J., Smith, C., & Bakalar, R. S. (2007). Personal health records: Empowering consumers. *Journal of Healthcare Information Management*, *21*(1), 76–86. PMID:17299929

Bandura, A. (2006). Guide for constructing self-efficacy scales. In T. Urban & F. Pajares (Eds.), *Self-efficacy Beliefs of Adolescents*. Charlotte, NC: Information Age Publishing.

Banitsas, K. A., Perakis, K., Tachakra, S., & Koutsouris, D. (2006). Use of 3G mobile phone links for teleconsultation between a moving ambulance and a hospital base station. *Journal of Telemedicine and Telecare*, *12*(1), 23–26. doi:10.1258/135763306775321335 PMID:16438775

Banitsas, K., Perakis, K., Koutsouris, D., Konis, G., & Tachakra, S. (2005). Ambulance 3G. *Conference Proceedings; ... Annual International Conference of the IEEE Engineering in Medicine and Biology Society. IEEE Engineering in Medicine and Biology Society. Conference*, *1*, 371–374. doi:10.1109/IEMBS.2005.1616422 PMID:17282191

Barlow, J., Wright, C., Sheasby, J., Turner, A., & Hainsworth, J. (2002). Self management approaches for people with chronic conditions: A review. *Patient Education and Counseling*, *48*(2), 177–187. doi:10.1016/S0738-3991(02)00032-0 PMID:12401421

Barnato, A. E., Llewellyn-Thomas, H. A., Peters, E. M., Siminoff, L., Collins, E. D., & Barry, M. J. (2007). Communication and Decision Making in Cancer Care: Setting Research Priorities for Decision Support/Patients' Decision Aids. *Medical Decision Making*, *27*(5), 626–634. doi:10.1177/0272989X07306788 PMID:17873249

Barnes, J., Duffy, A., Hamnett, N., McPhail, J., Seaton, C., Shokrollahi, K., ... Pritchard Jones, R. (2014). The Mersey Burns App: Evolving a model of validation. *Emergency Medicine Journal*. doi:10.1136/emermed-2013-203416 PMID:25371408

Barrera, M. Jr, Glasgow, R. E., McKay, H. G., Boles, S. M., & Feil, E. G. (2002). Do internet-based support interventions change perceptions of social support?: An experimental trial of approaches for supporting diabetes self management. *American Journal of Community Psychology*, *30*(5), 637–654. doi:10.1023/A:1016369114780 PMID:12188054

Bartlett, S. J., Lukk, P., Butz, A., Lampros-Klein, F., & Rand, C. S. (2002). Enhancing medication adherence among inner-city children with asthma: Results from pilot studies. *The Journal of Asthma*, *39*(1), 47–54. doi:10.1081/JAS-120000806 PMID:11883739

Barton, A. J. (2010). Using mobile health technology to enhance patient-centered care. *Clinical Nurse Specialist CNS*, *24*(5), 233–234. PMID:20716974

Basch, E., Deal, A. M., Kris, M. G., Scher, H. I., Hudis, C. A., Sabbatini, P., ... Schrag, D. (2016). Symptom monitoring with patient-reported outcomes during routine cancer treatment: A randomized controlled trial. *Journal of Clinical Oncology*, *34*(6), 557–565. doi:10.1200/JCO.2015.63.0830 PMID:26644527

Bashshur, R., Shannon, G., Krupinski, E., & Grigsby, J. (2011). Policy: The taxonomy of telemedicine. *Telemedicine Journal and e-Health*, *17*(6), 484–494. doi:10.1089/tmj.2011.0103 PMID:21718114

Bates, M. J. (2009). Information Behavior. In M. J. Bates & M. N. Maack (Eds.), *Encyclopedia of Library and Information Sciences* (3rd ed.). New York, NY: CRC Press. doi:10.1081/E-ELIS3-120043263

Bateson, G. (1970). A systems approach. *International Journal of Psychiatry*, *9*, 242–244. PMID:5482974

Baudendistel, I., Winkler, E., Kamradt, M., Brophy, S., Längst, G., Eckrich, F., ... Ose, D. (2015). The patients' active role in managing a personal electronic health record: A qualitative analysis. *Supportive Care in Cancer*, *23*(9), 2613–2621. doi:10.100700520-015-2620-1 PMID:25652149

Bauer, S., de Niet, J., Timman, R., & Kordy, H. (2010). Enhancement of care through self-monitoring and tailored feedback via text messaging and their use in the treatment of childhood overweight. *Patient Education and Counseling*, *79*(3), 315–319. doi:10.1016/j.pec.2010.03.014 PMID:20418046

Bayne, S., & Ross, J. (2007). The 'digital native' and 'digital immigrant': a dangerous opposition. *Annual Conference of the Society for Research into Higher Education.*

Beasley, J. M., Riley, W. T., Davis, A., & Singh, J. (2008). Evaluation of a PDA-based dietary assessment and intervention program: A randomized controlled trial. *Journal of the American College of Nutrition*, *27*(2), 280–286. doi:10.1080/07315724.2008.10719701 PMID:18689560

Beaver, K., Bogg, J., & Luker, K. (1999). Decision making role preferences and information needs: A comparison of colorectal and breast cancer. *Health Expectations*, *2*(4), 266–276. doi:10.1046/j.1369-6513.1999.00066.x PMID:11281903

Bellina, L., Azzolina, G., Nucatola, I., Maggio, A., Consiglio, F., Ingrassia, R., ... Carrabino, R. (2014). M-phone impact on practical training: Role of m-phone as part of the educative method for training local health workers of rural areas of developing countries. *Health and Technology*, *4*(3), 289–294. doi:10.100712553-013-0073-4

Bellina, L., & Missoni, E. (2009). Mobile cell-phones (M-phones) in telemicroscopy: Increasing connectivity of isolated laboratories. *Diagnostic Pathology*, *4*(1), 19. doi:10.1186/1746-1596-4-19 PMID:19545373

Bender, J. L., Yue, R. Y. K., To, M. J., Deacken, L., & Jadad, A. R. (2013). A lot of action, but not in the right direction: Systematic review and content analysis of smartphone applications for the prevention, detection, and management of cancer. *Journal of Medical Internet Research*, *15*(12), e287. doi:10.2196/jmir.2661 PMID:24366061

Benedetti, F. (2011). *The Patient's Brain: The neuroscience behind the doctor-patient relationship*. Oxford, UK: Oxford University Press.

Bentley, L., Dittman, K., & Whitten, J. (2004). *System analysis and design methods*. McGraw-Hill Higher Education.

Bergrath, S., Rossaint, R., Lenssen, N., Fitzner, C., & Skorning, M. (2013). Prehospital digital photography and automated image transmission in an emergency medical service - an ancillary retrospective analysis of a prospective controlled trial. *Scandinavian Journal of Trauma, Resuscitation and Emergency Medicine*, *21*(1), 3. doi:10.1186/1757-7241-21-3 PMID:23324531

Berkovsky, S., Freyne, J., & Oinas-Kukkonen, H. (2012). Influencing individually: Fusing personalization and persuasion. *ACM Transactions on Interactive Intelligent Systems*, *2*(2), 1–8. doi:10.1145/2209310.2209312

Bernetti, L., Nuzzaco, G., Muscia, F., Gamboni, A., Zedde, M., Eusebi, P., ... Corea, F. (2018). Stroke networks and telemedicine: An Italian national survey. *Neurology International*, *10*(1), 7599. doi:10.4081/ni.2018.7599 PMID:29844893

Beutel, A., Prakash, B. A., Rosenfeld, R., & Faloutsos, C. (2012). Interacting viruses in networks: Can both survive? *KDD: Proceedings / International Conference on Knowledge Discovery & Data Mining. International Conference on Knowledge Discovery & Data Mining*, *12*, 426–434. doi:10.1145/2339530.2339601

Bhargave, R., & Johnmar, F. (n.d.). *ePatient 2015. 15 Surprising Trends Changing Health Care*. Retrieved 5 10, 2015, from epatient2015: www.epatient2015.com

Bhatt, K., Pourmand, A., & Sikka, N. (2018). Targeted Applications of Unmanned Aerial Vehicles (Drones) in Telemedicine. *Telemedicine Journal and e-Health*, tmj.2017.0289. doi:10.1089/tmj.2017.0289 PMID:29489441

Bielecki, M. (2012). *Leveraging Mobile Health Technology for Patient Recruitment: An Emerging Opportunity*. Northbrook, IL: Blue Chip Patient Recruitment.

Biermann, E., Dietrich, W., & Standl, E. (2000). Telecare of diabetic patients with intensified insulin therapy. A randomized clinical trial. *Studies in Health Technology and Informatics*, *77*, 327–332. PMID:11187566

Blood pressure statistics. (2018). Retrieved from https://www.belmarrahealth.com/understanding-blood-pressure-readings-is-key-to-overall-well-being/

Blount, M., Batra, V. M., Capella, A. N., Ebling, M. R., Jerome, W. F., Martin, S. M., ... Wright, S. P. (2007). Remote health-care monitoring using personal care connect. *IBM Systems Journal*, *46*(1), 95–115. doi:10.1147j.461.0095

Bodenheimer, T., Lorig, K., Holman, H., & Grumbach, K. (2002). Patient self-management of chronic disease in primary care. *Journal of the American Medical Association*, *288*(19), 2469–2475. doi:10.1001/jama.288.19.2469 PMID:12435261

Bogoch, I. I., Koydemir, H. C., Tseng, D., Ephraim, R. K. D., Duah, E., Tee, J., ... Ozcan, A. (2017). Evaluation of a Mobile Phone-Based Microscope for Screening of Schistosoma haematobium Infection in Rural Ghana. *The American Journal of Tropical Medicine and Hygiene*, *96*(6), 1468–1471. doi:10.4269/ajtmh.16-0912 PMID:28719262

Bolle, S. R., Johnsen, E., & Gilbert, M. (2011). Video calls for dispatcher-assisted cardiopulmonary resuscitation can improve the confidence of lay rescuers--surveys after simulated cardiac arrest. *Journal of Telemedicine and Telecare*, *17*(2), 88–92. doi:10.1258/jtt.2010.100605 PMID:21139017

Boone, K. W. (2011). *The CDA Tm Book*. Springer Science & Business Media. doi:10.1007/978-0-85729-336-7

Boon, M. E., Kok, L. P., & Under, J. (1993). Neural network processing can provide means to catch errors that slip through human screening of pap smears. *Diagnostic Cytopathology*, *9*(4), 411–416. doi:10.1002/dc.2840090408 PMID:8261846

Borve, A., Terstappen, K., Sandberg, C., & Paoli, J. (2013). Mobile teledermoscopy-there's an app for that! *Dermatology Practical & Conceptual*, *3*(2), 41–48. doi:10.5826/dpc.0302a05 PMID:23785643

Boulos, M. N. K., Brewer, A. C., Karimkhani, C., Buller, D. B., & Robert, P. (2014). Mobile medical and health apps : State of the art, concerns, regulatory control and certification. *Online Journal of Public Health Informatics*, *5*(3), 1–23. PMID:24683442

Boulos, M. N., Brewer, A. C., Karimkhani, C., Buller, D. B., & Dellavalle, R. P. (2014). Mobile medical and health apps: State of the art, concerns, regulatory control and certification. *Online Journal of Public Health Informatics*, *5*(3), 229. doi:10.5210/ojphi.v5i3.4814 PMID:24683442

Boutilier, J. J., Brooks, S. C., Janmohamed, A., Byers, A., Buick, J. E., Zhan, C., ... Chan, T. C. Y. (2017). Optimizing a Drone Network to Deliver Automated External Defibrillators. *Circulation*, *135*(25), 2454–2465. doi:10.1161/CIRCULATIONAHA.116.026318 PMID:28254836

Bradley, C., & Blenkinsopp, A. (1996). Over the counter drugs: The future for self medication. *BMJ (Clinical Research Ed.)*, *312*(7034), 835–837. doi:10.1136/bmj.312.7034.835 PMID:8608296

BRAVEHEALTH. (2016). *Patient Centric Approach for an Integrated, Adaptive, Context Aware Remote Diagnosis and Management of Cardiovascular Diseases* (European Commission, CORDIS, Projects & Results Service). Retrieved Dec 2, 2016, from http://cordis.europa.eu/project/rcn/102204_en.html

Brender, J., & McNair, P. (1996). User requirements on the future laboratory information systems. *Computer Methods and Programs in Biomedicine*, *50*(2), 87–93. doi:10.1016/0169-2607(96)01738-Q PMID:8875016

Brennan, L. K., Kreuter, M. W., Caburnay, C. A., & Wilshire, B. L. (1998). *Linking smokers to smoking cessation programs: does perceived importance of specific program characteristics predict cessation?* Paper presented at the Society of Behavioral Medicine Conference, New Orleans, LA.

Brennan, P. F., & Safran, C. (2005). Empowered consumers. In D. Lewis, G. Eysenbach, R. Kukafka, P. Z. Stavri, & H. Jimison (Eds.), *Consumer Health Informatics: informing consumers and improving health care*. New York, NY: Springer. doi:10.1007/0-387-27652-1_2

Breslauer, D. N., Maamari, R. N., Switz, N. A., Lam, W. A., & Fletcher, D. A. (2009). Mobile phone based clinical microscopy for global health applications. *PLoS One*, *4*(7), e6320. doi:10.1371/journal.pone.0006320 PMID:19623251

Brettle, D. S. (2007). Display considerations for hospital-wide viewing of soft copy images. *The British Journal of Radiology*, *80*(955), 503–507. doi:10.1259/bjr/26436784 PMID:17704314

Brinkrolf, P., Scheer, D., Hasebrook, J., & Hahnenkamp, K. (2017). Land|Rettung: Zukunftsfeste notfallmedizinische Neuausrichtung eines Landkreises. In Amelung (Ed.), Innovationsfonds (pp. 140-145). MWV.

Briscoe, D., Adair, C. F., Thompson, L. D., Tellado, M. V., Buckner, S. B., Rosenthal, D. L., & O'Leary, T. J. (2000). Telecytologic diagnosis of breast fine needle aspiration biopsies. Intraobserver concordance. *Acta Cytologica*, *44*(2), 175–180. doi:10.1159/000326357 PMID:10740603

Broach, J., Hart, A., Griswold, M., Lai, J., Boyer, E. W., Skolnik, A. B., & Chai, P. R. (2018). Usability and Reliability of Smart Glasses for Secondary Triage During Mass Casualty Incidents. *Proc Annu Hawaii Int Conf Syst Sci*, 2018, 1416-1422.

Brochhausen, M., Spear, A. D., Cocos, C., Weiler, G., Martín, L., Anguita, A., ... Sfakianakis, S. (2011). The ACGT Master Ontology and its applications–Towards an ontology-driven cancer research and management system. *Journal of Biomedical Informatics*, *44*(1), 8–25. doi:10.1016/j.jbi.2010.04.008 PMID:20438862

Brokmann, J. C., Conrad, C., Rossaint, R., Bergrath, S., Beckers, S. K., Tamm, M., ... Hirsch, F. (2016). Treatment of Acute Coronary Syndrome by Telemedically Supported Paramedics Compared With Physician-Based Treatment: A Prospective, Interventional, Multicenter Trial. *Journal of Medical Internet Research, 18*(12), e314. doi:10.2196/jmir.6358 PMID:27908843

Brokmann, J. C., Rossaint, R., Hirsch, F., Beckers, S. K., Czaplik, M., Chowanetz, M., ... Bergrath, S. (2016). Analgesia by telemedically supported paramedics compared with physician-administered analgesia: A prospective, interventional, multicentre trial. *European Journal of Pain (London, England), 20*(7), 1176–1184. doi:10.1002/ejp.843 PMID:26914284

Brokmann, J. C., Rossaint, R., Muller, M., Fitzner, C., Villa, L., Beckers, S. K., & Bergrath, S. (2017). Blood pressure management and guideline adherence in hypertensive emergencies and urgencies: A comparison between telemedically supported and conventional out-of-hospital care. *Journal of Clinical Hypertension (Greenwich, Conn.), 19*(7), 704–712. doi:10.1111/jch.13026 PMID:28560799

Brug, J., Campbell, M., & van Assema, P. (1999). The application and impact of computer-generated personalized nutrition education: A review of the literature. *Patient Education and Counseling, 36*(2), 145–156. doi:10.1016/S0738-3991(98)00131-1 PMID:10223019

Brug, J., Oenema, A., & Campbell, M. (2003). Past, present, and future of computer-tailored nutrition education. *The American Journal of Clinical Nutrition, 77*(4), 1028S–1034S. doi:10.1093/ajcn/77.4.1028S PMID:12663313

Brug, J., Oenema, A., & Ferreira, I. (2005). Theory, evidence and Intervention Mapping to improve behavior nutrition and physical activity interventions. *The International Journal of Behavioral Nutrition and Physical Activity, 2*(2). PMID:15807898

Brug, J., Steenhaus, I., van Assema, P., & de Vries, H. (1996). The impact of computer-tailored nutrition intervention. *Preventive Medicine, 25*(3), 236–242. doi:10.1006/pmed.1996.0052 PMID:8781000

Brug, J., van Assema, P., Kok, G., Lenderink, T., & Glanz, K. (1994). Self-rated dietary fat intake: Association with objective assessment of fat, psychosocial factors, and intention to change. *Journal of Nutrition Education, 26*(5), 218–223. doi:10.1016/S0022-3182(12)80890-9

Buchbinder, R. (2008). Self-management education en masse: effectiveness of the Back Pain: Don't Take It Lying Down mass media campaign. *The Medical Journal of Australia, 189*(10Suppl), S29–S32. PMID:19143582

Bull, F. C., & Jamrozik, K. (1998). Advice on exercise from a family physician can help sedentary patients to become active. *American Journal of Preventive Medicine, 15*(2), 85–94. doi:10.1016/S0749-3797(98)00040-3 PMID:9713663

Burger, R. (1991). Computer Viruses and Data Protection. *Abacus.*

Burke, L. E., Conroy, M. B., Sereika, S. M., Elci, O. U., Styn, M. A., Acharya, S. D., ... Glanz, K. (2011). The effect of electronic self-monitoring on weight loss and dietary intake: A randomized behavioral weight loss trial. *Obesity (Silver Spring, Md.), 19*(2), 338–344. doi:10.1038/oby.2010.208 PMID:20847736

Burney, S. M. A., Nadeem, M., & Zain, A. (2010). Information and Communication Technology in Healthcare Management Systems: Prospects for Developing countries. *International Journal of Computers and Applications, 4*, 1.

Burns, M., & Mohr, D. (in press). eHealth, telehealth, and Telemedicine. In Encyclopedia of Behavioral Medicine. Springer.

Burns, M., Begale, M., Duffecy, J., Gergle, D., Karr, C., Giangrande, E., & DC., M. (2011). Harnessing context sensing to develop a mobile intervention for depression. *J Med Internet Res, 13*(3).

Burns, M. N., Begale, M., Duffecy, J., Gergle, D., Karr, C. J., Giangrande, E., & Mohr, D. C. (2011). Harnessing context sensing to develop a mobile intervention for depression. *Journal of Medical Internet Research, 13*(3), e55. doi:10.2196/jmir.1838 PMID:21840837

Buscher, C., & Schilberg, D. (n.d.). *TemRas Telemedizinische Rettungsassistenzsystem.* Retrieved 04.06.2013, from http://www.temras.de/

Calleja-Castillo, J. M., & Gonzalez-Calderon, G. (2018). WhatsApp in Stroke Systems: Current Use and Regulatory Concerns. *Frontiers in Neurology, 9*, 388. doi:10.3389/fneur.2018.00388 PMID:29904369

Callender, C., & Thompson, D. (2018). Family TXT: Feasibility and Acceptability of a mHealth Obesity Prevention Program for Parents of Pre-Adolescent African American Girls. *Children (Basel), 5*(6). doi:10.3390/children5060081 PMID:29921811

Callese, T. E., Richards, C. T., Shaw, P., Schuetz, S. J., Paladino, L., Issa, N., & Swaroop, M. (2015). Trauma system development in low- and middle-income countries: A review. *The Journal of Surgical Research, 193*(1), 300–307. doi:10.1016/j.jss.2014.09.040 PMID:25450600

Campbell, M. K., DeVellis, B. M., Strecher, V. J., Ammerman, A. S., DeVellis, R. F., & Sandler, R. S. (1994). Improving dietary behavior: The effectiveness of tailored messages in primary care settings. *American Journal of Public Health, 84*(5), 783–787. doi:10.2105/AJPH.84.5.783 PMID:8179049

Campbell, M. K., & Quintiliani, L. M. (2006). Tailored interventions in public health. Where does tailoring fit in interventions to reduce health disparities? *The American Behavioral Scientist, 49*(6), 775–793. doi:10.1177/0002764205283807

Canale, S. (2013). *The Bravehealth Software Architecture for the Monitoring of Patients Affected by CVD.* Fifth International Conference on eHealth, Telemedicine, and Social Medicine (eTELEMED 2013).

CAREGIVERSPRO-MMD. (2016). *Self-management interventions and mutual assistance community services, helping patients with dementia and caregivers connect with others for evaluation, support and inspiration to improve the care experience* (EU Project Official web site). Retrieved Jan 18, 2017, from caregiversprommd-project.eu/

Casas, L., Castaneda, B., & Treuillet, S. (2011). *Imaging technologies applied to chronic wounds: a survey.* ACM.

Casebeer, L. L., Strasser, S. M., Spettell, C. M., Wall, T. C., Weissman, N., Ray, M. N., & Allison, J. J. (2003). Designing tailored Web-based instruction to improve practicing physicians' preventive practices. *Journal of Medical Internet Research, 5*(3), e20. doi:10.2196/jmir.5.3.e20 PMID:14517111

Case, D. O. (2012). *Looking for Information. A Survey of Research on Information Seeking, Needs, and Behavior.* Bingley, UK: Emerald.

Cavoukian, A. (2011). *Privacy by design in law, policy and practice: a white paper for regulators, decision-makers and policy-makers.* Retrieved from http://www.ontla.on.ca/library/repository/mon/25008/312239.pdf

Cawsey, A., Grasso, F., & Jones, R. B. (1999). A conversational model for health promotion on the World Wide Web. Artificial intelligence in medicine. *Proceedings of the Joint European Conference on Artificial Intelligence in Medicine and Medical Decision Making.*

CDC. (2009). *The power of prevention: Chronic disease...the public health challenge of the 21st century.* National Center for Chronic Disease Prevention and Health Promotion. National Center for Chronic Disease Prevention and Health Promotion.

Chakraborty, C., Gupta, B., & Ghosh, S. K. (2014). Mobile metadata assisted community database of chronic wound. *International Journal of Wound Medicine, 6*, 34–42. doi:10.1016/j.wndm.2014.09.002

Chambers, R. (2006). Guest editorial: The role of the health professional in supporting self care. *Quality in Primary Care*, *14*, 129–131.

Chao, J. T. II, Loescher, L. J., Soyer, H. P., & Curiel-Lewandrowski, C. (2013). Barriers to mobile teledermoscopy in primary care. *Journal of the American Academy of Dermatology*, *69*(5), 821–824. doi:10.1016/j.jaad.2012.10.039 PMID:24124819

Chaplais, E., Naughton, G., Thivel, D., Courteix, D., & Greene, D. (2015). Smartphone Interventions for Weight Treatment and Behavioral Change in Pediatric Obesity: A Systematic Review. *Telemedicine Journal and e-Health*, *21*(10), 822–830. doi:10.1089/tmj.2014.0197 PMID:26290954

Chatman, E. A., & Pendleton, V. E. M. (1995). Knowledge gap, information-seeking and the poor. *The Reference Librarian*, *23*(49/50), 135–145. doi:10.1300/J120v23n49_10

Chau, P. Y. K., & Hu, P. J. (2004). Technology Implementation for Telemedicine Programs. *Communications of the ACM*, *47*(2), 87–92. doi:10.1145/966389.966396

Chen, M., Gonzalez, S., Vasilakos, A., Cao, H., & Leung, V. (2011). *Body area networks: A survey*, Springer. *Mobile Networks and Applications*, *16*(2), 171–193. doi:10.100711036-010-0260-8

Chinmay, C., Bharat, G., & Soumya, K. G. (2013). *A review on telemedicine-based WBAN framework for patient monitoring*. Telemedicine and e-health, Marry Ann Liebert *Inc*.

Chinmay, C., & Gupta, B. (2016). Adaptive Filtering Technique for Chronic Wound Image analysis under Tele-Wound Network. *International Journal of Communication, Navigation, Sensing and Services*, *1*, 57–76.

Chinmay, C., Gupta, B., & Ghosh, S. K. (2016), *Mobile Telemedicine Systems for Remote Patient's Chronic Wound Monitoring*. IGI.

Chochliouros, I. (n.d.). *Live Video-to-Video Supporting Interactive City Infrastructure*. Retrieved 03.06.2013, from http://www.livecity-psp.eu/

Chochliouros, I., Stephanakis, I., Spiliopoulou, A., Sfakianakis, E., & Ladid, L. (2012). Developing Innovative Live Video-to-Video Communications for Smarter European Cities. In L. Iliadis, I. Maglogiannis, H. Papadopoulos, K. Karatzas, & S. Sioutas (Eds.), *Artificial Intelligence Applications and Innovations* (Vol. 382, pp. 279–289). Springer Berlin Heidelberg. doi:10.1007/978-3-642-33412-2_29

Cho, J. H., Chang, S. A., Kwon, H. S., Choi, Y.-H., Ko, S.-H., Moon, S.-D., ... Yoon, K.-H. (2006). Long-term effect of the internet-based glucose monitoring system on HbA1c reduction and glucose stability: A 30-month follow up study for diabetes management with a ubiquitous medical care system. *Diabetes Care*, *29*(12), 2625–2631. doi:10.2337/dc05-2371 PMID:17130195

Choudhri, A. F., Carr, T. M. III, Ho, C. P., Stone, J. R., Gay, S. B., & Lambert, D. L. (2012). Handheld device review of abdominal CT for the evaluation of acute appendicitis. *Journal of Digital Imaging*, *25*(4), 492–496. doi:10.100710278-011-9431-9 PMID:22146833

Choudhri, A. F., Norton, P. T., Carr, T. M. III, Stone, J. R., Hagspiel, K. D., & Dake, M. D. (2013). Diagnosis and treatment planning of acute aortic emergencies using a handheld DICOM viewer. *Emergency Radiology*, *20*(4), 267–272. doi:10.100710140-013-1118-8 PMID:23525945

CHRONIOUS. (2008). *An Open, Ubiquitous and Adaptive Chronic Disease Management Platform for COPD and Renal Insufficiency*. Retrieved from www.chronious.eu

Claesson, A., Svensson, L., Nordberg, P., Ringh, M., Rosenqvist, M., Djarv, T., ... Hollenberg, J. (2017). Drones may be used to save lives in out of hospital cardiac arrest due to drowning. *Resuscitation, 114*, 152–156. doi:10.1016/j.resuscitation.2017.01.003 PMID:28110000

Clarke, J., Proudfoot, J., Birch, M. R., Whitton, A. E., Parker, G., Manicavasagar, V., ... Hadzi-Pavlovic, D. (2014). Effects of mental health self-efficacy on outcomes of a mobile phone and web intervention for mild-to-moderate depression, anxiety and stress: Secondary analysis of a randomised controlled trial. *BMC Psychiatry, 14*(1), 272. doi:10.118612888-014-0272-1 PMID:25252853

Clark, N. M. (2003). Management of chronic disease by patients. *Annual Review of Public Health, 24*(1), 289–313. doi:10.1146/annurev.publhealth.24.100901.141021 PMID:12415147

Cochand-Priollet, B., Koutroumbas, K., Megalopoulou, T. M., Pouliakis, A., Sivolapenko, G., & Karakitsos, P. (2006). Discriminating benign from malignant thyroid lesions using artificial intelligence and statistical selection of morphometric features. *Oncology Reports, 15*, 1023–1026. PMID:16525694

Cole, C., & Leide, J. E. (2006). A cognitive framework for human information behavior: The place of metaphor in human information organizing behavior. In A. Spink & C. Cole (Eds.), *New Directions in Human Information Behavior* (pp. 171–202). Dordrecht, Germany: Springer. doi:10.1007/1-4020-3670-1_10

Cole-Lewis, H., & Kershaw, T. (2010). Text Messaging as a Tool for Behavior Change in Disease Prevention and Management. *Epidemiologic Reviews, 32*(1), 56–69. doi:10.1093/epirev/mxq004 PMID:20354039

Collado-Borrell, R., Escudero-Vilaplana, V., Ribed-Sánchez, A., Ibáñez-García, S., Herranz-Alonso, A., & Sanjurjo-Sáez, M. (2016). Smartphone applications for cancer patients; what we know about them. *Farmacia Hospitalaria, 40*(1), 25–35. PMID:26882831

Collins, B. (2011). iPad and cytopathology: Content creation and delivery. *CytoJournal, 8*(16c). http://www.ncbi.nlm.nih.gov/pmc/articles/PMC3230889/

Commodity12. (2011). *Continuous multi-parametric and multi-layered analysis of diabetes type 1 & 2*. Retrieved from www.commodity12.eu

Consolvo, S., Everitt, K. M., Smith, I., & Landay, J. A. (2006). Design requirements for technologies that encourage physical activity. In *Proceedings of CHI 2006*. Montréal, Canada. ACM Press.

Contrada, R. J., & Goyal, T. M. (2004). Individual differences, health and illness: the role of emotional traits and generalized expectancies. In The SAGE Handbook of Health Psychology (pp. 143–169). London, UK: SAGE Publications Ltd.

Cordina, M., McElnay, J. C., & Hughes, C. M. (2001). Assessment of a community pharmacy-based program for patients with asthma. *Pharmacotherapy, 21*(10), 1196–1203. doi:10.1592/phco.21.15.1196.33894 PMID:11601666

CORDIS, European Community - Community Research and Development Information. (n.d.). *EC CORDIS Projects & Results Service*. Retrieved December 3, 2016, from http://data.europa.eu/euodp/en/data

Coster, S. (2000). Monitoring blood glucose control in diabetes mellitus: A systematic review. *Health Technology Assessment, 4*(12). PMID:10944740

Crowe, A., Linder, A., Hameed, O., Salih, C., Roberson, J., Gidley, J., & Eltoum, I. A. (2011). The impact of implementation of the Bethesda System for Reporting Thyroid Cytopathology on the quality of reporting, "risk" of malignancy, surgical rate, and rate of frozen sections requested for thyroid lesions. *Cancer Cytopathology, 119*(5), 315–321. doi:10.1002/cncy.20174 PMID:21751427

Cucciniello, M., Guerrazzi, C., Nasi, G., & Ongaro, E. (2015). Coordination mechanisms for implementing Complex Innovations in the Health Care Sector. *Public Management Review, 17*(7), 1040–1060. doi:10.1080/14719037.2015.1029348

Cucciniello, M., & Nasi, G. (2014). Transparency for trust in government: How effective is formal transparency? *International Journal of Public Administration, 37*(13), 911–921. doi:10.1080/01900692.2014.949754

Cucoranu, I. C., Parwani, A. V., & Pantanowitz, L. (2014). Digital whole slide imaging in cytology. *Archives of Pathology & Laboratory Medicine, 138*(3), 300. doi:10.5858/arpa.2013-0270-LE PMID:24576021

Cummins, N. M., Dixon, M., Garavan, C., Landymore, E., Mulligan, N., & O'Donnell, C. (2013). Can advanced paramedics in the field diagnose patients and predict hospital admission? *Emergency Medicine Journal, 30*(12), 1043–1047. doi:10.1136/emermed-2012-201899 PMID:23407377

Cunha, J. P. S., Cunha, B., Xavier, W., Ferreira, N., & Meireles, L. (2010). *Vital-Jacket®: A wearable wireless vital signs monitor for patients' mobility in cardiology and sports.* IEETA/Dep. Electron. Telecommunication & Information, *4th International Conference on Pervasive Computing Technologies for Healthcare (PervasiveHealth).*

Cunningham, A. J., Lockwood, G. A., & Cunningham, J. A. (1991). A relationship between perceived self-efficacy and quality of life in cancer patients. *Patient Education and Counseling, 17*(1), 71–78. doi:10.1016/0738-3991(91)90052-7 PMID:1997998

Curaudeau, G. A., Sharma, N., & Rovin, R. A. (2011). Development of an iPhone application for sideline concussion testing. *Neurosurgical Focus, 31*(5), E4. doi:10.3171/2011.8.FOCUS11186 PMID:22044103

Currell, R., & Urquhart, C. (2004). Nursing record systems: effects on nursing practice and health care outcomes. *Cochrane Review, 2.*

Currie, L. M. (2005). Evaluation frameworks for nursing informatics. *International Journal of Medical Informatics, 74*(11), 908–916. doi:10.1016/j.ijmedinf.2005.07.007 PMID:16099711

Curtis, D., Shih, E., Bailey, J., Stair, T., & Greenes, R.A. (2008). Physiological signal monitoring in the waiting areas of an emergency room. *International Procedings of BodyNets,* 1-8.

Cuzzell. (1988). The new RYB color code. *The American Journal of Nursing, 88*(10), 1342–1346. PMID:3177488

Czaplik, M., Bergrath, S., Rossaint, R., Thelen, S., Brodziak, T., Valentin, B., ... Brokmann, J. C. (2014). Employment of telemedicine in emergency medicine. Clinical requirement analysis, system development and first test results. *Methods of Information in Medicine, 53*(2), 99–107. doi:10.3414/ME13-01-0022 PMID:24477815

D'Ambrosio, M. V., Bakalar, M., Bennuru, S., Reber, C., Skandarajah, A., Nilsson, L., ... Fletcher, D. A. (2015). Point-of-care quantification of blood-borne filarial parasites with a mobile phone microscope. *Science Translational Medicine, 7*(286), 286re284. doi:10.1126citranslmed.aaa3480 PMID:25947164

Dagal, A., Greer, S. E., & McCunn, M. (2014). International disparities in trauma care. *Current Opinion in Anaesthesiology, 27*(2), 233–239. doi:10.1097/ACO.0000000000000049 PMID:24514036

Dally, D. L., Dahar, W., Scott, A., Roblin, D., & Khoury, A. T. (2002). The impact of a health education program targeting patients with high visit rates in a managed care organization. *American Journal of Health Promotion, 17*(2), 101–111. doi:10.4278/0890-1171-17.2.101 PMID:12471862

Daou, R. A. Z., Aad, E., Nakhle, F., Hayek, A., & Horscok, J. (2015). Patient Vital Signs Monitoring via Android Application. *Proceedings of International Conference on Advances in Biomedical Engineering (ICABME).* 10.1109/ICABME.2015.7323278

Davies, N. J., Kinman, G., Thomas, R. J., & Bailey, T. (2008). Information satisfaction in breast and prostate cancer patients: Implications for quality of life. *Psycho-Oncology*, *17*(10), 1048–1052. doi:10.1002/pon.1305 PMID:18203242

Davison, B. J., Kirk, P., Degner, L. F., & Hassard, T. H. (1999). Information and patient participation in screening for prostate cancer. *Patient Education and Counseling*, *37*(3), 255–263. doi:10.1016/S0738-3991(98)00123-2 PMID:14528551

Davison, B. J., Parker, P. A., & Goldenberg, S. L. (2004). Patients' preferences for communicating a prostate cancer diagnosis and participating in medical decision making. *BJU International*, *93*(1), 47–51. doi:10.1111/j.1464-410X.2004.04553.x PMID:14678366

De Clercq, P. A., Hasman, A., & Wolffenbuttel, B. H. (2003). A consumer health record for supporting the patient-centered management of chronic diseases. *Medical Informatics and the Internet in Medicine*, *28*(2), 117–127. doi:10.1080/14639230310001600506 PMID:14692588

de Iongh, A., Fagan, P., Fenner, J., & Kidd, L. (2015). *A practical guide to self-management support: Key components for successful implementation.* London: The Health Foundation.

de Lusignan, S., Wells, S., Johnson, P., Meredith, K., & Leatham, E. (2001). Compliance and effectiveness of 1 year's home telemonitoring. The report of a pilot study of patients with chronic heart failure. *European Journal of Heart Failure*, *3*(6), 723–730. doi:10.1016/S1388-9842(01)00190-8 PMID:11738225

de Onis, M., Blössner, M., & Borghi, E. (2010). Global prevalence and trends of overweight and obesity among preschool children. *The American Journal of Clinical Nutrition*, *92*(5), 1257–1264. doi:10.3945/ajcn.2010.29786 PMID:20861173

Decipher, P. C. P. (2013). *Mobile health for European citizens.* Retrieved from www.decipherpcp.eu

Deena, M., & Muhammad, A. (2012). A survey of challenges and applications of wireless body area network (WBAN) and role of a virtual doctor server in existing architecture. *IEEE 3rd International Conference on Intelligent Systems Modelling and Simulation*, 214-219.

Degner, L., Krisjanson, L. J., Bowman, D., Sloan, J. A., Carriere, K. C., O'Neil, J., ... Mueller, B. (1997). Informational needs and decisional preferences in women with breast cancer. *Journal of the American Medical Association*, *277*(18), 1485–1492. doi:10.1001/jama.1997.03540420081039 PMID:9145723

DeHaes, H., & Koedoot, N. (2003). Patient centred decision making in palliative cancer treatment: A world of paradoxes. *Patient Education and Counseling*, *50*(1), 43–49. doi:10.1016/S0738-3991(03)00079-X PMID:12767584

Delisle Nystrom, C., Sandin, S., Henriksson, P., Henriksson, H., Maddison, R., & Lof, M. (2018). A 12-month follow-up of a mobile-based (mHealth) obesity prevention intervention in pre-school children: The MINISTOP randomized controlled trial. *BMC Public Health*, *18*(1), 658. doi:10.118612889-018-5569-4 PMID:29793467

Della Mea, V., Cataldi, P., Pertoldi, B., & Beltrami, C. A. (2000). Combining dynamic and static robotic telepathology: A report on 184 consecutive cases of frozen sections, histology and cytology. *Analytical Cellular Pathology*, *20*(1), 33–39. doi:10.1155/2000/734943 PMID:11007436

Deloitte Consulting. (2013). *European Interoperability Framework for eHealth.* ISA. doi:10.2759/14325

Deloitte. (2014a). *Healthcare and Life Sciences Predictions 2020: A bold future?* Deloitte Centre for Health Solutions.

Deloitte. (2014b). *The four dimensions of effective health: People, places, payment, purpose.* Deloitte.

Demichelis, F., Della Mea, V., Forti, S., Dalla Palma, P., & Beltrami, C. A. (2002). Digital storage of glass slides for quality assurance in histopathology and cytopathology. *Journal of Telemedicine and Telecare*, *8*(3), 138–142. doi:10.1177/1357633X0200800303 PMID:12097174

Denis, F., Lethrosne, C., Pourel, N., Molinier, O., Pointreau, Y., Domont, J., ... Letellier, C. (2017). Randomized trial comparing a web-mediated follow-up with routine surveillance in lung cancer patients. *JNCI. Journal of the National Cancer Institute, 109*(9). doi:10.1093/jnci/djx029 PMID:28423407

Department of Economic and Social Affairs, Population Division. (2001). World Population Ageing: 1950-2050. New York: United Nations.

Department of Economic and Social Affairs, Population Division. (2007). World Population Ageing 2007. New York: United Nations.

Department of Health Department of Health. (2001). *The Expert Patient: a new approach to chronic disease management for the 21st century*. London: Department of Health.

Department of Health. (2000). *The NHS Plan. A plan for investment. A plan for reform*. London: Department of Health.

Department of Health. (2005a). *Supporting People with Long Term Conditions: an NHS and Social Care Model to support local innovation and integration*. London: Department of Health.

Department of Health. (2005b). *Self Care: A real choice*. London: Department of Health.

Department of Health. (2006a). *Our Health, Our Say*. London: Department of Health.

Derr, R. L. (1983). A conceptual analysis of information need. *Information Processing & Management, 19*(5), 273–278. doi:10.1016/0306-4573(83)90001-8

Dey, P., Logasundaram, R., & Joshi, K. (2013). Artificial neural network in diagnosis of lobular carcinoma of breast in fine-needle aspiration cytology. *Diagnostic Cytopathology, 41*(2), 102–106. doi:10.1002/dc.21773 PMID:21987420

Dhukaram A. V. (2011). *End-User Perception Towards Pervasive Cardiac Healthcare Services: Benefits, Acceptance, Adoption, Risks, Security, Privacy and Trust*. Dublin, Ireland: PervasiveHealth.

Diamantis, A., Magiorkinis, E., & Koutselini, H. (2014). 50 years after the death of George Nicholas Papanicolaou (1883-1962): Evaluation of his scientific work. *Acta Medico-Historica Adriatica: AMHA, 12*(1), 181–188. PMID:25310617

Dick, W. F. (2003). Anglo-American vs. Franco-German emergency medical services system. *Prehosp Disaster Med, 18*(1), 29-35.

Diekmann, O., & Heesterbeek, J. A. (2000). *Mathematical Epidemiology of Infectious Diseases: Model Building, Analysis and Interpretation*. New York: John Wiley & Sons, Incorporated.

Dijkstra, A., & De Vries, H. (1999). The development of computer-generated tailored interventions. *Patient Education and Counseling, 36*(2), 193–203. doi:10.1016/S0738-3991(98)00135-9 PMID:10223023

Dijkstra, A., De Vries, H., & Roijackers, J. (1998a). Computerized tailored feedback to change cognitive determinants of smoking: A Dutch field experiment. *Health Education Research, 13*(2), 197–206. doi:10.1093/her/13.2.197 PMID:10181018

Dijkstra, A., De Vries, H., & Roijackers, J. (1998b). Longterm effectiveness of computer-generated tailored feedback in smoking cessation. *Health Education Research, 13*(2), 207–214. doi:10.1093/her/13.2.207 PMID:10181019

Dill, A., Brown, P., Ciambrone, D., & Rakowski, W. (1995). The meaning and practice of self care by older adults: A qualitative assessment. *Research on Aging, 17*(1), 8–41. doi:10.1177/0164027595171002

Do C. H. A. N. G. E. (2015). *Do CHANGE: Do Cardiac Health Advanced New Generation Ecosystem*. Retrieved Jan 11, 2017, from www.do-change.eu

Docherty, A., Owens, A., Asadi-Lari, M., Petchey, R., Williams, J., & Carter, Y. H. (2008). Knowledge and information needs of informal caregivers in palliative care: A qualitative systematic review. *Palliative Medicine*, *22*(2), 153–171. doi:10.1177/0269216307085343 PMID:18372380

Dodd, M. J., Janson, S., Facione, N., Faucett, J., Froelicher, E. S., Humphreys, J., ... Taylor, D. (2001). Advancing the science of symptom management. *Journal of Advanced Nursing*, *335*(5), 668–676. doi:10.1046/j.1365-2648.2001.01697.x PMID:11298204

Dogac, A. (2012). Interoperability in eHealth systems. *Proceedings of the VLDB Endowment International Conference on Very Large Data Bases*, *5*(12), 2026–2027. doi:10.14778/2367502.2367568

Drozdov, I., Ouzounis, C. A., Shah, A. M., & Tsoka, S. (2011). Functional Genomics Assistant (FUGA): A toolbox for the analysis of complex biological networks. *BMC Research Notes*, *4*(1), 462. doi:10.1186/1756-0500-4-462 PMID:22035155

E., H. K., & M., S. J. (2010). Ecological momentary interventions: Incorporating mobile technology into psychosocial and health behaviour treatments. *British Journal of Health Psychology, 15*(1), 1-39. doi:10.1348/135910709X466063

Eastman, C., & Marzillier, J. S. (1984). Theoretical and Methodological Difficulties in Bandura's Self-Efficacy Theory. *Cognitive Therapy and Therapy*, *8*(3), 213–229. doi:10.1007/BF01172994

EC Horizon 2020. (n.d.). *Workprogramme 2018-2020 Evaluation Rules.* Retrieved from Research & Innovation Participant Portal: http://ec.europa.eu/research/participants/data/ref/h2020/other/wp/2018-2020/annexes/h2020-wp1820-annex-h-esacrit_en.pdf

EC. (2014). *Green Paper on mobile Health.* Brussels: European Commission.

EC. (2015). *European Commission, Digital Agenda for Europe. A Europe 2020 Initiative.* Retrieved 5 15, 2015, from European Commission: http://ec.europa.eu/digital-agenda/en/connected-continent-legislative-package

EC. (2015). *Horizon 2020. The EU Framework Programme for Research and Innovation.* Retrieved 5 15, 2015, from European Commission: https://ec.europa.eu/programmes/horizon2020/

eHealth Network. (2015). *Refined eHealth European interoperability framework.* Retrieved from http://ec.europa.eu/health//sites/health/files/ehealth/docs/ev_20151123_co03_en.pdf

eHGI. (2012). *Discussion Paper on Semantic and Technical Interoperability.* eHealth Governance Initiative (eHGI).

Ekman, I., Swedberg, K., Taft, C., Lindseth, A., Norberg, A., Brink, E., ... Sunnerhagen, K. S. (2011). Person-centered care—Ready for prime time. *European Journal of Cardiovascular Nursing, 10*(4), 248–251. doi:10.1016/j.ejcnurse.2011.06.008 PMID:21764386

eKuore. (2017). *eKuore Pro: electronic stethoscope for health professionals.* Retrieved Feb 4, 2017, from www.ekuore.com/en/

Elsevier. (2015). *Robbins Pathology Flash Cards.* Retrieved 15 April, 2015, from https://itunes.apple.com/us/app/robbins-pathology-flash-cards/id367031323?mt=8

Elwyn, G., Frosch, D. L., & Kobrin, S. (2015). Implementing shared decision-making: Consider all the consequences. *Implementation Science; IS, 11*(1), 114. doi:10.118613012-016-0480-9 PMID:27502770

EmERGE. (2015). *Creating mHealth solutions to facilitate remote access to health care providers and increase adherence for People Living with HIV (PLHIV).* Retrieved Jan 14, 2017, from www.emergeproject.eu

Empower. (2011). *Support of Patient Empowerment by an intelligent self-management pathway for patients.* Retrieved from www.empower-fp7.eu

Eng, T. R. (2002). E-health research and evaluation: Challenges and opportunities. *Journal of Health Communication, 7*(4), 267–272. doi:10.1080/10810730290001747 PMID:12356287

Enwald, H. P., & Huotari, M. L. (2010). Preventing the obesity epidemic by second generation tailored health communication: An interdisciplinary review. *Journal of Medical Internet Research, 12*(2), e24. doi:10.2196/jmir.1409 PMID:20584698

Epstein, R. M., Franks, P., Fiscella, K., Shields, C. G., Meldrum, S. C., Kravitz, R. L., & Duberstein, P. R. (2005). Measuring patient-centered communication in patient physician consultations: Theoretical and practical issues. *Social Science & Medicine, 61*(7), 1516–1528. doi:10.1016/j.socscimed.2005.02.001 PMID:16005784

Eriksson-Backa, K. (2008). Access to health information: perceptions of barriers among elderly in a language minority. *Information Research, 13*(4).

Eshkeiti, A. M., Joyce, B. B., Narakathu, S., Emamian, S. G. R., Avuthu, J., & Atashbar, M. Z. (2014). A novel self-supported printed flexible strain sensor for monitoring body movement and temperature. Proceedings of IEEE SENSORS.

EU FP7-ICT. (2014). *EU FP7-ICT (Information and Communication Technologies) Workprogramme*. Retrieved April 7, 2015, from http://cordis.europa.eu/fp7/ict/home_en.html

Eugster, M. J., Schmid, M., Binder, H., & Schmidberger, M. (2013). Grid and cloud computing methods in biomedical research. *Methods of Information in Medicine, 52*(1), 62–64. PMID:23318694

European Commision. (2018, April 25). *EC - Digital Single Market*. Retrieved from Communication on enabling the digital transformation of health and care in the Digital Single Market; empowering citizens and building a healthier society: https://ec.europa.eu/digital-single-market/en/news/communication-enabling-digital-transformation-health-and-care-digital-single-market-empowering

European Commission. (2012). *General Data Protection Regulation: Proposal for a Regulation of the European Parliament and of the Council.* Retrieved Dec 9, 2016, from EC Justice, Data protection: ec.europa.eu/justice/data-protection/document/review2012/com_2012_11_en.pdf

European Commission. (2016). *Horizon 2020, Work Programme 2016 - 2017, 5.i. Information and Communication Technologies.* Retrieved Jan 8, 2017, from ec.europa.eu/research/participants/data/ref/h2020/wp/2016_2017/main/h2020-wp1617-leit-ict_en.pdf

European Commission. (2016). *Horizon 2020, Work Programme 2016 - 2017, 8. Health, demographic change and well-being.* Retrieved Jan 6, 2017, from ec.europa.eu/research/participants/data/ref/h2020/wp/2016_2017/main/h2020-wp1617-health_en.pdf

European Parliament and the Council of 12 July 2002. (2002). *Directive 2002/58/EC: Processing of personal data and the protection of privacy in the electronic communications sector.* Retrieved Jan 12, 2017, from eur-lex.europa.eu/eli/dir/2002/58/oj

European Parliament and the Council of 24 October 1995. (1995). *Directive 95/46/EC: Protection of individuals with regard to the processing of personal data and the free movement of such data.* Retrieved Jan 8, 2017, from data.europa.eu/eli/dir/1995/46/oj

European Parliament. (2000). *Charter of Fundamental Rights Of The European Union (2000/C 364/01).* Retrieved Jan 8, 2017, from Official Journal of the European Communities: www.europarl.europa.eu/charter/pdf/text_en.pdf

European Society of R. (2018). ESR paper on the proper use of mobile devices in radiology. *Insights Imaging, 9*(2), 247-251. doi:10.100713244-017-0589-7

European Union Agency for Network and Information Security. (2018). *Handbook on security of personal data processing*. Retrieved from https://www.enisa.europa.eu/publications/handbook-on-security-of-personal-data-processing

Evans, W. D. (2006). How social marketing works in health care. *British Medical Journal, 332*(7551), 1207–1210. PMID:16710002

Eysenbach, G. (2001). What is e-health? *Journal of Medical Internet Research, 3*(2), e20. doi:10.2196/jmir.3.2.e20 PMID:11720962

Eysenbach, G. (2003). The impact of the Internet on cancer outcomes. *CA: a Cancer Journal for Clinicians, 53*(6), 356–370. doi:10.3322/canjclin.53.6.356 PMID:15224975

Eyuboglu, E., & Schulz, P. J. (2016). Do health literacy and patient empowerment affect self-care behaviour? A survey study among Turkish patients with diabetes. *BMJ Open, 6*(3), e010186. doi:10.1136/bmjopen-2015-010186 PMID:26975936

Fagerberg, J., & Kurkinen, L. (n.d.). *mHealth and Home Monitoring.* Berg Insight. Gothenburg: M2M Research Series. *Berg Insight AB.*

Farella, E., Pieracci, A., Benini, L., Rocchi, L., & Acquaviva, A. (2008). Interfacing human and computer with wireless body area sensor networks: The WiMoCA solution. *Multimedia Tools and Applications, 38*(3), 337–363. doi:10.100711042-007-0189-5

Faridi, Z., Liberti, L., Shuval, K., Northrup, V., Ali, A., & Katz, D. L. (2008). 'Evaluating the impact of mobile telephone technology on type 2 diabetic patients' self management: The NICHE pilot study.'. *Journal of Evaluation in Clinical Practice, 14*(3), 465–469. doi:10.1111/j.1365-2753.2007.00881.x PMID:18373577

Felzen, M., Brokmann, J. C., Beckers, S. K., Czaplik, M., Hirsch, F., Tamm, M., ... Bergrath, S. (2017). Improved technical performance of a multifunctional prehospital telemedicine system between the research phase and the routine use phase - an observational study. *Journal of Telemedicine and Telecare, 23*(3), 402–409. doi:10.1177/1357633X16644115 PMID:27080747

Fenlon, D., & Foster, C. (2009). Self management support: a review of the evidence. Southampton, Macmillan Research Unit, University of Southampton.

Fidel, R. (2012). *Human Information Interaction: An Ecological Approach to Information Behavior.* Cambridge, MA: MIT Press. doi:10.7551/mitpress/9780262017008.001.0001

Field, A. S., Schmitt, F., & Vielh, P. (2017). IAC Standardized Reporting of Breast Fine-Needle Aspiration Biopsy Cytology. *Acta Cytologica, 61*(1), 3–6. doi:10.1159/000450880 PMID:27806362

Fife, E., & Pereira, F. (2011). Digital home health and mHealth: prospects and challenges for adoption in the U.S. FITCE 50th Congress (FITCE), 1-11.

Filho, F., Menezes, N., Filho, F., Soares, G., Solla, D. J. F., Argôlo, F. C., ... Lopes, R. D. (2018). Implementation of a Regional Network for ST-Segment–Elevation Myocardial Infarction (STEMI) Care and 30-Day Mortality in a Low- to Middle-Income City in Brazil: Findings From Salvador's STEMI Registry (RESISST). *Journal of the American Heart Association, 7*(14). doi:10.1161/jaha.118.008624 PMID:29980522

Finkelstein, J., Hripcsak, G., & Cabrera, M. (1998). Telematic system for monitoring of asthma severity in patients' homes. *Studies in Health Technology and Informatics, 52*(Pt 1), 272–276. PMID:10384460

Fiordelli, M., Diviani, N., & Schulz, P. J. (2013). Mapping mHealth research: a decade of evolution. *J Med Internet Res, 15*(5). doi:10.2196/jmir.2430

Fogg, B. J. (2003). *Persuasive Technology: Using Computers to Change What We Think and Do*. New York, NY: Morgan Kaufmann. doi:10.1016/B978-155860643-2/50011-1

Fontelo, P., Faustorilla, J., Gavino, A., & Marcelo, A. (2012). Digital pathology - implementation challenges in low-resource countries. *Analytical Cellular Pathology (Amsterdam)*, *35*(1), 31–36. doi:10.1155/2012/125695 PMID:22233702

Forster, A., Smith, J., & Young, J. (2004). *Information provision for stroke patients and their caregivers (Cochrane Review)*. Chichester, UK: John Wiley & Sons.

Fourie, I. (2008). Information needs and information behaviour of patients and their family members in a cancer palliative care setting: an exploratory study of an existential context from different perspectives. *Information Research, 13*(4).

Fowsantear, W., Argo, E., Pattinson, C., & Cash, P. (2013). Comparative proteomics of Helicobacter species: The discrimination of gastric and enterohepatic Helicobacter species. *Journal of Proteomics*. doi:10.1016/j.jprot.2013.07.016 PMID:23899588

Franschman, G., Peerdeman, S. M., Greuters, S., Vieveen, J., Brinkman, A. C. M., Christiaans, H. M. T., ... Boer, C. (2009). Prehospital endotracheal intubation in patients with severe traumatic brain injury: Guidelines versus reality. *Resuscitation*, *80*(10), 1147–1151. doi:10.1016/j.resuscitation.2009.06.029 PMID:19632024

Fraser, H., Bailey, C., Sinha, C., Mehl, G., & Labrique, A. (2011). *Call to action on global eHealth evaluation: consensus statement of the WHO Global eHealth Evaluation Meeting, Bellagio, September 2011*. The Bellagio eHealth Evaluation Group.

Freshwater, E., & Crouch, R. (n.d.). Technology for trauma: testing the validity of a smartphone app for pre-hospital clinicians. *International Emergency Nursing, 23*(1), 32-37. doi:10.1016/j.ienj.2014.04.003

Friedman, J. (2014). Rhode Island Hospital launches country's first Google Glass study in emergency department. *R I Med J (2013)*, *97*(4), 47.

Friedman, C. P., & Wyatt, J. (2006). *Evaluation methods in medical informatics* (2nd ed.). New York: Springer.

Friis, L. S., Elverdam, B., & Schmidt, K. G. (2003). The patient's perspective. *Supportive Care in Cancer*, *11*(3), 162–170. PMID:12618926

Frost & Sullivan. (2012). *U.S. Hospital Health Data Analytics Market: Growing EHR Adoption Fuels A New Era in Analytics*. Retrieved 11 18, 2013, from Frost & Sullivan: http://www.frost.com/c/10046/sublib/display-report.do?id=NA03-01-00-00-00

FTC. (2013). *Mobile Privacy Disclosures. Building Trust Through Transparency*. Federal Trade Commission.

FTC. (2015). *Privacy and Security*. Retrieved 5 15, 2015, from Federal trade Commission. Protecting America's Consumers: http://business.ftc.gov/privacy-and-security

Fulciniti, F., Yanoh, K., Karakitsos, P., Watanabe, J., Di Lorito, A., Margari, N., ... Hirai, Y. (2018). The Yokohama system for reporting directly sampled endometrial cytology: The quest to develop a standardized terminology. *Diagnostic Cytopathology*, *46*(5), 400–412. doi:10.1002/dc.23916 PMID:29479846

Fu, M. R., LeMone, P., & McDaniel, R. (2004). An integrated approach to an analysis of symptom management in patients with cancer. *Oncology Nursing Forum*, *31*(1), 65–70. doi:10.1188/04.ONF.65-70 PMID:14722589

Fung, K. M., Hassell, L. A., Talbert, M. L., Wiechmann, A. F., Chaser, B. E., & Ramey, J. (2012). Whole slide images and digital media in pathology education, testing, and practice: The Oklahoma experience. *Analytical Cellular Pathology (Amsterdam)*, *35*(1), 37–40. doi:10.1155/2012/103857 PMID:21965282

Funnell, M. M., & Anderson, R. M. (2000). The problem with compliance in diabetes. *Journal of the American Medical Association*, *284*(13), 1709. doi:10.1001/jama.284.13.1709-JMS1004-6-1 PMID:11015809

Funnell, M. M., & Anderson, R. M. (2003). Patient empowerment: A look back, a look ahead. *The Diabetes Educator*, *29*(3), 454–464. doi:10.1177/014572170302900310 PMID:12854337

Gaba, D. M. (2007). The future vision of simulation in healthcare. *Simulation in Healthcare*, *2*(2), 126–135. doi:10.1097/01.SIH.0000258411.38212.32 PMID:19088617

Gagnon, M., Inhorn, S., Hancock, J., Keller, B., Carpenter, D., Merlin, T., ... Whalen, R. (2004). Comparison of cytology proficiency testing: Glass slides vs. virtual slides. *Acta Cytologica*, *48*(6), 788–794. doi:10.1159/000326447 PMID:15581163

Gao, T., Massey, T., Selvo, L., Crawford, D., Chen, B., Lorincz, K., ... Welsh, M. (2007). The advanced health and disaster AID network: A light-weight wireless medical system for triage. *IEEE Transactions on Biomedical Circuits and Systems*, *1*(3), 203–216. doi:10.1109/TBCAS.2007.910901 PMID:23852414

Garrison, J. A., Schardt, C., & Kochi, J. K. (2000). Web-based distance continuing education: A new way of thinking for students and instructors. *Bulletin of the Medical Library Association*, *88*(3), 211–217. PMID:10928706

Gens, F. (2011). *Top 10 Predictions. IDC Predictions 2012: Competing for 2020.* IDC. Retrieved December 5, 2013, from IDC: http://cdn.idc.com/research/Predictions12/Main/downloads/IDCTOP10Predictions2012.pdf

Georga, E. I., Protopappas, V. C., Bellos, C. V., & Fotiadis, D. I. (2014). Wearable systems and mobile applications for diabetes disease management. *Health and Technology*, *4*(2), 101–112. doi:10.100712553-014-0082-y

Georgiou, A., & Westbrook, J. I. (2006). Computerised Order Entry Systems and Pathology Services - A Synthesis of the Evidence. *The Clinical Biochemist. Reviews / Australian Association of Clinical Biochemists*, *27*(2), 79–87. PMID:17077878

Gerber, D. E., Laccetti, A. L., Chen, B., Yan, J., Cai, J., Gates, S., ... Lee, S. J. C. (2014). Predictors and intensity of online access to electronic medical records among patients with cancer. *Journal of Oncology Practice / American Society of Clinical Oncology*, *10*(5), e307–e312. doi:10.1200/JOP.2013.001347 PMID:25006222

Germann, J. N., Kirschenbaum, D. S., & Rich, B. H. (2007). Child and Parental Self-Monitoring as Determinants of Success in the Treatment of Morbid Obesity in Low-Income Minority Children. *Journal of Pediatric Psychology*, *32*(1), 111–121. doi:10.1093/jpepsy/jsl007 PMID:16775083

Gethin, G., & Cowman, S. (2005). Wound measurement comparing the use of acetate tracings and Visitrak digital planimetry. *Journal of Clinical Nursing*, *15*(4), 422–427. doi:10.1111/j.1365-2702.2006.01364.x PMID:16553755

Ghaznavi, F., Evans, A., Madabhushi, A., & Feldman, M. (2013). Digital imaging in pathology: Whole-slide imaging and beyond. *Annual Review of Pathology*, *8*(1), 331–359. doi:10.1146/annurev-pathol-011811-120902 PMID:23157334

Ghorai, K., Akter, S., Khatun, F., & Ray, P. (2014). mHealth for Smoking Cessation Programs: A Systematic Review. *Journal of Personalized Medicine*, *4*(3), 412–423. doi:10.3390/jpm4030412 PMID:25563359

Gibson, P. G., Powell, H., & Coughlan, J. (2004). *Limited (information only) patient education programs for adults with asthma (Cochrane Review).* Chichester, UK: John Wiley & Sons.

Giovagnoli, M. R., Cenci, M., Olla, S. V., & Vecchione, A. (2002). Cervical false negative cases detected by neural network-based technology. Critical review of cytologic errors. *Acta Cytologica*, *46*(6), 1105–1109. doi:10.1159/000327115 PMID:12462090

Girault, A., Ferrua, M., Lalloué, B., Sicotte, C., Fourcade, A., Yatim, F., ... Minvielle, E. (2015). Internet-based technologies to improve cancer care coordination: Current use and attitudes among cancer patients. *European Journal of Cancer, 51*(4), 551–557. doi:10.1016/j.ejca.2014.12.001 PMID:25661828

Glanz, K., Lewis, F. M., & Rimer, B. K. (Eds.). (1997). *Health Behavior and Health Education.* San Francisco, CA: Jossey-Bass Publishers.

Glaser, J. (2011). Cloud computing can simplify HIT infrastructure management. *Healthcare Financial Management, 65*(8), 52–55. PMID:21866720

Glasgow, N. J., Ponsonby, A. L., & Yates, R. (2003). Proactive asthma care in childhood: General practice based randomised controlled trial. *BMJ (Clinical Research Ed.), 327*(7416), 659. doi:10.1136/bmj.327.7416.659 PMID:14500440

Glasgow, R. E., Peeples, M., & Skovlund, S. E. (2008). Where is the patient in diabetes performance measures? *Diabetes Care, 31*(5), 1046–1050. doi:10.2337/dc07-1845 PMID:18445728

GlobalData. (2012). *Snapshot: The US cloud computing market for medical imaging.* Retrieved 22/08/2013, from http://www.medicaldevice-network.com/features/featuresnapshot-the-us-cloud-computing-market-for-medical-imaging

Glynn, L. G., Hayes, P. S., Casey, M., Glynn, F., Alvarez-Iglesias, A., Newell, J., ... Murphy, A. W. (2013). SMART MOVE - a smartphone-based intervention to promote physical activity in primary care: Study protocol for a randomized controlled trial. *Trials, 14*(1), 157. doi:10.1186/1745-6215-14-157 PMID:23714362

Goacher, E., Randell, R., Williams, B., & Treanor, D. (2017). The Diagnostic Concordance of Whole Slide Imaging and Light Microscopy: A Systematic Review. *Archives of Pathology & Laboratory Medicine, 141*(1), 151–161. doi:10.5858/arpa.2016-0025-RA PMID:27399211

Goncalves, J., Cordeiro, L., Batista, P., & Monteiro, E. (2012). LiveCity: A Secure Live Video-to-Video Interactive City Infrastructure. In L. Iliadis, I. Maglogiannis, H. Papadopoulos, K. Karatzas, & S. Sioutas (Eds.), *Artificial Intelligence Applications and Innovations* (Vol. 382, pp. 260–267). Springer Berlin Heidelberg. doi:10.1007/978-3-642-33412-2_27

Goode, A. S. M. (2008). *A vendor-neutral library and viewer for wholeslide images* (Vol. Tech Rep CMU-CS-08-136.). Pittsburgh, PA: School of Computer Science, Carnegie Mellon University.

Gorini, A., Masiero, M., & Pravettoni, G. (2016). Patient decision aids for prevention and treatment of cancer diseases: Are they really personalised tools? *European Journal of Cancer Care, 25*(6), 936–960. doi:10.1111/ecc.12451 PMID:26856816

Gottrup, F., Holstein, P., Jorgensen, B., Lohmann, M., & Karlsmar, T. (2001). A new concept of a multidisciplinary wound healing center and a national expert function of wound healing. *Archives of Surgery, 136*(7), 765–772. doi:10.1001/archsurg.136.7.765 PMID:11448387

Grand View Research. (2017). *mHealth App Market By Type (Fitness, Lifestyle Management, Nutrition & Diet, Women's Health, Healthcare Providers, Disease Management) And Segment Forecasts, 2018 - 2025.* Grand View Research.

Grasso, F. (1998). Exciting avocados and dull pears: combining behavioral and argumentative theory for producing effective advice. In *Proceedings of the 20th Annual Meeting of the Cognitive Science Society* (pp. 436-41). Hillsdale, NJ: Erlbaum Associates.

Greenbaum, D., & Gerstein, M. (2011). The role of cloud computing in managing the deluge of potentially private genetic data. *The American Journal of Bioethics, 11*(11), 39–41. doi:10.1080/15265161.2011.608242 PMID:22047125

Greenfield, McManus, & Wilson. (2007). Self care – has DIY gone too far? *The British Journal of General Practice, 57*, 907–908. PMID:17132376

Grilli, R., Ramsay, C., & Minozzi, S. (2004). *Mass media interventions: effects on health services utilisation (Cochrane Review)*. Chichester, UK: John Wiley & Sons.

Grunerbl A. (2014). Smartphone Based Recognition of States and State Changes in Bipolar Disorder Patients. *IEEE Journal of Biomedical and Health Informatics, 19*(1), 140-148.

GSMA & PwC. (2012). *Touching lives through mobile health - Assessment of the global market opportunity*. PriceWaterhouseCoopers.

Gupta, S., Chang, P., Anyigbo, N., & Sabharwal, A. (2011). mobileSpiro: accurate mobile spirometry for self-management of asthma. *Proceedings of the First ACM Workshop on Mobile Systems, Applications, and Services for Healthcare.*

Guru, M., & Ragib, H., & Khan, R. (2017). Towards Non-Intrusive Continuous Healthcare Monitoring with the smart Hospital growth. *Proceedings of 14th IEEE Annual Consumer Communications & Networking Conference (CCNC).*

Gustafson, D. H., & Wyatt, J. C. (2004). Evaluation of ehealth systems and services. *BMJ (Clinical Research Ed.), 328*(7449), 1150. doi:10.1136/bmj.328.7449.1150 PMID:15142895

Gutman, D. A., Cobb, J., Somanna, D., Park, Y., Wang, F., Kurc, T., ... Cooper, L. A. (2013). Cancer Digital Slide Archive: An informatics resource to support integrated in silico analysis of TCGA pathology data. *Journal of the American Medical Informatics Association, 20*(6), 1091–1098. doi:10.1136/amiajnl-2012-001469 PMID:23893318

Guzik, P., & Malik, M. (2016). ECG by mobile technologies. *Journal of Electrocardiology, 49*(6), 894–901. doi:10.1016/j.jelectrocard.2016.07.030 PMID:27524474

Haapala, I., Barengo, N. C., Biggs, S., Surakka, L., & Manninen, P. (2009). Weight loss by mobile phone: A 1-year effectiveness study. *Public Health Nutrition, 12*(12), 2382–2391. doi:10.1017/S1368980009005230 PMID:19323865

Haghpanah, S., Bogie, K., Wang, X., Banks, P. G., & Ho, C. H. (2006). Reliability of electronic versus manual wound measurement techniques. *Archives of Physical Medicine and Rehabilitation, 87*(10), 1396–1402. doi:10.1016/j.apmr.2006.06.014 PMID:17023252

Halligan, B. D., Geiger, J. F., Vallejos, A. K., Greene, A. S., & Twigger, S. N. (2009). Low cost, scalable proteomics data analysis using Amazon's cloud computing services and open source search algorithms. *Journal of Proteome Research, 8*(6), 3148–3153. doi:10.1021/pr800970z PMID:19358578

Hall, K. D., & Jordan, P. N. (2008). Modeling weight-loss maintenance to help prevent body weight regain. *The American Journal of Clinical Nutrition, 88*(6), 1495–1503. doi:10.3945/ajcn.2008.26333 PMID:19064508

Han, J., & Kamber, M. (Eds.). (2006). *Data mining: Concepts and techniques*. Morgan Kaufmann.

Hartman, D. J. (2016). Mobile Technology for the Practice of Pathology. *Advances in Anatomic Pathology, 23*(2), 118–124. doi:10.1097/PAP.0000000000000093 PMID:26849818

Hassan, M. M., Hossain, M. S., Alamri, A., Hossain, M. A., Al-Qurishi, M., Aldukhayyil, Y., & Ahmed, D. T. (2012). *A cloud-based serious games framework for obesity*. Paper presented at the Proceedings of the 1st ACM multimedia international workshop on Cloud-based multimedia applications and services for e-health, Nara, Japan.

Hawkins, R. P., Kreuter, M., Resnicow, K., Fishbein, M., & Dijkstra, A. (2008). Understanding tailoring in communicating about health. *Health Education Research, 23*(3), 454–466. doi:10.1093/her/cyn004 PMID:18349033

Haymart, M. R., Cayo, M., & Chen, H. (2009). Papillary thyroid microcarcinomas: Big decisions for a small tumor. *Annals of Surgical Oncology*, *16*(11), 3132–3139. doi:10.124510434-009-0647-6 PMID:19653044

Health Level Seven International. (2018). *Homepage*. Retrieved from http://www.hl7.org/

Health on the Move. (2017). *Health on the move: Exploring the ethical, social, and political underpinnings of portable devices for healthcare and lifestyle*. Retrieved Feb 3, 2017, from http://cordis.europa.eu/project/rcn/187888_en.html

Heart rate precautions. (2018). Retrieved from https://www.webmd.com/heart-disease/what-to-do-heart-races#1

Heart rate statistics. (2015). Retrieved from http://www.statcan.gc.ca/pub/82-626-x/2013001/t004-eng.html

HEARTEN. (2015). *A co-operative mHEALTH environment targeting adherence and management of patients suffering from Heart Failure Table of Content*. Retrieved from www.hearten.eu

Heinrich, C., & Kuiper, R. A. (2012). Using handheld devices to promote medication adherence in chronic illness. *The Journal for Nurse Practitioners*, *8*(4), 288–293. doi:10.1016/j.nurpra.2011.10.010

Help4Mood. (2011). *A Computational Distributed System to Support the Treatment of Patients with Major Depression*. Retrieved from help4mood.info

Hethcote, H. W. (2000). The mathematics of infectious diseases. *SIAM Review*, *42*(4), 599–653. doi:10.1137/S0036144500371907

Hewitt, M., Greenfield, S., & Stovall, E. (Eds.). (2005). *From cancer patient to cancer survivor: lost in transition*. National Academies Press.

Hibbard, J. H., & Cunningham, P. J. (2008). How engaged are consumers in their health and health care, and why does it matter? *Research Brief*, (8), 1–9.

Hibbard, J. H., & Mahoney, E. (2010). Toward a theory of patient and consumer activation. *Patient Education and Counseling*, *78*(3), 377–381. doi:10.1016/j.pec.2009.12.015 PMID:20188505

Hickey, T., Dean, K., & Holstein, B. (1986). Emerging trends in gerontology and geriatrics: Implications for the self-care of the elderly. *Social Science & Medicine*, *23*(12), 1363–1369. doi:10.1016/0277-9536(86)90299-6 PMID:3823991

Higgins, J. P., & Green, S. (2006). Cohrane handbook for systematic reviews of interventions 4.2.6. In *The Cochrane Library, Issue 4*. Chichester, UK: JohnWiley & Sons, Ltd.

Hill, J. O., Wyatt, H. R., Reed, G. W., & Peters, J. C. (2003). Obesity and the Environment: Where Do We Go from Here? *Science*, *299*(5608), 853–855. doi:10.1126cience.1079857 PMID:12574618

HIMSS. (2014). *3rd Annual HIMSS Analytics Mobile Survey*. HIMSS Analytics.

HIMSS. (2015). *Healtcare Information and Management Systems Society*. Retrieved 5 13, 2015, from HIMSS transforming health through IT: http://www.himss.org/

Hipp, J. D., Lucas, D. R., Emmert-Buck, M. R., Compton, C. C., & Balis, U. J. (2011). Digital slide repositories for publications: Lessons learned from the microarray community. *The American Journal of Surgical Pathology*, *35*(6), 783–786. doi:10.1097/PAS.0b013e31821946b6 PMID:21552111

Hirsch, D., Robenshtok, E., Bachar, G., Braslavsky, D., & Benbassat, C. (2015). The Implementation of the Bethesda System for Reporting Thyroid Cytopathology Improves Malignancy Detection Despite Lower Rate of Thyroidectomy in Indeterminate Nodules. *World Journal of Surgery*, *39*(8), 1959–1965. doi:10.100700268-015-3032-6 PMID:25809059

Hirschorn, D. S., Krupinski, E. A., & Flynn, M. J. (2014). PACS displays: How to select the right display technology. *Journal of the American College of Radiology*, *11*(12), 1270–1276. doi:10.1016/j.jacr.2014.09.016 PMID:25467904

HL7 International (2015). *HL7 CDA ® Release 2 Implementation Guide: Reporting to Public Health Cancer Registries from Ambulatory Healthcare Providers*. Release 1, DSTU Release 1.1 – US Realm.

HL7 International. (2018). *FHIR Release 3*. Retrieved from http://www.hl7.org/fhir/

Hoffman-Goetz, L., & Donelle, L. (2007). Chat room computer-mediated support on health issues for aboriginal women. *Health Care for Women International*, *28*(4), 397–418. doi:10.1080/07399330601180057 PMID:17454185

Holmstrom, I., & Roing, M. (2010). The relation between patient-centredness and patient empowerment: A discussion on concepts. *Patient Education and Counseling*, *79*(2), 167–172. doi:10.1016/j.pec.2009.08.008 PMID:19748203

Howie, J. G. R., Heaney, D., & Maxwell, M. (2004). Quality, core values and the general practice consultation: Issues of definition, measurement and delivery. *Family Practice*, *21*(4), 458–468. doi:10.1093/fampra/cmh419 PMID:15249538

Huang, Y. N., Peng, X. C., Ma, S., Yu, H., Jin, Y. B., Zheng, J., & Fu, G. H. (2018). Development of Whole Slide Imaging on Smartphones and Evaluation With ThinPrep Cytology Test Samples: Follow-Up Study. *JMIR mHealth and uHealth*, *6*(4), e82. doi:10.2196/mhealth.9518 PMID:29618454

Hubbard, G., Kidd, L., Donaghy, E., MacDonald, C., Simpson, M., Haig, A., & Walker, S. (2005). *Phase 1 Report: Literature Review: Involvement of people affected by cancer in research, policy and planning and practice*. University of Stirling.

Hubert, G., Müller-Barna, P., & Audebert, H. (2014). Recent advances in TeleStroke: A systematic review on applications in prehospital management and Stroke Unit treatment or TeleStroke networking in developing countries. *International Journal of Stroke*, *9*(8), 968–973. doi:10.1111/ijs.12394 PMID:25381687

Hull, P., Emerson, S. J., Quirk, E. M., Canedo, R. J., Jones, L. J., Vylegzhanina, V., ... Husaini, A. B. (2017). A Smartphone App for Families With Preschool-Aged Children in a Public Nutrition Program: Prototype Development and Beta-Testing. *JMIR mHealth and uHealth*, *5*(8), e102. doi:10.2196/mhealth.7477 PMID:28768611

Humphrey, N. (2002). *The mind made flesh*. Oxford, UK: Oxford University Press.

Hurling, R., Catt, M., De Boni, M., Fairley, B. W., Hurst, T., Murray, P., ... Sodhi, J. S. (2007). Using Internet and Mobile Phone Technology to Deliver an Automated Physical Activity Program: Randomized Controlled Trial. *Journal of Medical Internet Research*, *9*(2), e7. doi:10.2196/jmir.9.2.e7 PMID:17478409

Iconomou, G., Viha, A., Koutras, A., Vagenakis, A. G., & Kalofonos, H. P. (2002). Information needs and awareness of diagnosis in patients with cancer receiving chemotherapy: A report from Greece. *Palliative Medicine*, *16*(4), 315–321. doi:10.1191/0269216302pm574oa PMID:12132544

ICT4Depression. (2015). *User-friendly ICT Tools to Enhance Self-Management and Effective*. Retrieved from www.ICT4DEPRESSION.eu

iManageCancer. (2015). *Empowering patients and strengthening self-management in cancer diseases*. Retrieved Jan 10, 2017, from imanagecancer.eu

IMS. (2013). *Patient Apps for Improved Healthcare: From Novelty to Mainstream*. IMS Institute for Healthcare Informatics.

Integrating the Healthcare Enterprise. (2018). *Homepage*. Retrieved from http://www.ihe.net/

International Agency for Research on Cancer. (2015). *World cancer report 2014*. Retrieved from https://www.iarc.fr/en/publications/pdfs-online/wcr/2003/WorldCancerReport.pdf

International Diabetes Federation. (2006). *Diabetes Atlas* (3rd ed.). Brussels: Author.

International Organization for Standardization. (2012). *ISO 15189:2012. Medical laboratories – Requirements for quality and competence*. Geneva: International Organization for Standardization.

International Organization for Standardization. (2014). *ISO/IEC 25000:2014, Systems and software engineering -- Systems and software Quality Requirements and Evaluation (SQuaRE) -- Guide to SQuaRE. ISO/ IEC JTC 1/ SC 7, Software and systems engineering*. Retrieved from https://www.iso.org/standard/64764.html

International Telecommunication Union (ITU). (2014). *The World in 2014. ICT facts and Figures*. Geneva: International Telecommunication Union.

INTERSTRESS. (2010). *Interreality in the Management and Treatment of Stress-Related Disorders*. Retrieved from www.interstress.eu

IQVIA Institute for Human and Data Science. (2017). *The Growing Value of Digital Health: Evidence and Impact on Human Health and the Healthcare System*. Institute Report.

ISA. (n.d.). *eHealth European Interoperability Framework*. Interoperability Solutions for European Pyblic Administration.

Ishikawa, H., Hashimoto, H., & Kiuchi, T. (2013). The evolving concept of 'patient-centeredness' in patient-physician communication research. *Social Science & Medicine*, *96*, 147–153. doi:10.1016/j.socscimed.2013.07.026 PMID:24034962

iSIM Project. (2015). Retrieved from http://www.cs.uoregon.edu/research/mds/iSIM/

ITU Statistics. (2018). Retrieved from Global and regional ICT data (2005-2017): www.itu.int/en/ITU-D/Statistics/Pages/stat/default.aspx

Izadi-Mood, N., Sarmadi, S., & Sanii, S. (2013). Quality control in cervicovaginal cytology by cytohistological correlation. *Cytopathology*, *24*(1), 33–38. doi:10.1111/j.1365-2303.2011.00926.x PMID:21929578

Jain, T., Sibley, A., Stryhn, H., & Hubloue, I. (2018). Comparison of Unmanned Aerial Vehicle Technology Versus Standard Practice in Identification of Hazards at a Mass Casualty Incident Scenario by Primary Care Paramedic Students. *Disaster Medicine and Public Health Preparedness*, *1-4*. doi:10.1017/dmp.2017.129 PMID:29382398

Janda, M., Loescher, L. J., Banan, P., Horsham, C., & Soyer, H. P. (2014). Lesion selection by melanoma high-risk consumers during skin self-examination using mobile teledermoscopy. *JAMA Dermatology*, *150*(6), 656–658. doi:10.1001/jamadermatol.2013.7743 PMID:24522284

Jantien Vrijmoet-Wiersma, C. M., van Klink, J. M., Kolk, A. M., Koopman, H. M., Ball, L. M., & Maarten Egeler, R. (2008). Assessment of parental psychological stress in pediatric cancer: A review. *Journal of Pediatric Psychology*, *33*(7), 694–706. doi:10.1093/jpepsy/jsn007 PMID:18287109

Jantunen, I., Laine, H., Huuskonen, P., Trossen, D., & Ermolov, V. (2008). Smart sensor architecture for mobile-terminal-centric ambient intelligence. *Sensors and Actuators*, *142*(1), 352–360. doi:10.1016/j.sna.2007.04.014

Jason, W. P., Benny, P. L. L., Oliver, W., Morris, S., Nick, P., Ara, D., Chris, T., & Guang, Z.Y. (2004). Ubiquitous monitoring environment for wearable and implantable sensors (UbiMon). *UbiComp'04, The 6th International Conference on Ubiquitous Computing, Poster Proc.*, 1-2.

Jemal, A., Bray, F., Center, M. M., Ferlay, J., Ward, E., & Forman, D. (2011). Global cancer statistics. *CA: a Cancer Journal for Clinicians*, *61*(2), 69–90. doi:10.3322/caac.20107 PMID:21296855

Jerant, A., von Frederichs-Fitzwater, M., & Moore, M. (2005). Patient's perceived barriers to active self-management of chronic conditions. *Patient Education and Counseling*, *57*(3), 300–307. doi:10.1016/j.pec.2004.08.004 PMID:15893212

Jialdasani, R., Desai, S., Gupta, M., Kothari, A., Deshpande, R., Shet, T., ... Chinoy, R. (2006). An analysis of 46 static telecytology cases over a period of two years. *Journal of Telemedicine and Telecare*, *12*(6), 311–314. doi:10.1258/135763306778558132 PMID:17022840

Jiang, S., Cao, Y., Iyengar, S., Kuryloski, P., Jafari, R., Xue, Y., ... Wicker, S. (2008). CareNet: an integrated wireless sensor networking environment for remote healthcare. *International Conference on Body Area Networks*, *9*, 1-3.

Jin, Z., Oresko, J., Huang, S., & Cheng, A. C. (2009). HeartToGo: a personalized medicine technology for cardiovascular disease prevention and detection. *Proceedings of IEEE/NIH LiSSA*, 80-83.

Johnsen, E., & Bolle, S. R. (2008). To see or not to see--better dispatcher-assisted CPR with video-calls? A qualitative study based on simulated trials. *Resuscitation*, *78*(3), 320–326. doi:10.1016/j.resuscitation.2008.04.024 PMID:18583015

Johnson, J. D., Andrews, J. E., & Allard, S. (2001). A model for understanding and affecting cancer genetics information seeking. *Library & Information Science Research*, *23*(4), 335–349. doi:10.1016/S0740-8188(01)00094-9

Johnson, J. D., & Case, D. O. (2012). *Health Information Seeking*. New York, NY: Peter Lang Publishing.

Johnson, P. T., Zimmerman, S. L., Heath, D., Eng, J., Horton, K. M., Scott, W. W., & Fishman, E. K. (2012). The iPad as a mobile device for CT display and interpretation: Diagnostic accuracy for identification of pulmonary embolism. *Emergency Radiology*, *19*(4), 323–327. doi:10.100710140-012-1037-0 PMID:22450843

Jones, C., & Shao, B. (2011). *The Net Generation and Digital Natives. Implications for Higher Education*. The Open University.

Jones, P., & Melei, A. I. (1993). Health is empowerment. *Advances in Nursing Science*, *15*(3), 1–14. doi:10.1097/00012272-199303000-00003 PMID:8434899

Jovanov, E. (2005). Wireless technology and system integration in body area networks for m-health applications. *Proceedings of the IEEE Engineering in Medicine and Biology, 27th Annual International Conference*, *7*, 7158-7160.

Kafalı, Ö. (2013). COMMODITY12: A smart e-health environment for diabetes management. *Journal of Ambient Intelligence and Smart Environments*, *5*, 479–502.

Karakitsos, P., Cochand-Priollet, B., Pouliakis, A., Guillausseau, P. J., & Ioakim-Liossi, A. (1999). Learning vector quantizer in the investigation of thyroid lesions. *Analytical and Quantitative Cytology and Histology*, *21*(3), 201–208. PMID:10560492

Karakitsos, P., Megalopoulou, T. M., Pouliakis, A., Tzivras, M., Archimandritis, A., & Kyroudes, A. (2004). Application of discriminant analysis and quantitative cytologic examination to gastric lesions. *Analytical and Quantitative Cytology and Histology*, *26*(6), 314–322. PMID:15678613

Karakitsos, P., Stergiou, E. B., Pouliakis, A., Tzivras, M., Archimandritis, A., Liossi, A. I., & Kyrkou, K. (1996). Potential of the back propagation neural network in the discrimination of benign from malignant gastric cells. *Analytical and Quantitative Cytology and Histology*, *18*(3), 245–250. PMID:8790840

Katehakis, D. G., Kondylakis, H., Koumakis, L., Kouroubali, A., & Marias, K. (2017). Integrated care solutions for the citizen: Personal health record functional models to support interoperability. *EJBI*, *13*(1), 41–56.

Katehakis, D. G., & Tsiknakis, M. (2006). *Electronic Health Record. Wiley Encyclopedia of Biomedical Engineering*. Hoboken, NJ: John Wiley & Sons, Inc.

Keeling, M. J., & Rohani, P. (2008). *Modeling Infectious Diseases in Humans and Animals*. Princeton University Press.

Keller, P. (2006). Regulatory Focus and Efficacy of Health Messages. *The Journal of Consumer Research*, *33*(June), 109–114. doi:10.1086/504141

Kelsey, M. M., Zaepfel, A., Bjornstad, P., & Nadeau, K. J. (2014). Age-Related Consequences of Childhood Obesity. *Gerontology*, *60*(3), 222–228. doi:10.1159/000356023 PMID:24434909

Kempe, D., Kleinberg, J. M., & Tardos, É. (2003). *Maximizing the spread of influence through a social network*. SIGKDD.

Kennedy, A., Robinson, A., Hann, M., Thompson, D., & Wilkin, D. (2003). A cluster-randomised controlled trial of a patient-centred guidebook for patients with ulcerative colitis: Effect on knowledge, anxiety and quality of life. *Health & Social Care in the Community*, *11*(1), 64–72. doi:10.1046/j.1365-2524.2003.00399.x PMID:14629234

Kephart, J. O., & White, S. R. (1993). Measuring and modeling computer virus prevalence. *IEEE Computer Society Symposium on Research in Security and Privacy*, 2-15. 10.1109/RISP.1993.287647

Kerem, Y., Eastvold, J. S., Faragoi, D., Strasburger, D., Motzny, S. E., & Kulstad, E. B. (2014). The role of prehospital electrocardiograms in the recognition of ST-segment elevation myocardial infarctions and reperfusion times. *The Journal of Emergency Medicine*, *46*(2), 202–207. doi:10.1016/j.jemermed.2013.08.084 PMID:24268634

Kermack, W. O., & McKendrick, A. G. (1927). A contribution to the Mathematical Theory of Epidemics. *Proceedings of the Royal Society of London. Series A, Containing Papers of a Mathematical and Physical Character*, *115*(772), 700–711. doi:10.1098/rspa.1927.0118

Kerr, M. E. (1988). *Family evaluation: an approach based on Bowen theory*. New York: Norton.

Kessel, K. A., Vogel, M. M., Kessel, C., Bier, H., Biedermann, T., Friess, H., ... Combs, S. E. (2017). Mobile health in oncology: A patient survey about app-assisted cancer care. *JMIR mHealth and uHealth*, *5*(6), e81. doi:10.2196/mhealth.7689 PMID:28615159

Khaylis, A., Yiaslas, T., Bergstrom, J., & Gore-Felton, C. (2010). A Review of Efficacious Technology-Based Weight-Loss Interventions: Five Key Components. *Telemedicine Journal and e-Health*, *16*(9), 931–938. doi:10.1089/tmj.2010.0065 PMID:21091286

Khurana, K. K. (2012). Telecytology and its evolving role in cytopathology. *Diagnostic Cytopathology*, *40*(6), 498–502. doi:10.1002/dc.22822 PMID:22619124

King, A. C., Ahn, D. K., Oliveira, B. M., Atienza, A. A., Castro, C. M., & Gardner, C. D. (2008). Promoting Physical Activity Through Hand-Held Computer Technology. *American Journal of Preventive Medicine*, *34*(2), 138–142. doi:10.1016/j.amepre.2007.09.025 PMID:18201644

Kirschenbaum, D. S., Germann, J. N., & Rich, B. H. (2005). Treatment of morbid obesity in low-income adolescents: Effects of parental self-monitoring. *Obesity Research*, *13*(9), 1527–1529. doi:10.1038/oby.2005.187 PMID:16222054

Kiselev, A. R., Gridnev, V. I., Shvartz, V. A., Posnenkova, O. M., & Dovgalevsky, P. Y. (2012). Active ambulatory care management supported by short message services and mobile phone technology in patients with arterial hypertension. *Journal of the American Society of Hypertension*, *6*(5), 346–355. doi:10.1016/j.jash.2012.08.001 PMID:22995803

Klack, L., Ziefle, M., Wilkowska, W., & Kluge, J. (2013). Telemedical versus conventional heart patient monitoring: A survey study with German physicians. *International Journal of Technology Assessment in Health Care*, *29*(4), 378–383. doi:10.1017/S026646231300041X PMID:24290330

Klasnja, P., Hartzler, A., Powell, C., Phan, G., & Pratt, W. (2010). Health weaver mobile: Designing a mobile tool for managing personal health information during cancer care. *AMIA ... Annual Symposium Proceedings - AMIA Symposium. AMIA Symposium*, *2010*, 392–396. PMID:21347007

Kleber, C., Giesecke, M., Tsokos, M., Haas, N., Schaser, K., Stefan, P., & Buschmann, C. (2012). Overall Distribution of Trauma-related Deaths in Berlin 2010: Advancement or Stagnation of German Trauma Management? *World Journal of Surgery*, *36*(9), 2125–2130. doi:10.100700268-012-1650-9 PMID:22610265

Koch, T., Jenkin, P., & Kralik, D. (2004). Chronic illness self management: Locating the 'self'. *Journal of Advanced Nursing*, *48*(5), 484–492. doi:10.1111/j.1365-2648.2004.03237.x PMID:15533086

Kolbe, J. (2002). The influence of socioeconomic and psychological factors on patient adherence to self management strategies: Lessons learned in asthma. *Disease Management & Health Outcomes*, *10*(9), 551–570. doi:10.2165/00115677-200210090-00004

Kondoh, H., Teramoto, K., Kawai, T., Mochida, M., & Nishimura, M. (2013). Development of the regional EPR and PACS sharing system on the infrastructure of cloud computing technology controlled by patient identifier cross reference manager. *Studies in Health Technology and Informatics*, *192*, 1073. PMID:23920847

Kondoh, H., Teramoto, K., Kawai, T., Mochida, M., & Nishimura, M. (2013). Development of the Regional EPR and PACS Sharing System on the Infrastructure of Cloud Computing Technology Controlled by Patient Identifier Cross Reference Manager. *Studies in Health Technology and Informatics*, *192*, 1073. PMID:23920847

Kondylakis, H., Bucur, A., Dong, F., Renzi, C., Manfrinati, A., Graf, N., . . . Kiefer, S. (2017a). iManageCancer: Developing a Platform for Empowering Patients and Strengthening Self-Management in Cancer Diseases. *Computer-Based Medical Systems (CBMS), IEEE 30th International Symposium*, 755-760.

Kondylakis, H., Spanakis, E. G., Sfakianakis, S., Sakkalis, V., Tsiknakis, M., Marias, K., . . . Dong, F. (2015). Digital patient: Personalized and translational data management through the MyHealthAvatar EU project. *Engineering in Medicine and Biology Society (EMBC), 2015 37th Annual International Conference of the IEEE,* 1397-1400.

Kondylakis, H., Koumakis, L., Hänold, S., Nwankwo, I., Forgó, N., Marias, K., & Graf, N. (2017b). Donor's support tool: Enabling informed secondary use of patient's biomaterial and personal data. *International Journal of Medical Informatics*, *97*, 282–292. doi:10.1016/j.ijmedinf.2016.10.019 PMID:27919386

Kondylakis, H., Koumakis, L., Tsiknakis, M., & Marias, K. (2018). Implementing a data management infrastructure for big healthcare data. *IEEE EMBS International Conference on Biomedical & Health Informatics (BHI)*, 361-364.

Konganti, K., Wang, G., Yang, E., & Cai, J. J. (2013). SBEToolbox: A Matlab Toolbox for Biological Network Analysis. *Evolutionary Bioinformatics Online*, *9*, 355–362. doi:10.4137/EBO.S12012 PMID:24027418

Konstantas, D., & Herzog, R. (2003). Continuous monitoring of vital constants for mobile users: the MobiHealth approach. *25th Annual International Conference of the IEEE EMBS*, 3728-3731.

Korber, A., Rietkoo, T. J., Grabbe, S., & Dissemond, J. (2006). Three-dimensional documentation of wound healing: First results of a new objective method for measurement. *Journal of the German Society of Dermatology*, *4*(10), 848–854. PMID:17010174

Kotronoulas, G., Kearney, N., Maguire, R., Harrow, A., Di Domenico, D., Croy, S., & MacGillivray, S. (2014). What is the value of the routine use of patient-reported outcome measures toward improvement of patient outcomes, processes of care, and health service outcomes in cancer care? A systematic review of controlled trials. *Journal of Clinical Oncology*, *32*(14), 1480–1501. doi:10.1200/JCO.2013.53.5948 PMID:24711559

Koumakis, L., Kondylakis, H., Katehakis, D. G., Iatraki, G., Argyropaidas, P., Hatzimina, M., & Marias, K. (2018). A content-aware analytics framework for open health data. Precision Medicine Powered by pHealth and Connected Health, 59–64.

Koumpouros, I. (2012). Information and Communication Technologies & Society. Athens: New Technologies Publications.

Koumpouros, Y. (2016). A Systematic Review on Existing Measures for the Subjective Assessment of Rehabilitation and Assistive Robot Devices. *Journal of Healthcare Engineering*, 10. doi:10.1155/2016/1048964

Koumpouros, Y., & Georgoulas, A. (2016). mHealth R&D activities in Europe. In E. A. Moumtzoglou (Ed.), M-Health Innovations for Patient-Centered Care (pp. 22-27). IGI Global.

Koumpouros, Y. (2014). Big Data in Healthcare. In A. Moumtzoglou & A. Kastania (Eds.), *Cloud Computing Applications for Quality Health care Delivery. A volume in the Advances in Healthcare Information Systems and Administration Book Series* (pp. 35–59). IGI Global.

Krebs, P., Prochaska, J. O., & Rossi, J. S. (2010). Defining what works in tailoring: A meta-analysis of computer-tailored interventions for health behavior change. *Preventive Medicine*, *51*(3–4), 214–221. doi:10.1016/j.ypmed.2010.06.004 PMID:20558196

Kreuter, M. W., Farrell, D., Olevich, L., & Brennan, L. (1999). *Tailoring health messages: Customizing communication with computer technology*. Mahwah, NJ: Erlbaum.

Kreuter, M. W., & Strecher, V. J. (1996). Do tailored behavior change messages enhance the effectiveness of health risk appraisals? Results from a randomized trial. *Health Education Research*, *11*(1), 97–105. doi:10.1093/her/11.1.97 PMID:10160231

Kreuter, M. W., & Wray, R. J. (2003). Tailored and Targeted Health Communication: Strategies for Enhancing Information Relevance. *American Journal of Health Behavior*, *27*(1), S227–S232. doi:10.5993/AJHB.27.1.s3.6 PMID:14672383

Krishnamurthy, S., Mathews, K., McClure, S., Murray, M., Gilcrease, M., Albarracin, C., ... Liang, K. (2013). Multi-Institutional Comparison of Whole Slide Digital Imaging and Optical Microscopy for Interpretation of Hematoxylin-Eosin-Stained Breast Tissue Sections. *Archives of Pathology & Laboratory Medicine*, *137*(12), 1733–1739. doi:10.5858/arpa.2012-0437-OA PMID:23947655

Krishna, S., Boren, S. A., & Balas, E. A. (2009). Healthcare via cell phones: A systematic review. *Telemedicine Journal and e-Health*, *15*(3), 231–240. doi:10.1089/tmj.2008.0099 PMID:19382860

Kroeze, W., Werkman, A., & Brug, J. (2006). A systematic review of randomized trials on the effectiveness of computer-tailored education on physical activity and dietary behaviors. *Annals of Behavioral Medicine*, *31*(3), 205–223. doi:10.120715324796abm3103_2 PMID:16700634

Krohn, R., & Metcalf, D. (2012). *mHealth: From Smartphones to Smart Systems*. HIMSS.

Kruger, D. F., White, K., Galpern, A., Mann, K., Massirio, A., McLellan, M., & Stevenson, J. (2003). Effect of modem transmission of blood glucose data on telephone consultation time, clinic work flow, and patient satisfaction for patients with gestational diabetes mellitus. *Journal of the American Academy of Nurse Practitioners*, *15*(8), 371–375. doi:10.1111/j.1745-7599.2003.tb00410.x PMID:14509102

Krzysztofek, M. (2017). *Post-reform personal data protection in the European Union: general data protection regulation (EU) 2016/679*. EU.

KSI - Knowledge Sourcing Intelligence LLP. (2017). *Mobile Health (mHealth) App Market - Industry Trends, Opportunities and Forecasts to 2023*. Author.

Kubono, K. (2004). Quality management system in the medical laboratory--ISO15189 and laboratory accreditation. *Rinsho Byori*, *52*(3), 274–278. PMID:15137330

Kuo, A. M. (2011). Opportunities and challenges of cloud computing to improve health care services. *Journal of Medical Internet Research, 13*(3), e67. doi:10.2196/jmir.1867 PMID:21937354

Kuo, T. T., Kim, H. E., & Ohno-Machado, L. (2017). Blockchain distributed ledger technologies for biomedical and health care applications. *Journal of the American Medical Informatics Association, 24*(6), 1211–1220. doi:10.1093/jamia/ocx068 PMID:29016974

Kushi, L. H., Doyle, C., McCullough, M., Rock, C. L., Demark-Wahnefried, W., Bandera, E. V., ... Gansler, T. (2012). American Cancer Society Guidelines on nutrition and physical activity for cancer prevention: Reducing the risk of cancer with healthy food choices and physical activity. *CA: a Cancer Journal for Clinicians, 62*(1), 30–67. doi:10.3322/caac.20140 PMID:22237782

Kushniruk, A. W., Patel, V. L., & Cimino, J. J. (1997). Usability testing in medical informatics: cognitive approaches to evaluation of information systems and user interfaces. *Proceedings of the AMIA Annual Fall Symposium*, 218-222.

Kussaibi, H., Macary, F., Kennedy, M., Booker, D., Brodsky, V., Schrader, T., ... Daniel, C. (2010). HL7 CDA implementation guide for structured anatomic pathology reports methodology and tools. *Studies in Health Technology and Informatics, 160*(Pt 1), 289–293. PMID:20841695

Kvåle, K., & Bondevik, M. (2008). What is important for patient centred care? A qualitative study about the perceptions of patients with cancer. *Scandinavian Journal of Caring Sciences, 22*(4), 582–589. doi:10.1111/j.1471-6712.2007.00579.x PMID:19000089

Labrique, A., Vasudevan, L., Kochi, E., & Mehl, G. (2013). mHealth innovations as health system strengthening tools: 12 common applications and visual framework. *Global Health, Science and Practice, 1*(2), 160–171. doi:10.9745/GHSP-D-13-00031 PMID:25276529

Lafata, J. E., Baker, A. M., Divine, G. W., McCarthy, B. D., & Xi, H. (2002). The use of computerized birthday greeting reminders in the management of diabetes. *Journal of General Internal Medicine, 17*(7), 521–530. doi:10.1046/j.1525-1497.2002.10901.x PMID:12133142

Laffel, L. M., Vangsness, L., Connell, A., Goebel-Fabbri, A., Butler, D., & Anderson, B. J. (2003). Impact of ambulatory, family-focused teamwork intervention on glycemic control in youth with type 1 diabetes. *The Journal of Pediatrics, 142*(4), 409–416. doi:10.1067/mpd.2003.138 PMID:12712059

Laktabai, J., Platt, A., Menya, D., Turner, E. L., Aswa, D., Kinoti, S., & O'Meara, W. P. (2018). A mobile health technology platform for quality assurance and quality improvement of malaria diagnosis by community health workers. *PLoS One, 13*(2), e0191968. doi:10.1371/journal.pone.0191968 PMID:29389958

Lam, Q., Ajzner, E., Campbell, C. A., & Young, A. (2016). Critical Risk Results - An Update on International Initiatives. *EJIFCC, 27*(1), 66–76. PMID:27683507

Landis, J. R., & Koch, G. G. (1977). The measurement of observer agreement for categorical data. *Biometrics, 33*(1), 159–174. doi:10.2307/2529310 PMID:843571

Larson, P. J., Carrieri-Kohlman, V., Dodd, M. J., Douglas, M., Faucett, J., Froelicher, E. S., ... Underwood, P. (1994). A model for symptom management. *Image--the Journal of Nursing Scholarship, 26*, 154–164. PMID:7829111

Latifi, R. (2010). *Telemedicine for Trauma, Emergencies, and Disaster Management.* Norwood: Artech House.

Latifi, R., Weinstein, R. S., Porter, J. M., Ziemba, M., Judkins, D., Ridings, D., ... Leyva, F. (2007). Telemedicine and telepresence for trauma and emergency care management. *Scandinavian Journal of Surgery, 96*(4), 281–289. doi:10.1177/145749690709600404 PMID:18265854

Laulkar, R., & Daimiwal, N. (2012). Acquisition of PPG signal for diagnosis of parameters related to heart. *Proceedings of 1st international symposium on physics and technology of sensors(ISPTS).*

Lee, E. S., Kim, I. S., Choi, J. S., Yeom, B. W., Kim, H. K., Han, J. H., ... Leong, A. S. (2003). Accuracy and reproducibility of telecytology diagnosis of cervical smears. A tool for quality assurance programs. *American Journal of Clinical Pathology, 119*(3), 356–360. doi:10.1309/7YTVAG4XNR48T75H PMID:12645336

Lee, J. E., Lee, D. E., Kim, K., Shim, J. E., Sung, E., Kang, J.-H., & Hwang, J.-Y. (2017). Development of tailored nutrition information messages based on the transtheoretical model for smartphone application of an obesity prevention and management program for elementary-school students. *Nutrition Research and Practice, 11*(3), 247–256. doi:10.4162/nrp.2017.11.3.247 PMID:28584582

Lee, J., Kim, S., Kim, P., Liu, X., Lee, T., Kim, K. M., ... Kang, W. K. (2013). A novel proteomics-based clinical diagnostics technology identifies heterogeneity in activated signaling pathways in gastric cancers. *PLoS One, 8*(1), e54644. doi:10.1371/journal.pone.0054644 PMID:23372746

Lee, Y., Shin, S. Y., Kim, J. Y., Kim, J. H., Seo, D. W., Joo, S., ... Bates, D. W. (2015). Evaluation of Mobile Health Applications Developed by a Tertiary Hospital as a Tool for Quality Improvement Breakthrough. *Healthcare Informatics Research, 21*(4), 299–306. doi:10.4258/hir.2015.21.4.299 PMID:26618037

Lehto, T. (2013). *The Importance of Persuasive Systems Design in Enhancing Consumers´ Perceptions and Adoption of Health Behavior Change Support Systems* (Doctoral dissertation). University of Oulu, Department of Information Processing Science.

Leica Microsystems. (2011). *Leica Microsystems Launches Free Digital Pathology App for iPad and iPhone.* Retrieved 10 April, 2015, from http://www.leica-microsystems.com/news-media/news/news-details/article/leica-microsystems-launches-free-digital-pathology-app-for-ipad-and-iphone/

Lenz, E., Pugh, L., Milligan, R., Gift, A., & Suppe, E. (1997). The middle range theory of unpleasant symptoms: An update. *Advances in Nursing Science, 19*(3), 14–27. doi:10.1097/00012272-199703000-00003 PMID:9055027

Lenz, E., Suppe, E., Pugh, L., & Milligan, R. (1995). Collaborative development of middle range nursing theories: Toward a theory of unpleasant symptoms. *Advances in Nursing Science, 17*(3), 1–13. doi:10.1097/00012272-199503000-00003 PMID:7778887

Leprevost, F. V., Lima, D. B., Crestani, J., Perez-Riverol, Y., Zanchin, N., Barbosa, V. C., & Carvalho, P. C. (2013). Pinpointing differentially expressed domains in complex protein mixtures with the cloud service of PatternLab for Proteomics. *Journal of Proteomics, 89*, 179–182. doi:10.1016/j.jprot.2013.06.013 PMID:23796493

Leventhal, H., Benyamini, Y., Brownlee, S., Diefenbach, M., Leventhal, E. A., Patrick-Miller, L., & Robitaille, C. (1997). Illness representations: theoretical foundations. In K. J. Petrie & J. A. Weinman (Eds.), *Perceptions of Health and Illness: Current Research and Applications* (pp. 19–45). Harwood Academic Publishers.

Leventhal, H., Leventhal, E. A., & Cameron, L. (2001). Representations, procedures and affect in illness self regulation: a perceptual-cognitive model. In A. Baum, T. Revenson, & J. Singer (Eds.), *Handbook of Health Psychology* (pp. 19–47). New York: Earlbaum.

Leventhal, H., Nerenz, D. R., & Steel, D. J. (1984). Illness representations and coping with health threats. In A. Baum, S. E. Taylor, & J. E. Singer (Eds.), Handbook of Psychology and Health (Vol. 4, pp. 219–252). Hillsdale, NJ: Erlbaum.

Levine, A. I., DeMaria, S., Schwartz, A. D., & Sim, A. J. (2013). *The Comprehensive Textbook of Healthcare Simulation.* Springer. doi:10.1007/978-1-4614-5993-4

Levin, L. S., & Idler, E. L. (1983). Self-care in health. *Annual Review of Public Health*, *4*(1), 181–201. doi:10.1146/annurev.pu.04.050183.001145 PMID:6860437

Levin, L. S., Katz, A., & Holst, E. (1977). *Self-Care: Lay Initiatives in Health*. New York Prodist.

Lieberman, D. A. (2012). Video Games for Diabetes Self-Management: Examples and Design Strategies. *Journal of Diabetes Science and Technology*, *6*(4), 802–806. doi:10.1177/193229681200600410 PMID:22920805

Li, G., Zhao, F., & Cui, Y. (2013). Proteomics using mammospheres as a model system to identify proteins deregulated in breast cancer stem cells. *Current Molecular Medicine*, *13*(3), 459–463. PMID:23331018

Lin, M., Rezaie, S., & Husain, I. (2014). Top 10 mobile apps in Emergency Medicine. *Emergency Medicine Journal*, *31*(5), 432–433. doi:10.1136/emermed-2014-203607 PMID:24567149

Linn, L. A., & Koo, M. B. (2016). Blockchain for health data and its potential use in health it and health care related research. In *ONC/NIST Use of Blockchain for Healthcare and Research Workshop*. Gaithersburg, MD: ONC/NIST.

Litwin, S. E. (2014). Childhood Obesity and Adulthood Cardiovascular Disease*: Quantifying the Lifetime Cumulative Burden of Cardiovascular Risk Factors. *Journal of the American College of Cardiology*, *64*(15), 1588–1590. doi:10.1016/j.jacc.2014.07.962 PMID:25301462

Liu, W.-T., Wang, C.-H., Lin, H.-C., Lin, S.-M., Lee, K.-Y., Lo, Y.-L., ... Kuo, H.-P. (2008). Efficacy of a cell phone-based exercise programme for COPD. *The European Respiratory Journal*, *32*(3), 651–659. doi:10.1183/09031936.00104407 PMID:18508824

Lorig, K. R., Ritter, P. L., Laurent, D. D., & Fries, J. F. (2004). Long-term randomized controlled trials of tailored-print and small-group arthritis self management interventions. *Medical Care*, *42*(4), 346–354. doi:10.1097/01.mlr.0000118709.74348.65 PMID:15076811

Lorig, K., & Holman, H. (2003). Self-Management Education: History, Definition, Outcomes, and Mechanisms. *Annals of Behavioral Medicine*, *26*(1), 1–7. doi:10.1207/S15324796ABM2601_01 PMID:12867348

Lossius, H. M., Roislien, J., & Lockey, D. J. (2012). Patient safety in pre-hospital emergency tracheal intubation: A comprehensive meta-analysis of the intubation success rates of EMS providers. *Critical Care (London, England)*, *16*(1), R24. doi:10.1186/cc11189 PMID:22325973

Lupse, O. S., Vida, M., & Stoicu-Tivadar, L. (2012). Cloud computing technology applied in healthcare for developing large scale flexible solutions. *Studies in Health Technology and Informatics*, *174*, 94–99. PMID:22491119

Lustria, M. L., Cortese, J., Noar, S. M., & Glueckauf, R. L. (2009). Computer-tailored health interventions delivered over the Web: Review and analysis of key components. *Patient Education and Counseling*, *74*(2), 156–173. doi:10.1016/j.pec.2008.08.023 PMID:18947966

Lutfey, K. E., & Wishner, W. J. (1999). Beyond "compliance" is "adherence". Improving the prospect of diabetes care. *Diabetes Care*, *22*(4), 635–639. doi:10.2337/diacare.22.4.635 PMID:10189544

Madden, K., Flowers, L., Salani, R., Horowitz, I., Logan, S., Kowalski, K., ... Mohammed, S. I. (2009). Proteomics-based approach to elucidate the mechanism of antitumor effect of curcumin in cervical cancer. *Prostaglandins, Leukotrienes, and Essential Fatty Acids*, *80*(1), 9–18. doi:10.1016/j.plefa.2008.10.003 PMID:19058955

Mahbub, I., Pullano, S. A., Wang, H., Islam, S. K., Fiorillo, S., To, G., & Mahfouz, M. R. (2017). A Low- Power Wireless Piezoelectric Sensor-Based Respiration Monitoring System Realized in CMOS Process. *IEEE Sensors Journal*, *17*(6), 1858–1864. doi:10.1109/JSEN.2017.2651073

Maher, E. J. (2013). Managing the consequences of cancer treatment and the English National Cancer Survivorship Initiative. *Acta Oncologica*, *52*(2), 225–232. doi:10.3109/0284186X.2012.746467 PMID:23237053

Mailloux, L. U., Kapikian, N., Napolitano, B., Mossey, R. T., Bellucci, A. G., Wilkes, B. M., ... Miller, I. J. (1996). Home hemodialysis: Patient outcomes during a 24-year period of time from 1970 through 1993. *Advances in Renal Replacement Therapy*, *3*(2), 112–119. doi:10.1016/S1073-4449(96)80050-1 PMID:8814916

Malcolm, S. (2013). *Smartphone apps, permissions and privacy concerns and next steps.* TEKDESK: A division of the community opportunity and innovation network. Retrieved from http://rebootpeterborough.ca/wp-content/uploads/2013/04/Smartphone-Apps-Permissions-and-Privacy-Report.pdf, 1-93.

Maly, R. C., Abrahamse, A. F., Hirsch, S. H., & ... . (1996). What influences physician practice behavior? An interview study of physicians who received consultative geriatric assessment recommendations. *Archives of Family Medicine*, *5*(8), 448–454. doi:10.1001/archfami.5.8.448 PMID:8797548

Mameli, C., Brunetti, D., Colombo, V., Bedogni, G., Schneider, L., Penagini, F., ... Zuccotti, G. V. (2018). Combined use of a wristband and a smartphone to reduce body weight in obese children: Randomized controlled trial. *Pediatric Obesity*, *13*(2), 81–87. doi:10.1111/ijpo.12201 PMID:27900849

Manahan, M. N., Soyer, H. P., Loescher, L. J., Horsham, C., Vagenas, D., Whiteman, D. C., ... Janda, M. (2015). A pilot trial of mobile, patient-performed teledermoscopy. *British Journal of Dermatology*, *172*(4), 1072–1080. doi:10.1111/bjd.13550 PMID:25418126

Mandel, J. C., Kreda, D. A., Mandl, K. D., Kohane, I. S., & Ramoni, R. B. (2016). SMART on FHIR: A standards-based, interoperable apps platform for electronic health records. *Journal of the American Medical Informatics Association*, *23*(5), 899–908. doi:10.1093/jamia/ocv189 PMID:26911829

Mankar, N. B., & Nagdeve, U. T. (2013). *Comparison of different imaging techniques used for chronic wounds.* IJRET. *International Journal of Research in Engineering and Technology*, *2*(7), 68–70. doi:10.15623/ijret.2013.0207009

Marchevsky, A. M., Tsou, J. A., & Laird-Offringa, I. A. (2004). Classification of individual lung cancer cell lines based on DNA methylation markers: Use of linear discriminant analysis and artificial neural networks. *The Journal of Molecular Diagnostics*, *6*(1), 28–36. doi:10.1016/S1525-1578(10)60488-6 PMID:14736824

Marcos, C. (2015, Apr 15). Solving the interoperability challenge of a distributed complex patient guidance system: A data integrator based on HL7's Virtual Medical Record standard. *J Am Med Inform Assoc.*

Marcus, B. H., Emmons, K. M., Simkin-Silverman, L. R., Linnan, L. A., Taylor, E. R., Bock, B. C., ... Abrams, D. B. (1998). Evaluation of motivationally tailored versus standard self-help physical activity interventions at the workplace. *American Journal of Health Promotion*, *12*(4), 246–253. doi:10.4278/0890-1171-12.4.246 PMID:10178617

Margari, N., Pouliakis, A., Anoinos, D., Terzakis, E., Koureas, N., Chrelias, C., ... Karakitsos, P. (2016). A reporting system for endometrial cytology: Cytomorphologic criteria-Implied risk of malignancy. *Diagnostic Cytopathology*, *44*(11), 888–901. doi:10.1002/dc.23605 PMID:27653446

Markidou, S., Karakitsos, P., & Pouliakis, A. (1999). Telecytology. In O. Ferrer-Roca & M. Sosa-Iudicissa (Eds.), *Handbook of Telemedicine* (Vol. 54). Amsterdam: IOS press.

Markin, R. S., & Whalen, S. A. (2000). Laboratory automation: Trajectory, technology, and tactics. *Clinical Chemistry*, *46*(5), 764–771. PMID:10794775

Markopoulos, C., Karakitsos, P., Botsoli-Stergiou, E., Pouliakis, A., Gogas, J., Ioakim-Liossi, A., & Kyrkou, K. (1997). Application of back propagation to the diagnosis of breast lesions by fine needle aspiration. *The Breast*, *6*(5), 293–298. doi:10.1016/S0960-9776(97)90008-4

Martínez-Pérez, B., De La Torre-Díez, I., & López-Coronado, M. (2015). Privacy and security in mobile health apps: A review and recommendations. *Journal of Medical Systems*, *39*(1), 181. doi:10.100710916-014-0181-3 PMID:25486895

Martin, S. J., Chen, G., Dattilo, J., & Johnson, C. T. (2015). Physicians' Knowledge Regarding Tablet- and Handheld-Based Applications in Gynecology and Obstetrics. *Obstetrics and Gynecology*, *125*(Suppl 1), 119S–120S. doi:10.1097/01.AOG.0000463206.49148.98

Martin, T. (2012). Assessing mHealth: Opportunities and barriers to patient engagement. *Journal of Health Care for the Poor and Underserved*, *23*(3), 935–941. doi:10.1353/hpu.2012.0087 PMID:24212144

Massone, C., Brunasso, A. M., Campbell, T. M., & Soyer, H. P. (2009). Mobile teledermoscopy--melanoma diagnosis by one click? *Seminars in Cutaneous Medicine and Surgery*, *28*(3), 203–205. doi:10.1016/j.sder.2009.06.002 PMID:19782945

Massone, C., Brunasso, A. M., Hofmann-Wellenhof, R., Gulia, A., & Soyer, H. P. (2010). Teledermoscopy: Education, discussion forums, teleconsulting and mobile teledermoscopy. *Giornale Italiano di Dermatologia e Venereologia*, *145*(1), 127–132. PMID:20197751

Maurer, U., Rowe, A., Smailagic, A., & Siewiorek, P. (2006). eWatch: a wearable sensor and notification platform. *Proceedings of International Workshop on BSN, Wearable and Implanted Body Sensor Networks*, 144-145.

McCorkle, R., Ercolano, E., Lazenby, M., Schulman-Green, D., Schilling, L. S., Lorig, K., & Wagner, E. H. (2011). Self-management: Enabling and empowering patients living with cancer as a chronic illness. *CA: a Cancer Journal for Clinicians*, *61*(1), 50–62. doi:10.3322/caac.20093 PMID:21205833

McGuire, S. (2016). World Cancer Report 2014. Geneva, Switzerland: World Health Organization.

McKenzie, P. J. (2002). Communcation barriers and information-seeking counterstrategies in accounts of practitioner-patient encounters. *Library & Information Science Research*, *24*(1), 31–47. doi:10.1016/S0740-8188(01)00103-7

McKinsey & GSMA. (2010). *mHealth: A new vision for healthcare.* McKinsey & Company, Inc. and GSMA.

McKnight, J., Babineau, B., & Gahm, J. (2011). *North American Health Care Provider Information Market Size & Forecast.* ESG-Enterprise Strategy Group.

McLean, R., Jury, C., Bazeos, A., & Lewis, S. M. (2009). Application of camera phones in telehaematology. *Journal of Telemedicine and Telecare*, *15*(7), 339–343. doi:10.1258/jtt.2009.090114 PMID:19815902

McRoy, S. W., Liu-Perez, A., & Ali, S. S. (1998). Interactive computerized health care education. *Journal of the American Medical Informatics Association*, *5*(4), 347–356. doi:10.1136/jamia.1998.0050347 PMID:9670132

Mead, N., & Bower, P. (2000). Patient-centredness: A conceptual framework and review of the empirical literature. *Social Science & Medicine*, *51*(7), 1087–1110. doi:10.1016/S0277-9536(00)00098-8 PMID:11005395

Medical Library Association. (2003). *Health Information Literacy: Definitions.* Retrieved April 20, 2015, from https://www.mlanet.org/resources/healthlit/define.html

Melbye, S., Hotvedt, M., & Bolle, S. (2014). Mobile videoconferencing for enhanced emergency medical communication - a shot in the dark or a walk in the park? -- A simulation study. *Scandinavian Journal of Trauma, Resuscitation and Emergency Medicine*, *22*(1), 35. doi:10.1186/1757-7241-22-35 PMID:24887256

Menendez-Jandula, B., Souto, J. C., Oliver, A., Montserrat, I., Quintana, M., Gich, I., ... Fontcuberta, J. (2005). Comparing self management of oral anticoagulant therapy with clinic management: A randomized trial. *Annals of Internal Medicine, 142*(1), 1–10. doi:10.7326/0003-4819-142-1-200501040-00006 PMID:15630104

Meszaros, L. (2014). *Johns Hopkins Atlas of Pancreatic Cytopathology*. Retrieved 10 February, 2015, from http://www.mdlinx.com/endocrinology/mobile-app-center/mobile-app-detail.cfm?app_id=1221

METABO. (2008). *Controlling Chronic Diseases related to Metabolic Disorders*. Retrieved from www.metabo-eu.org

Metelmann, B., Metelmann, C., Morris, D., Cordeiro, L., Chochliouros, I., von der Heyden, M., . . . Wendt, M. (2014). *Live Video Transmission to Improve Emergency Medicine* [Videoübertragung in Echtzeit zur Verbesserung der Notfallmedizin]. Paper presented at the VDE-Kongress 2014 - Smart Cities, Frankfurt am Main, Germany.

Metelmann, C., Metelmann, B., Morris, D., Cordeiro, L., Chochliouros, I., von der Heyden, M., . . . Wendt, M. (2014). *The Potential of Telemedicine for Patients at Home* [Potenziale der Telemedizin bei Patienten in der Häuslichkeit]. Paper presented at the VDE-Kongress 2014 - Smart Cities, Frankfurt am Main, Germany.

Metelmann, B., Metelmann, C., Meissner, K., Wendt, M., Goncalves, J., Gilligan, P., & von der Heyden, M. (2014). The Potential of Telemedicine. In L. Iliadis, I. Maglogiannis, H. Papadopoulos, S. Sioutas, & C. Makris (Eds.), *Artificial Intelligence Applications and Innovations* (Vol. 437, pp. 30–37). Springer Berlin Heidelberg.

Metelmann, C., Metelmann, B., Wendt, M., Meissner, K., & von der Heyden, M. (2014). LiveCity: The Impact of Video Communication on Emergency Medicine. *International Journal of Electronic Government Research, 10*(3), 47–65. doi:10.4018/ijegr.2014070104

mHealth4Africa. (2015). *Community-based ICT for Maternal Healthcare in Africa*. Retrieved Jan 21, 2017, from www.mhealth4afrika.eu

mHealthAlliance & VitalWaveConsulting. (2013). *Sustainable Financing for Mobile Health (mHealth): Options and opportunities for mHealth financial models in low and middle-income countries*. mHealth Alliance.

mHealthAlliance. (2012). *Baseline Evaluation of the mHealth Ecosystem and the Performance of the mHealth Alliance*. mHealth Alliance.

mHealthCompetenceCentre. (2014). *News*. Retrieved 5 10, 2015, from mHealth Competence Centre: http://www.mobilehealthglobal.com/in-the-news/news/41/the-mhealth-app-market-will-reach-26-bilion-usd-revenue-by-2017-says-himss-europe-report

MHRA, Medicines and Healthcare Products Regulatory Agency. (2014). *Medical device stand-alone software including apps*. Retrieved from https://www.gov.uk/government/publications/medical-devices-software-applications-apps

Michie, S., Miles, J., & Weinman, J. (2003). Patient-centredness in chronic illness: What is it and does it matter? *Patient Education and Counseling, 51*(3), 197–206. doi:10.1016/S0738-3991(02)00194-5 PMID:14630376

Milenkovic,, A., Otto, C., & Jovanov. (2006). Wireless sensor networks for personal health monitoring: Issues and an implementation. *Current Communication, 29*, 13–14.

Miluzzo, E., Lane, N., Fodor, K., Peterson, R., Lu, H., Musolesi, M., . . . Campbell, A. (2008). Sensing meets mobile social networks: The design, implementation and evaluation of the CenceMe application. In *SenSys '08 Proceedings of the 6th ACM conference on Embedded network sensor systems* (pp. 337-350). ACM.

Miranda, J. J., Moscoso, M. G., Toyama, M., Cavero, V., Diez-Canseco, F., & Ovbiagele, B. (2018). Role of mHealth in overcoming the occurrence of post-stroke depression. *Acta Neurologica Scandinavica*, *137*(1), 12–19. doi:10.1111/ane.12832 PMID:28901543

Mirza, H., & El-Masri, S. (2013). National Electronic Medical Records integration on Cloud Computing System. *Studies in Health Technology and Informatics*, *192*, 1219. PMID:23920993

Miyamoto, S., Dharmar, M., Fazio, S., Tang-Feldman, Y., & Young, H. M. (2018). mHealth Technology and Nurse Health Coaching to Improve Health in Diabetes: Protocol for a Randomized Controlled Trial. *JMIR Research Protocols*, *7*(2), e45. doi:10.2196/resprot.9168 PMID:29449200

Mobasheri, M. H., Johnston, M., King, D., Leff, D., Thiruchelvam, P., & Darzi, A. (2014). Smartphone breast applications - What's the evidence? *The Breast*, *23*(5), 4–10. doi:10.1016/j.breast.2014.07.006 PMID:25153432

MobiGuide. (2011). *Guiding Patients Anytime, Everywhere*. Retrieved from www.mobiguide-project.eu

Modzelewski, K. L., Stockman, M. C., & Steenkamp, D. W. (2018). Rethinking the Endpoints of mHealth Intervention Research in Diabetes Care. *Journal of Diabetes Science and Technology*, *12*(2), 389–392. doi:10.1177/1932296817733007 PMID:28952379

Mohammed, Y., Mostovenko, E., Henneman, A. A., Marissen, R. J., Deelder, A. M., & Palmblad, M. (2012). Cloud parallel processing of tandem mass spectrometry based proteomics data. *Journal of Proteome Research*, *11*(10), 5101–5108. doi:10.1021/pr300561q PMID:22916831

Mohr, D., Burns, M., Schueller, S., Clarke, G., & Klinkman, M. (2013). Behavioral Intervention Technologies: Evidence review and recommendations for future research in mental health. *General Hospital Psychiatry, Special Section: Health Information Technology and Mental Health Services Research: A Path Forward, 35*, 332-338.

Mollison, D. (1995). *The structure of Epidemic Models*. Cambridge University Press.

MONARCA. (2010). *MONitoring, treAtment and pRediCtion of bipolAr Disorder Episodes*. Retrieved from www.monarca-project.eu

MONILET. (2015). *Monitoring Bracelet for Health Use*. Retrieved Jan 12, 2017, from http://cordis.europa.eu/project/rcn/194665_en.html

Montgomery, K., Mundt, C., Tellier, A., Udoh, V., Berker, R., Giovangrandi, L., … Kovacs, G. (2004). Lifeguard – a personal physiological monitor for extreme environments. *IEEE International Conference of EMBS.*

Moore, G. E. (1965). Cramming more components onto integrated circuits. *Electronics Magazine*, 4.

Moreo, K. (2005). Understanding and overcoming the challenges of effective case management for patients with chronic wounds. *The Case Manager*, *16*(2), 62–67. doi:10.1016/j.casemgr.2005.01.014 PMID:15818347

Moroz, P. J., & Spiegel, D. A. (2014). The World Health Organization's action plan on the road traffic injury pandemic: Is there any action for orthopaedic trauma surgeons? *Journal of Orthopaedic Trauma*, *28*(Suppl 1), S11–S14. doi:10.1097/BOT.0000000000000105 PMID:24857989

Morris, M., & Guilak, F. (2009). Mobile heart health: Project highlight. *IEEE Pervasive Computing*, *8*(2), 57–61. doi:10.1109/MPRV.2009.31

Morrison, A. (2001). Effectiveness of printed patient educational materials in chronic illness: A systematic review of controlled trials. *J Manag Pharm Care*, *1*(1), 51–62. doi:10.1300/J234v01n01_07

Mosier, J., Joseph, B., & Sakles, J. C. (2013). Telebation: Next-generation telemedicine in remote airway management using current wireless technologies. *Telemedicine Journal and e-Health, 19*(2), 95–98. doi:10.1089/tmj.2012.0093 PMID:23215736

Mouli, K. C., & Sesadri, U. (2013). Single to Multi Clouds for Security in Cloud Computing by using Secret Key Sharing. *International Journal of Computers and Technology, 10*(4), 1539–1545. doi:10.24297/ijct.v10i4.3254

Moumtzoglou, A. (2014). Redefining Patient-Centered Care. *International Journal of Reliable and Quality E-Healthcare, 3*(2), iv–v.

Moumtzoglou, A., & Pouliakis, A. (2015). Mapping Population Health Management Roadmap into Cervical Cancer Screening Programs. *International Journal of Reliable and Quality E-Healthcare, 4*(3), 1–18. doi:10.4018/IJRQEH.2015070101

Moving Life. (2011). *MObile eHealth for the VINdication of Global LIFEstyle change and disease management solutions*. Retrieved from www.moving-life.eu

m-Resist. (2015). *Mobile Therapeutic Attention for Patients with Treatment Resistant Schizophrenia*. Retrieved from www.mresist.eu

Multiple analog inputs on only one analog pin. (2016). Retrieved from http://www.instructables.com/id/Multiple-Analog-Inputs-on-Only-One-Analoge-Pin/

Mun, S. K., Elsayed, A. M., Tohme, W. G., & Wu, Y. C. (1995). Teleradiology/telepathology requirements and implementation. *Journal of Medical Systems, 19*(2), 153–164. doi:10.1007/BF02257066 PMID:7602247

Murray-Johnson, L., & Witte, K. (2003). Looking toward the future: health message design strategies. In T. L. Thompson, A. M. Dorsey, K. I. Miller, & R. Parrott (Eds.), *Handbook of Health Communication*. Mahwah, NJ: Lawrence Erlbaum Associates Inc.

Mustoe, T. (2004). Understanding chronic wounds: A unifying hypothesis on their pathogenesis and implications for therapy. *American Journal of Surgery, 187*(5), 65–70. doi:10.1016/S0002-9610(03)00306-4 PMID:15147994

Mustoe, T. A., O'Shaughnessy, K., & Kloeters, O. (2006). Chronic wound pathogenesis and current treatment strategies: A unifying hypothesis. *Plastic and Reconstructive Surgery, 117*, 35–41. doi:10.1097/01.prs.0000225431.63010.1b PMID:16799373

Muth, T., Peters, J., Blackburn, J., Rapp, E., & Martens, L. (2013). ProteoCloud: A full-featured open source proteomics cloud computing pipeline. *Journal of Proteomics, 88*, 104–108. doi:10.1016/j.jprot.2012.12.026 PMID:23305951

Muto, N. (2012). *Basic smartphone workshop*. Retrieved from http://www.saultcareercentre.ca/wp-content/uploads/2012/09/PREVIEW-SMARTPHONE.pdf, *1-5*.

myAirCoach. (2015). *Analysis, modelling and sensing of both physiological and environmental factors for the customized and predictive self-management of Asthma*. Retrieved Jan 14, 2017, from http://www.myaircoach.eu

MyCyFAPP. (2015). *My App for Cystic Fibrosis*. Retrieved Jan 14, 2017, from http://www.mycyfapp.eu

MySQL. (2018). *MySQL NDB Cluster: High Availability*. Retrieved December 6th, 2017, from https://www.mysql.com/products/cluster/availability.html

Nagy, G. K., & Newton, L. E. (2006). Cytopathology proficiency testing: Where do we go from here? *Diagnostic Cytopathology, 34*(4), 257–264. doi:10.1002/dc.20361 PMID:16544329

Nahl, D., & Bilal, D. (2007). *Information and Emotion: The Emergent Affective Paradigm in Information Behavior Research and Theory*. Medford, NJ: Information Today.

Nakamura, T., Yokota, Y., Terakawa, J., Reeder, W., Voit, T., Someya, & Sekino, M. (2016). Development of flexible and wide-range polymer-based temperature sensor for human bodies. *Proceedings of IEEE-EMBS International Conference on Biomedical and Health Informatics (BHI).*

Napolitano, M. A., Hayes, S., Bennett, G. G., Ives, A. K., & Foster, G. D. (2013). Using Facebook and text messaging to deliver a weight loss program to college students. *Obesity (Silver Spring, Md.)*, *21*(1), 25–31. doi:10.1002/oby.20232 PMID:23505165

Narczyk, P., Siwiec, K., & Pleskacz, W. A. (2016). Precision human body temperature measurement based on thermistor sensor. *Proceedings of IEEE 19th International Symposium on Design and Diagnostics of Electronic Circuits& Systems (DDECS)*. 10.1109/DDECS.2016.7482451

Nasi, G., Cucciniello, M., & Guerrazzi, C. (2015). The role of mobile technologies in health care processes: The case of cancer supportive care. *Journal of Medical Internet Research*, *17*(2), e26. doi:10.2196/jmir.3757 PMID:25679446

National Center for Chronic Disease Prevention and Health Promotion, Division of Cancer Prevention and Control. (2014). *Implementation Guide for Ambulatory Healthcare Provider Reporting to Central Cancer Registries, HL7 Clinical Document Architecture (CDA), Release 1.1*. IHE International. Retrieved from https://www.cdc.gov/phin/resources/guides/documents/implementation_guide_for_ambulatory_healthcare_provider_reporting_to_central_cancer_registries_march_2014.pdf

Nawyn, J., Intille, S. S., & Larson, K. (2006). Embedding behavior modification strategies intoa consumer electronic device: a case study. In *Proceedings of UbiComp 2006, Ubiquitous Computing: 8th International Conference*. Berlin: Springer. 10.1007/11853565_18

Nayar, R., & Wilbur, D. (2015). *The Bethesda system for reporting cervical cytology: definitions, criteria, and explanatory notes* (2nd ed.). New York: Springer.

Nemeth, M., Sprigle, S., & Gajjala, A. (2010). Clinical usability of a wound measurement device. *36th Annual American Spinal Injury Conference*, 1-17.

Nephron+. (2010). *ICT enabled Wearable Artificial Kidney and Personal Renal Care System*. Retrieved from www.nephronplus.eu

Neve, M., Morgan, P. J., Jones, P. R., & Collins, C. E. (2010). Effectiveness of web-based interventions in achieving weight loss and weight loss maintenance in overweight and obese adults: A systematic review with meta-analysis. *Obesity Reviews*, *11*(4), 306–321. doi:10.1111/j.1467-789X.2009.00646.x PMID:19754633

Newbould, J., Taylor, D., & Bury, M. (2006). Lay-led self-management in chronic illness: A review of the evidence. *Chronic Illness*, *2*(4), 249–261. doi:10.1177/17423953060020040401 PMID:17212872

Newman, M. (2002). Spread of epidemic disease on networks. *Physical Review Letters*, *66*, 1–11. PMID:12241447

Nezami, B. T., Lytle, L. A., & Tate, D. F. (2016). A randomized trial to reduce sugar-sweetened beverage and juice intake in preschool-aged children: Description of the Smart Moms intervention trial. *BMC Public Health*, *16*(1), 837. doi:10.118612889-016-3533-8 PMID:27542357

Nezami, B. T., Ward, D. S., Lytle, L. A., Ennett, S. T., & Tate, D. F. (2017). A mHealth randomized controlled trial to reduce sugar-sweetened beverage intake in preschool-aged children. *Pediatric Obesity*. doi:10.1111/ijpo.12258 PMID:29119719

Ng, C. H., & Yeo, J. F. (2004). The role of Internet and personal digital assistant in oral and maxillofacial pathology. *Annals of the Academy of Medicine, Singapore*, *33*(4Suppl), 50–52. PMID:15389308

Ng, M., Fleming, T., Robinson, M., Thomson, B., Graetz, N., Margono, C., ... Gakidou, E. (2014). Global, regional, and national prevalence of overweight and obesity in children and adults during 1980–2013: A systematic analysis for the Global Burden of Disease Study 2013. *Lancet*, *384*(9945), 766–781. doi:10.1016/S0140-6736(14)60460-8 PMID:24880830

NIH. (n.d.). *National Institutes of Health. Office of Behavioral and Social Sciences Research*. Retrieved 5 14, 2015, from NIH. Office of Behavioral and Social Sciences Research: http://obssr.od.nih.gov/scientific_areas/methodology/mhealth/

Nilsen, J. E. (2012). *Improving quality of care in the Emergency Medical Communication Centres (EMCC)*. Paper presented at the Konferanse for medisinsk nødmeldetjeneste, Sola, Norway.

Noar, S. M., Harrington, N. G., & Aldrich, R. S. (2009). The role of message tailoring in the development of persuasive health communication messages. In C. S. Beck (Ed.), *Communication Yearbook 33* (pp. 73–133). New York, NY: Routledge.

Noar, S. M., Harrington, N. G., Van Stee, S. K., & Aldrich, R. S. (2011). Tailored Health Communication to Change Lifestyle Behaviors. *American Journal of Lifestyle Medicine*, *5*(2), 112–122. doi:10.1177/1559827610387255

NoHoW. (2015). *Evidence-based tools for weight loss maintenance*. Retrieved Jan 8, 2017, from nohow.eu/

Nollen, N. L., Hutcheson, T., Carlson, S., Rapoff, M., Goggin, K., Mayfield, C., & Ellerbeck, E. (2013). Development and functionality of a handheld computer program to improve fruit and vegetable intake among low-income youth. *Health Education Research*, *28*(2), 249–264. doi:10.1093/her/cys099 PMID:22949499

Nollen, N. L., Mayo, M. S., Carlson, S. E., Rapoff, M. A., Goggin, K. J., & Ellerbeck, E. F. (2014). Mobile Technology for Obesity Prevention: A Randomized Pilot Study in Racial- and Ethnic-Minority Girls. *American Journal of Preventive Medicine*, *46*(4), 404–408. doi:10.1016/j.amepre.2013.12.011 PMID:24650843

Norman, G. J., Zabinski, M. F., Adams, M. A., Rosenberg, D. E., Yaroch, A. L., & Atienza, A. A. (2007). A Review of eHealth Interventions for Physical Activity and Dietary Behavior Change. *American Journal of Preventive Medicine*, *33*(4), 336–345.e316. doi:10.1016/j.amepre.2007.05.007 PMID:17888860

Nutrigen Service. (2016). *Nutrigen service: Managing health through dietary needs, virtual consultations, and genetics*. Retrieved Jan 16, 2017, from cordis.europa.eu/project/rcn/205147_en.html

Nyatanga, L., & Dann, K. L. (2002). Empowerment in nursing: The role of philosophical and psychological factors. *Nursing Philosophy*, *3*(3), 134–139. doi:10.1046/j.1466-769X.2002.00107.x

NYMPHA-MD. (2014). *Next Generation Mobile Platforms for HeAlth, in Mental Disorders*. Retrieved from www.nympha-md-project.eu

O'Brien, M. J., Takahashi, M., Brugal, G., Christen, H., Gahm, T., Goodell, R. M., ... Winkler, C. (1998). Digital imagery/telecytology. International Academy of Cytology Task Force summary. Diagnostic Cytology Towards the 21st Century: An International Expert Conference and Tutorial. *Acta Cytologica*, *42*(1), 148–164. PMID:9479334

O'Malley, G., Clarke, M., Burls, A., Murphy, S., Murphy, N., & Perry, I. J. (2014). A smartphone intervention for adolescent obesity: Study protocol for a randomised controlled non-inferiority trial. *Trials*, *15*(1), 43. doi:10.1186/1745-6215-15-43 PMID:24485327

OAuth 2.0 (2018). *An open protocol to allow secure authorization in a simple and standard method from web, mobile and desktop applications*. Retrieved from https://oauth.net/

OECD. (2018). *Elderly population (indicator).* OECD. doi:10.1787/8d805ea1-en

Oenema, A., Brug, J., & Lechner, L. (2001). Web-based tailored nutrition education: Results of a randomized controlled trial. *Health Education Research, 16*(6), 647–660. doi:10.1093/her/16.6.647 PMID:11780705

Oermann, M. H., Webb, S. A., & Ashare, J. A. (2003). Outcomes of videotape instruction in clinic waiting area. *Orthopedic Nursing, 22*(2), 102–105. doi:10.1097/00006416-200303000-00006 PMID:12703393

Oh, H., Rizo, C., Enkin, M., Jadad, A., Powell, J., & Pagliari, C. (2005). What Is eHealth (3): A Systematic Review of Published Definitions. *Journal of Medical Internet Research, 7*(1), e1. doi:10.2196/jmir.7.1.e1 PMID:15829471

Oinas-Kukkonen, H. (2013). A foundation for the study of Behavior Change Support Systems. *Personal and Ubiquitous Computing, 17*(6), 1223–1235. doi:10.100700779-012-0591-5

Oliver, N., & Flores, F. (2006). HealthGear: a real-time wearable system for monitoring and analyzing physiological signals. *International Workshop on Wearable and Implanted Body Sensor Networks*, 3-5.

Omeni, O. C., Eljamaly, & Burdett, A.J. (2007). Energy efficient medium access protocol for wireless medical body area sensor networks. *Proceedings of the 4th IEEE EMBS*, 19-22.

Omoogun, Ramsurram, Guness, Seeam, Bellekens, & Seeam. (2017). Critical Patient eHealth Monitoring System using wearable sensors. *Proceedings of 1st International Conference on Next Generation Computing Applications.*

OpenSlide. (2015a). *OpenSlide Demo Site.* Retrieved 25 May, 2015, from http://www.openslide.org/demo

OpenSlide. (2015b). *OpenSlide homepage.* Retrieved 10 April, 2015, from http://www.openslide.org/

Orem, D. E. (1991). *Nursing: Concepts of Practice* (4th ed.). St Louis, MO: Mosby.

Orth, A., Wilson, E. R., Thompson, J. G., & Gibson, B. C. (2018). A dual-mode mobile phone microscope using the onboard camera flash and ambient light. *Scientific Reports, 8*(1), 3298. doi:10.103841598-018-21543-2 PMID:29459650

Osman, L. M., Calder, C., Godden, D. J., Friend, J. A., McKenzie, L., Legge, J. S., & Douglas, J. G. (2002). A randomised trial of self management planning for adult patients admitted to hospital with acute asthma. *Thorax, 57*(10), 869–874. doi:10.1136/thorax.57.10.869 PMID:12324673

Pai, A. L., Patiño-Fernández, A. M., McSherry, M., Beele, D., Alderfer, M. A., Reilly, A. T., ... Kazak, A. E. (2007). The Psychosocial Assessment Tool (PAT2. 0): Psychometric properties of a screener for psychosocial distress in families of children newly diagnosed with cancer. *Journal of Pediatric Psychology, 33*(1), 50–62. doi:10.1093/jpepsy/jsm053 PMID:17609228

PAL. (2015). *Personal Assistant for a healthy Lifestyle.* Retrieved from www.pal4u.eu

Palma, D., Goncalves, J., Cordeiro, L., Simoes, P., Monteiro, E., Magdalinos, P., & Chochliouros, I. (2013). Tutamen: An Integrated Personal Mobile and Adaptable Video Platform for Health and Protection. In H. Papadopoulos, A. Andreou, L. Iliadis, & I. Maglogiannis (Eds.), *Artificial Intelligence Applications and Innovations* (Vol. 412, pp. 442–451). Springer Berlin Heidelberg. doi:10.1007/978-3-642-41142-7_45

Pandher, P. S., & Bhullar, K. K. (2014). Smartphone applications for seizure management. *Health Informatics Journal.* doi:10.1177/1460458214540906 PMID:25038202

Pantanowitz, L., Henricks, W. H., & Beckwith, B. A. (2007). Medical laboratory informatics. *Clin Lab Med, 27*(4), 823-843. doi:10.1016/j.cll.2007.07.011

Pantanowitz, L., Hornish, M., & Goulart, R. A. (2009). The impact of digital imaging in the field of cytopathology. *CytoJournal*, *6*(1), 6. doi:10.4103/1742-6413.48606 PMID:19495408

Pantazopoulos, D., Karakitsos, P., Iokim-Liossi, A., Pouliakis, A., Botsoli-Stergiou, E., & Dimopoulos, C. (1998). Back propagation neural network in the discrimination of benign from malignant lower urinary tract lesions. *J Urol, 159*(5), 1619-1623. doi:10.1097/00005392-199805000-00057

Papanicolaou, G. (1928). *New Cancer Diagnosis.* Paper presented at the 3rd Race Bettrment Conference, Battle Creek.

Papanicolaou, G., & Traut, H. (1941). The diagnostic value of vaginal smears in carcinoma of the uterus. *American Journal of Obstetrics and Gynecology*, *42*(2), 193–206. doi:10.1016/S0002-9378(16)40621-6

Parkin, D. M., Boyd, L., & Walker, L. C. (2011). 16. The fraction of cancer attributable to lifestyle and environmental factors in the UK in 2010. *British Journal of Cancer*, *105*(S2), S77–S81. doi:10.1038/bjc.2011.489 PMID:22158327

Park, S., Parwani, A., Satyanarayanan, M., & Pantanowitz, L. (2012). Handheld computing in pathology. *Journal of Pathology Informatics*, *3*(1), 15–15. doi:10.4103/2153-3539.95127 PMID:22616027

Patel, R. P. (2012). Cloud computing and virtualization technology in radiology. [Review]. *Clinical Radiology*, *67*(11), 1095–1100. doi:10.1016/j.crad.2012.03.010 PMID:22607956

Paterson, B. L., & Sloan, J. (1994). A phenomenological study of the decision making experience of individuals with long standing diabetes. *Canadian Journal of Diabetes Care*, *18*(4), 10–19.

PATHway. (2017). *Technology-enabled behavioural change as a pathway towards better self-management of CVD.* Retrieved Feb 1, 2017, from www.pathway2health.eu/

Patton, G. G., & Thakore, S. (2013). Reducing inappropriate emergency department attendances--a review of ambulance service attendances at a regional teaching hospital in Scotland. *Emergency Medicine Journal*, *30*(6), 459–461. doi:10.1136/emermed-2012-201116 PMID:22802457

Pavlopoulos, S., Kyriacou, E., Berler, A., Dembeyiotis, S., & Koutsouris, D. (1998). A novel emergency telemedicine system based on wireless communication technology--AMBULANCE. *IEEE Transactions on Information Technology in Biomedicine*, *2*(4), 261–267. doi:10.1109/4233.737581 PMID:10719536

PD_Manager. (2015). *mHealth platform for Parkinson's Disease management.* Retrieved from www.parkinson-manager.eu

Pearlman, E. S., Wolfert, M. S., Miele, R., Bilello, L., & Stauffer, J. (2001). Utilization management and information technology: Adapting to the new era. *Clinical Leadership & Management Review*, *15*(2), 85–88. PMID:11299910

Pediatrics, A. A. (2011). Expert Panel on Integrated Guidelines for Cardiovascular Health and Risk Reduction in Children and Adolescents: Summary Report. *Pediatrics*, *128*(Supplement 5), S213–S256. doi:10.1542/peds.2009-2107C PMID:22084329

Pegasof4f. (2014). *Personalised Guidance Services for optimising lifestyle in teen-agers through awareness, motivation and engagement.* Retrieved from www.pegasof4f.eu

Peleg, M. (2013). Making healthcare more accessible, better, faster, and cheaper: the MobiGuide Project. *European Journal of ePractice: Issue on Mobile eHealth, 20*, 5-20.

Pentland, S. (2004). *Healthwear: medical technology becomes wearable.* Academic Press.

Perkins, G. D., Handley, A. J., Koster, R. W., Castren, M., Smyth, M. A., Olasveengen, T., ... Soar, J. (2015). European Resuscitation Council Guidelines for Resuscitation 2015: Section 2. Adult basic life support and automated external defibrillation. *Resuscitation, 95*, 81–99. doi:10.1016/j.resuscitation.2015.07.015 PMID:26477420

PERSONA. (2016). *PERSONAlised Health Monitoring System.* Retrieved Feb 1, 2017, from http://cordis.europa.eu/project/rcn/108629_en.html

Personal Connected Health Alliance. (2018). *Homepage.* Retrieved from http://www.pchalliance.org/

Pettigrew, K. E., Fidel, R., & Bruce, H. (2001). Conceptual frameworks in information behavior. *Annual Review of Information Science & Technology, 35*, 43–78.

Petty, R. E., & Cacioppo, J. T. (1986). The elaboration likelihood model of persuasion. *Advances in Experimental Psychology, 19*, 123–205. doi:10.1016/S0065-2601(08)60214-2

Philbrick, W. C. (2013). *mHealth and MNCH: State of the Evidence. Trends, Gaps, Stakeholder Needs, and Opportunities For Future Research on the Use of Mobile Technology to Improve Maternal, Newborn, and Child Health.* mHealth Alliance, UN Foundation. mHealth Alliance, UN Foundation.

Pinco, J., Goulart, R. A., Otis, C. N., Garb, J., & Pantanowitz, L. (2009). Impact of digital image manipulation in cytology. *Archives of Pathology & Laboratory Medicine, 133*(1), 57–61. doi:10.1043/1543-2165-133.1.57 PMID:19123737

Pirnstill, C. W., & Cote, G. L. (2015). Malaria Diagnosis Using a Mobile Phone Polarized Microscope. *Scientific Reports, 5*(1), 13368. doi:10.1038rep13368 PMID:26303238

Plassmann, P., & Jones, T. D. (1998). MAVIS: A non-invasive instrument to measure area and volume of wounds. *Medical Engineering & Physics, 20*(5), 332–338. doi:10.1016/S1350-4533(98)00034-4 PMID:9773686

Pouliakis, A., & Karakitsos, P. (2011). *Concepts of software design for population based cervical cencer screening.* Paper presented at the 36th European Congress of Cytology, Istanbul, Turkey.

Pouliakis, A., Margari, N., Archondakis, S., Karakitsou, E., & Karakitsos, P. (2016). Emerging Technologies Serving Cytopathology. Big Data, the Cloud and Mobile Computing. In I. E. Naqa (Ed.), Handbook of Research on Emerging Developments and Practices in Oncology. Hershey, PA: IGI Global.

Pouliakis, A., Archondakis, S., Karakitsou, E., & Karakitsos, P. (2014). Cloud Computing for Cytopathologists. In A. Moumtzoglou & A. Kastania (Eds.), *Cloud computing applications for quality health care delivery* (pp. 250–271). Hershey, PA: IGI Global. doi:10.4018/978-1-4666-6118-9.ch013

Pouliakis, A., Archondakis, S., Margari, N., & Karakitsos, P. (2016). From telecytology to mobile cytopathology: Past, present and future. In A. Moumtzoglou (Ed.), *M-Health Innovations for Patient-Centered Care.* Hershey, PA: IGI Global. doi:10.4018/978-1-4666-9861-1.ch012

Pouliakis, A., Athanasiadi, E., Karakitsou, E., Archondakis, S., Mourtzikou, A., Stamouli, M., ... Karakitsos, P. (2014). ISO 15189:2012 Management Requirements for Cytopathology Laboratory Information Systems. *International Journal of Reliable and Quality E-Healthcare, 3*(3), 37–57. doi:10.4018/ijrqeh.2014070103

Pouliakis, A., Iliopoulou, D., & Karakitsou, E. (2012). Design and Implementation Issues of an Information System Supporting Cervical Cancer Screening Programs. *Journal of Applied Medical Sciences, 1*(1), 61–91.

Pouliakis, A., Margari, N., Spathis, A., Kottaridi, C., Stamouli, M., Mourtzikou, A., ... Karakitsos, P. (2014). ISO 15189:2012 Technical Requirements for Cytopathology Laboratory Information Systems. *International Journal of Reliable and Quality E-Healthcare, 3*(3), 58–80. doi:10.4018/ijrqeh.2014070104

Pouliakis, A., Spathis, A., Kottaridi, C., Mourtzikou, A., Stamouli, M., Archondakis, S., & Karakitsos, P. (2014). Cloud Computing for BioLabs. In A. Moumtzoglou & A. Kastania (Eds.), *Cloud computing applications for quality health care delivery* (pp. 228–249). Hershey, PA: IGI Global. doi:10.4018/978-1-4666-6118-9.ch012

Pratt, M., Sarmiento, O. L., Montes, F., Ogilvie, D., Marcus, B. H., Perez, L. G., & Brownson, R. C. (2012). The implications of megatrends in information and communication technology and transportation for changes in global physical activity. *Lancet*, *380*(9838), 282–293. doi:10.1016/S0140-6736(12)60736-3 PMID:22818940

Pretlow, R. A., Stock, C. M., Allison, S., & Roeger, L. (2015). Treatment of child/adolescent obesity using the addiction model: A smartphone app pilot study. *Childhood Obesity*, *11*(3), 248–259. doi:10.1089/chi.2014.0124 PMID:25760813

Prevent, I. T. (2016). *The PreventIT Project: Improving health and active aging with mobile technology*. Retrieved Jan 16, 2017, from www.preventit.eu/

PriceWaterhouseCoopers. (2014). *Emerging mHealth: paths for growth*. PriceWaterhouseCoopers.

Prochaska, J. O., DiClemente, C. C., Velicer, W. F., & Rossi, J. S. (1993). Standardized, individualized, interactive and personalized self-help programs for smoking cessation. *Health Psychology*, *12*(5), 399–405. doi:10.1037/0278-6133.12.5.399 PMID:8223364

PSYCHE. (2010). *Personalised monitoring SYstems for Care in mental HEalth*. Retrieved from www.psyche-project.org

Pusztaszeri, M., Rossi, E. D., Auger, M., Baloch, Z., Bishop, J., Bongiovanni, M., . . . Faquin, W. C. (2016). The Bethesda System for Reporting Thyroid Cytopathology: Proposed Modifications and Updates for the Second Edition from an International Panel. Acta Cytol, 60(5), 399-405. doi:10.1159/000451020

PWC. (2012). *The power of the net generation*. PWC.

Qiang, C., Yamamichi, M., Hausman, V., & Altman, D. (2011). *Mobile Applications for the Health Sector. ICT Sector Unit*. The World Bank.

Raab, S. S., Zaleski, M. S., Thomas, P. A., Niemann, T. H., Isacson, C., & Jensen, C. S. (1996). Telecytology: Diagnostic accuracy in cervical-vaginal smears. *American Journal of Clinical Pathology*, *105*(5), 599–603. doi:10.1093/ajcp/105.5.599 PMID:8623769

Rachim, V. P., & Chung, W. Y. (2016). Wearable Noncontact Armband for Mobile ECG Monitoring System. *IEEE Transactions on Biomedical Circuits and Systems*, *10*(6), 1112–1118. doi:10.1109/TBCAS.2016.2519523 PMID:27214910

Raskovic, V., Denkovski, D., Atanasovski, V., & Gavrilovska, L. (2017). Cloud based solution for vital signs tracing. *Proceedings of 17th International conference on smart technologies*.

REACTION. (2010). *Remote Accessibility to Diabetes Management and Therapy in Operational healthcare Networks*. Retrieved from www.reaction-project.eu

Redman, B. K. (2005). The ethics of self management preparation for chronic illness. *Nursing Ethics*, *12*(4), 360–369. doi:10.1191/0969733005ne801oa PMID:16045244

Regenstrief Institute. (2018). LOINC: *The universal standard for identifying health measurements, observations, and documents*. Retrieved from https://loinc.org/

Reiter, E., & Sripanda, S. (2003). Acquiring correct knowledge from natural language generation. *Journal of Artificial Intelligence Research*, *18*, 491–516. doi:10.1613/jair.1176

Remmers, C., Hibbard, J., Mosen, D. M., Wagenfield, M., Hoye, R. E., & Jones, C. (2009). Is patient activation associated with future health outcomes and healthcare utilization among patients with diabetes? *The Journal of Ambulatory Care Management*, *32*(4), 320–327. doi:10.1097/JAC.0b013e3181ba6e77 PMID:19888008

RemPark. (2011). *Personal Health Device for the Remote and Autonomous Management of Parkinson's Disease*. Retrieved from www.rempark.eu

Renshaw, A. A. (2011). Quality improvement in cytology: Where do we go from here? *Archives of Pathology & Laboratory Medicine*, *135*(11), 1387–1390. doi:10.5858/arpa.2010-0606-RA PMID:22032562

research2guidance. (2012). *3rd mHealth Expert Survey*. research2guidance.

research2guidance. (2013). *Mobile Health Market Report 2013-2017. The commercialization of mHealth applications* (vol. 3). research2guidance.

research2guidance. (2015). *EU Countries' mHealth App Market Ranking 2015: Which EU countries are best for doing mHealth business*. research2guidance in partnership with mHealth Summit. research2guidance.

Respiratory rates statistics. (2018). Retrieved from https://www.aclsmedicaltraining.com/normal-values-in-children

Ribu, L., Holmen, H., Torbjornsen, A., Wahl, A. K., Grottland, A., Smastuen, M. C., ... Arsand, E. (2013). Low-intensity self-management intervention for persons with type 2 diabetes using a mobile phone-based diabetes diary, with and without health counseling and motivational interviewing: Protocol for a randomized controlled trial. *JMIR Research Protocols*, *2*(2), e34. doi:10.2196/resprot.2768 PMID:23978690

Richard, A., & Shea, K. (2011). Delineation of Self-care and AssociatedConcepts. *Journal of Nursing Scholarship*, *43*, 255–264. PMID:21884371

Richardson, A., & Ream, E. K. (1997). Self care behaviours initiated by chemotherapy patients in response to fatigue. *International Journal of Nursing Studies*, *34*(1), 35–43. doi:10.1016/S0020-7489(96)00031-4 PMID:9055119

Rienzo, M., Rizzo, F., Parati, G., Brambilla, F. M., & Castiglioni, P. (2005). MagIC system: A new textile-based wearable device for biological signal monitoring applicability in daily life and clinical setting. *Proceedings of the 27th Annual International IEEE EMBS Conference*, 7167–7169.

Riley, W. T., Cesar, A. M., & Rivera, D. E. (2014). *The importance of behavior theory in control system modeling of physical activity sensor data*. Paper presented at the 2014 36th Annual International Conference of the IEEE Engineering in Medicine and Biology Society.

Riley, W. T., & Rivera, D. E. (2014). Methodologies for optimizing behavioral interventions: Introduction to special section. *Translational Behavioral Medicine*, *4*(3), 234–237. doi:10.100713142-014-0281-0 PMID:25264463

Riley, W. T., Rivera, D. E., Atienza, A. A., Nilsen, W., Allison, S. M., & Mermelstein, R. (2011). Health behavior models in the age of mobile interventions: Are our theories up to the task? *Translational Behavioral Medicine*, *1*(1), 53–71. doi:10.100713142-011-0021-7 PMID:21796270

Rimer, B. K., Briss, P. A., Zeller, P. K., Chan, E. C., & Woolf, S. H. (2004). Informed decision making: What is its role in cancer screening? *Cancer*, *101*(5Suppl), 1214–1228. doi:10.1002/cncr.20512 PMID:15316908

Rimer, B. K., & Kreuter, M. W. (2006). Advancing tailored health communication: A persuasion and message effects perspective. *Journal of Communication*, *56*(s1), S184–S201. doi:10.1111/j.1460-2466.2006.00289.x

Rincon, E., Monteiro-Guerra, F., Rivera-Romero, O., Dorronzoro-Zubiete, E., Sanchez-Bocanegra, C. L., & Gabarron, E. (2017). Mobile Phone Apps for Quality of Life and Well-Being Assessment in Breast and Prostate Cancer Patients: Systematic Review. *JMIR mHealth and uHealth*, *5*(12), e187. doi:10.2196/mhealth.8741 PMID:29203459

Rippen, H., & Risk, A. (2000). eHealth Code of Ethics. *Journal of Medical Internet Research*, *2*(2), e9. doi:10.2196/jmir.2.2.e9

Roberts, K., Blethyn, K., Foreman, M., & Bleetman, A. (2009). Influence of air ambulance doctors on on-scene times, clinical interventions, decision-making and independent paramedic practice. *Emergency Medicine Journal*, *26*(2), 128–134. doi:10.1136/emj.2008.059899 PMID:19164630

Roberts, L., Little, P., Chapman, J., Cantrell, T., Pickering, R., & Langridge, J. (2010). The back home trial: General practitioner-supported leaflets may change back pain behavior. *Spine*, *27*(17), 1821–1828. doi:10.1097/00007632-200209010-00002 PMID:12221342

Robinson, T. N., Patrick, K., Eng, T. R., & Gustafson, D. (1998). An evidence-based approach to interactive health communication. *Journal of the American Medical Association*, *280*(14), 1264–1269. doi:10.1001/jama.280.14.1264 PMID:9786378

Robson, M. C., Cooper, D. M., Aslam, R., Gould, L. J., Harding, K. G., Margolis, D. J., ... Bryant, L. W. (2006). Guidelines for the treatment of venous ulcers. *Wound Repair and Regeneration*, *14*(6), 649–662. doi:10.1111/j.1524-475X.2006.00174.x PMID:17199831

Rodgers, A., Flowers, J., & Pencheon, D. (1999). Improving access needs a whole systems approach. *British Medical Journal*, *319*(7214), 866–867. doi:10.1136/bmj.319.7214.866 PMID:10506023

Roehrs, A., Da Costa, C. A., Da Rosa Righi, R., & De Oliveira, K. S. F. (2017). Personal health records: A systematic literature review. *Journal of Medical Internet Research*, *19*(1), e13. doi:10.2196/jmir.5876 PMID:28062391

Rogers, A., & Hay, S. (1998). Self-care and access to health care. In A. Rodgers & S. Hay (Eds.), *Opportunities for Improving Access to Care*. NHSE Anglia and Oxford Region Milton Keynes.

Rogers, E. M. (1986). *Communication Technology: The New Media in Society*. New York: The Free Press.

Rogers, R. W. (1985). Attitude Change and Information on Integration in Fear Appeals. *Psychological Reports*, *56*(1), 179–182. doi:10.2466/pr0.1985.56.1.179

Rojahn, S. (2014). *Why Some Doctors Like Google Glass So Much*. MIT Technology Review.

Roper, W. L. (1993). Health communication takes on new dimensions at CDC. *Public Health Reports*, *108*(2), 179–183. PMID:8385358

Rortgen, D., Bergrath, S., Rossaint, R., Beckers, S. K., Fischermann, H., Na, I. S., ... Skorning, M. (2013). Comparison of physician staffed emergency teams with paramedic teams assisted by telemedicine--a randomized, controlled simulation study. *Resuscitation*, *84*(1), 85–92. doi:10.1016/j.resuscitation.2012.06.012 PMID:22750663

Rosales Saurer, B., Mueller-Gorchs, M., & Kunze, C. (2009). Scenario-based design of an ICT platform for mobile information services in ambulatory care nursing. *Studies in Health Technology and Informatics*, *146*, 64–68. PMID:19592810

Rosenthal, A., Mork, P., Li, M. H., Stanford, J., Koester, D., & Reynolds, P. (2010). Cloud computing: A new business paradigm for biomedical information sharing. *Journal of Biomedical Informatics*, *43*(2), 342–353. doi:10.1016/j.jbi.2009.08.014 PMID:19715773

Ross, S. E., Moore, L. A., Earnest, M. A., Wittevrongel, L., & Lin, C.-T. (2004). Providing a web-based online medical record with electronic communication capabilities to patients with congestive heart failure: Randomized trial. *Journal of Medical Internet Research*, *6*(2), e12. doi:10.2196/jmir.6.2.e12 PMID:15249261

Roudsari, B., Nathens, A., Cameron, P., Civil, I., Gruen, R., Koepsell, T., ... Rivara, F. (2007). International comparison of prehospital trauma care systems. *Injury*, *38*(9), 993–1000. doi:10.1016/j.injury.2007.03.028 PMID:17640641

Roy, S., Pantanowitz, L., Amin, M., Seethala, R. R., Ishtiaque, A., Yousem, S. A., ... Hartman, D. J. (2014). Smartphone adapters for digital photomicrography. *Journal of Pathology Informatics*, *5*(1), 24. doi:10.4103/2153-3539.137728 PMID:25191623

Rudin, R. S., Fanta, C. H., Predmore, Z., Kron, K., Edelen, M. O., Landman, A. B., ... Bates, D. W. (2017). Core Components for a Clinically Integrated mHealth App for Asthma Symptom Monitoring. *Applied Clinical Informatics*, *8*(4), 1031–1043. doi:10.4338/ACI-2017-06-RA-0096 PMID:29241243

Rudnisky, C. J., Tennant, M. T., Weis, E., Ting, A., Hinz, B. J., & Greve, M. D. (2007). Web-based grading of compressed stereoscopic digital photography versus standard slide film photography for the diagnosis of diabetic retinopathy. *Ophthalmology*, *114*(9), 1748–1754. doi:10.1016/j.ophtha.2006.12.010 PMID:17368543

Ruland, C. M., Andersen, T., Jeneson, A., Moore, S., Grimsbø, G. H., Børøsund, E., & Ellison, M. C. (2013). Effects of an internet support system to assist cancer patients in reducing symptom distress: A randomized controlled trial. *Cancer Nursing*, *36*(1), 6–17. doi:10.1097/NCC.0b013e31824d90d4 PMID:22495503

Sahoo, P. K., Thakkar, H. K., & Lee, M. Y. (2017). A Cardiac Early Warning System with Multi Channel SCG and ECG Monitoring for Mobile Health. *Sensors (Basel)*, *17*(4), 711. doi:10.339017040711 PMID:28353681

Saini, D. K. (2012). Cyber Defense: Mathematical Modeling and Simulation. *International Journal of Applied Physics and Mathematics*, *2*(5), 312–315. doi:10.7763/IJAPM.2012.V2.121

Sakai, T., Kitamura, T., Nishiyama, C., Murakami, Y., Ando, M., Kawamura, T., ... Iwami, T. (2015). Cardiopulmonary resuscitation support application on a smartphone - randomized controlled trial. *Circulation Journal*, *79*(5), 1052–1057. doi:10.1253/circj.CJ-14-1258 PMID:25740350

Sakles, J. C., Mosier, J., Hadeed, G., Hudson, M., Valenzuela, T., & Latifi, R. (2011). Telemedicine and telepresence for prehospital and remote hospital tracheal intubation using a GlideScope videolaryngoscope: A model for tele-intubation. *Telemedicine Journal and e-Health*, *17*(3), 185–188. doi:10.1089/tmj.2010.0119 PMID:21443441

Sama, P. R., Eapen, Z. J., Weinfurt, K. P., Shah, B. R., & Schulman, K. A. (2014). An evaluation of mobile health application tools. *JMIR mHealth and uHealth*, *2*(2), e19. doi:10.2196/mhealth.3088 PMID:25099179

Samei, E., Badano, A., Chakraborty, D., Compton, K., Cornelius, C., Corrigan, K., ... Aapm, T. G. (2005). Assessment of display performance for medical imaging systems: Executive summary of AAPM TG18 report. *Medical Physics*, *32*(4), 1205–1225. doi:10.1118/1.1861159 PMID:15895604

Samoocha, D., Bruinvels, D. J., Elbers, N. A., Anema, J. R., & van der Beek, A. J. (2010). Effectiveness of web-based interventions on patient empowerment: A systematic review and meta-analysis. *Journal of Medical Internet Research*, *12*(2), e23. doi:10.2196/jmir.1286 PMID:20581001

Savolainen, R. (2008). *Everyday Information Practices. A Social Phenomenological Perspective*. Lanham, MD: Scarecrow.

Savolainen, R. (2009). Information use and information processing: Comparison of conceptualizations. *The Journal of Documentation*, *65*(2), 187–207. doi:10.1108/00220410910937570

Saw, S., Loh, T. P., Ang, S. B., Yip, J. W., & Sethi, S. K. (2011). Meeting regulatory requirements by the use of cell phone text message notification with autoescalation and loop closure for reporting of critical laboratory results. *American Journal of Clinical Pathology, 136*(1), 30–34. doi:10.1309/AJCPUZ53XZWQFYIS PMID:21685029

Schaffer, A. A., Simon, R., Desper, R., Richter, J., & Sauter, G. (2001). Tree models for dependent copy number changes in bladder cancer. *International Journal of Oncology, 18*(2), 349–354. PMID:11172603

Schepers, S. A., Sint Nicolaas, S. M., Maurice-Stam, H., Haverman, L., Verhaak, C. M., & Grootenhuis, M. A. (2018). Parental distress 6 months after a pediatric cancer diagnosis in relation to family psychosocial risk at diagnosis. *Cancer, 124*(2), 381–390. doi:10.1002/cncr.31023 PMID:28902391

Schiel, R., Kaps, A., & Bieber, G. (2012). Electronic health technology for the assessment of physical activity and eating habits in children and adolescents with overweight and obesity IDA. *Appetite, 58*(2), 432–437. doi:10.1016/j.appet.2011.11.021 PMID:22155072

Schwamm, L. H., Holloway, R. G., Amarenco, P., Audebert, H. J., Bakas, T., Chumbler, N. R., ... Wechsler, L. R. (2009). A review of the evidence for the use of telemedicine within stroke systems of care: A scientific statement from the American Heart Association/American Stroke Association. *Stroke, 40*(7), 2616–2634. doi:10.1161/STROKEAHA.109.192360 PMID:19423852

Schwarzer, R. (2008). Modeling health behavior change: How to predict and modify the adoption and maintenance of health behaviors. *Applied Psychology, 57*, 1–29.

Sciacovelli, L., Secchiero, S., Zardo, L., D'Osualdo, A., & Plebani, M. (2007). Risk management in laboratory medicine: Quality assurance programs and professional competence. *Clinical Chemistry and Laboratory Medicine, 45*(6), 756–765. doi:10.1515/CCLM.2007.165 PMID:17579529

ScoliosisManager. (2016). *Monitoring platform for scoliosis treatment to empower kids, parents, physicians and orthotists.* Retrieved Jan 15, 2017, from cordis.europa.eu/project/rcn/197418_en.html

Scottish Executive. (2003). *Partnership for Care: Scotland's Health White Paper.* Scottish Executive.

Scottish Executive. (2005a). *A National Service Framework for Service Change in the NHS in Scotland: Building a Health Service Fit for the Future.* Edinburgh, UK: Scottish Executive.

Scottish Executive. (2005b). *Delivering for Health.* Edinburgh, UK: Scottish Executive.

Seals, T. D., & Keith, M. R. (1997). Influence of patient information leaflets on anticonvulsant drug compliance in prison. *American Journal of Health-System Pharmacy, 54*(22), 2585–2587. PMID:9397219

Seguin, C., Blaquiere, G., Loundou, A., Michelet, P., & Markarian, T. (2018). Unmanned aerial vehicles (drones) to prevent drowning. *Resuscitation, 127*, 63–67. doi:10.1016/j.resuscitation.2018.04.005 PMID:29653153

Sepah, S. C., Jiang, L., & Peters, A. L. (2014). Translating the Diabetes Prevention Program into an Online Social Network:Validation against CDC Standards. *The Diabetes Educator, 40*(4), 435–443. doi:10.1177/0145721714531339 PMID:24723130

Sepah, S. C., Jiang, L., & Peters, A. L. (2015). Long-Term Outcomes of a Web-Based Diabetes Prevention Program: 2-Year Results of a Single-Arm Longitudinal Study. *Journal of Medical Internet Research, 17*(4), e92. doi:10.2196/jmir.4052 PMID:25863515

Sethares, K. A., & Elliott, K. (2004). The effect of a tailored message intervention on heart failure readmission rates, quality of life, and benefit and barrier beliefs in persons with heart failure. *Heart & Lung*, *33*(4), 249–260. doi:10.1016/j.hrtlng.2004.03.005 PMID:15252415

Shannon, P., Markiel, A., Ozier, O., Baliga, N. S., Wang, J. T., Ramage, D., ... Ideker, T. (2003). Cytoscape: A software environment for integrated models of biomolecular interaction networks. *Genome Research*, *13*(11), 2498–2504. doi:10.1101/gr.1239303 PMID:14597658

Shapiro, J. R., Bauer, S., Hamer, R. M., Kordy, H., Ward, D., & Bulik, C. M. (2008). Use of Text Messaging for Monitoring Sugar-sweetened Beverages, Physical Activity, and Screen Time in Children: A Pilot Study. *Journal of Nutrition Education and Behavior*, *40*(6), 385–391. doi:10.1016/j.jneb.2007.09.014 PMID:18984496

Sharifi, M., Dryden, E. M., Horan, C. M., Price, S., Marshall, R., Hacker, K., ... Taveras, E. M. (2013). Leveraging text messaging and mobile technology to support pediatric obesity-related behavior change: A qualitative study using parent focus groups and interviews. *Journal of Medical Internet Research*, *15*(12), e272. doi:10.2196/jmir.2780 PMID:24317406

Sharma, P., & Kamal, V. (2006). A novel application of mobile phone cameras in undergraduate pathology education. *Medical Teacher*, *28*(8), 745–746. PMID:17642089

Sharp, R. (2012). *Lacking regulation, many medical apps questionable at best.* Retrieved 5 15, 2015, from The New England Center for Investigative Reporting, Boston University: necir.org/2012/11/18/medical-apps/

Sheeran, P. (2005). Intention–Behavior Relations: A Conceptual and Empirical Review. In W. Stroebe & M. Hewstone (Eds.), *European Review of Social Psychology*. Chichester, UK: John Wiley & Sons. doi:10.1002/0470013478.ch1

Sheikh, A., Cresswell, K., Wright, A., & Bates, D. (2017). *Key Advances in Clinical Informatics: Transforming Health Care through Health Information Technology*. Academic Press.

Sheltami, T., Mahmoud, A., & Abu, A. (2006). Warning and monitoring medical system using sensor networks. *18th National Computer Conference*, 63-68.

Shen, Z., & Yang, Z. (2001). The problems and strategy relevant to the quality management of clinical laboratories. *Clinical Chemistry and Laboratory Medicine*, *39*(12), 1216–1218. doi:10.1515/CCLM.2001.194 PMID:11798079

Sherman, M. E., Dasgupta, A., Schiffman, M., Nayar, R., & Solomon, D. (2007). The Bethesda Interobserver Reproducibility Study (BIRST): A web-based assessment of the Bethesda 2001 System for classifying cervical cytology. *Cancer*, *111*(1), 15–25. doi:10.1002/cncr.22423 PMID:17186503

Sheyner, O. M. (2004). *Scenario Graphs and Attack Graphs*. Pittsburgh, PA: Carnegie Mellon University.

Shnayder, V., Chen, B., Lorincz, K., Jones, T., & Welsh, M. (2005). Sensor networks for medical care, *3rd International Conference on Embedded Networked Sensor Systems*. 10.1145/1098918.1098979

Siebenhofer, A., Rakovac, I., Kleespies, C., Piso, B., & Didjurgeit, U. (2008). Self-management of oral anticoagulation reduces major outcomes in the elderly. A randomized controlled trial. *Thrombosis and Haemostasis*, *100*(6), 1089–1098. PMID:19132235

Silhousette, T. M. (2010). *Advanced wound assessment and management system*. Retrieved from http://www.aranzmedical.com

Silva, D. (2014). *Helping measure person-centred care: A review of evidence about commonly used approaches and tools used to help measure person-centred care*. London: The Health Foundation.

Simoni, J. M., Huh, D., Frick, P. A., Pearson, C. R., Andrasik, M. P., Dunbar, P. J., & Hooton, T. M. (2009). Peer support and pager messaging to promote antiretroviral modifying therapy in Seattle: A randomized controlled trial. *JAIDS Journal of Acquired Immune Deficiency Syndromes*, *52*(4), 465–473. doi:10.1097/QAI.0b013e3181b9300c PMID:19911481

Skandarajah, A., Reber, C. D., Switz, N. A., & Fletcher, D. A. (2014). Quantitative imaging with a mobile phone microscope. *PLoS One*, *9*(5), e96906. doi:10.1371/journal.pone.0096906 PMID:24824072

Skeate, R. C., Wahi, M. M., Jessurun, J., & Connelly, D. P. (2007). Personal digital assistant-enabled report content knowledgebase results in more complete pathology reports and enhances resident learning. *Human Pathology*, *38*(12), 1727–1735. doi:10.1016/j.humpath.2007.05.019 PMID:17949779

Skinner, C. S., Strecher, V. J., & Hospers, H. (1994). Physician recommendations for mammography: Do tailored messages make a difference? *American Journal of Public Health*, *84*(1), 43–49. doi:10.2105/AJPH.84.1.43 PMID:8279610

Skoudis, E. (2004). *Malware Fighting malicious code. Computer Networking and Distribution Systems*. Prentice Hall.

SMART®. (2018). *An App Platform for Healthcare*. Retrieved from https://smarthealthit.org/

SMART4MD. (2015). *(S) Support (M) Monitoring (A) And (R) Reminder (T) Technology (4) for (M) Mild (D) Dementia*. Retrieved Jan 13, 2017, from www.smart4md.eu/

Smith, J. J., Morgan, P. J., Plotnikoff, R. C., Dally, K. A., Salmon, J., Okely, A. D., ... Lubans, D. R. (2014). Smart-Phone Obesity Prevention Trial for Adolescent Boys in Low-Income Communities: The ATLAS RCT. *Pediatrics*, *134*(3), e723–e731. doi:10.1542/peds.2014-1012 PMID:25157000

SNOMED International. (2018). *SNOMED CT: The Global Language of Healthcare*. Retrieved from https://www.snomed.org/snomed-ct

Snyder, R. J. (2005). Treatment of non-healing ulcers with allografts. *Clinics in Dermatology*, *23*(4), 388–395. doi:10.1016/j.clindermatol.2004.07.020 PMID:16023934

Soderhamn, O. (2000). Self care activity as a structure: A phenomenological approach. *Scandinavian Journal of Occupational Therapy*, *7*(4), 183–189. doi:10.1080/110381200300008724

Sofia, N., & Rabiah, A. (2011). Surveying the wireless body area network in the realm of wireless communication. *IEEE 7th International Conference on Information Assurance and Security*.

Sohn, J., Do, K. A., Liu, S., Chen, H., Mills, G. B., Hortobagyi, G. N., ... Gonzalez-Angulo, A. M. (2013). Functional proteomics characterization of residual triple-negative breast cancer after standard neoadjuvant chemotherapy. *Annals of Oncology: Official Journal of the European Society for Medical Oncology*, *24*(10), 2522–2526. doi:10.1093/annonc/mdt248 PMID:23925999

Solomon, D., Davey, D., Kurman, R., Moriarty, A., O'Connor, D., Prey, M., ... Young, N. (2002). The 2001 Bethesda System: Terminology for reporting results of cervical cytology. *Journal of the American Medical Association*, *287*(16), 2114–2119. doi:10.1001/jama.287.16.2114 PMID:11966386

SONY. (2010). *Sony Develops a "Rollable" OTFT*1-driven OLED Display that can wrap around a Pencil*. Retrieved 24 May, 2015, from http://www.sony.net/SonyInfo/News/Press/201005/10-070E/

Sound of Vision. (2015). *Sound of Vision: Natural sense of vision through acoustics and haptics*. Retrieved Jan 10, 2017, from www.soundofvision.net

Spat, S., Holl, B., Petritsch, G., Schaupp, L., Beck, P., & Pieber, T. R. (2013). Automatic system testing of a decision support system for insulin dosing using Google Android. *Studies in Health Technology and Informatics*, *186*, 187–191. PMID:23542995

Splendid. (2013). *Personalised Guide for Eating and Activity Behaviour for the Prevention of Obesity and Eating Disorders*. Retrieved from splendid-program.eu

Sprigle, S., Nirmal, P., Aditya, J., & Thad, S. (2006). Handheld, non-contact wound measurement device. *Clinical Symposium on Advances in Skin & Wound care*, 379.

Stallings, W. (2011). *Cryptography and network Security*. Pearson Education Inc.

Stamataki, M., Anninos, D., Brountzos, E., Georgoulakis, J., Panayiotides, J., Christoni, Z., ... Karakitsos, P. (2008). The role of liquid-based cytology in the investigation of thyroid lesions. *Cytopathology*, *19*(1), 11–18. doi:10.1111/j.1365-2303.2007.00512.x PMID:17986263

Statista. (2015). *Smartphone penetration worldwide 2008-2014*. Retrieved Jan 10, 2017, from Statista, The Statistics Portal: www.statista.com/statistics/218532/global-smartphone-penetration-since-2008/

Statista. (2015). *Value of the global mHealth (mobile health) market 2012-2020 (fee-based)*. Retrieved 5 7, 2015, from Statista. The Statistics Portal: http://www.statista.com/statistics/295771/mhealth-global-market-size/

Statista. (2016). *The Statistics Portal*. Retrieved 1 8, 2017, from Number of smartphone users worldwide from 2014 to 2020 (in billions): www.statista.com/statistics/330695/number-of-smartphone-users-worldwide/

Statista. (2018). *The Statistics Portal*. Retrieved from mHealth (mobile health) industry market size projection from 2012 to 2020 (in billion U.S. dollars): https://www.statista.com/statistics/295771/mhealth-global-market-size

Statista. (2018). *The Statistics portal*. Retrieved from Mobile phone users worldwide 2015-2020: https://www.statista.com/statistics/274774/forecast-of-mobile-phone-users-worldwide/

Steg, P., James, S., Atar, D., Badano, L., Lundqvist, C., Borger, M., ... Wallentin, L. (2012). ESC Guidelines for the management of acute myocardial infarction in patients presenting with ST-segment elevation: The Task Force on the management of ST-segment elevation acute myocardial infarction of the European Society of Cardiology (ESC). *European Heart Journal*. doi:10.1093/eurheartj/ehs215

Stephens, J., & Allen, J. (2013). Mobile phone interventions to increase physical activity and reduce weight: A systematic review. *The Journal of Cardiovascular Nursing*, *28*(4), 320–329. doi:10.1097/JCN.0b013e318250a3e7 PMID:22635061

Stergiou, N., Georgoulakis, G., Margari, N., Aninos, D., Stamataki, M., Stergiou, E., ... Karakitsos, P. (2009). Using a web-based system for the continuous distance education in cytopathology. *International Journal of Medical Informatics*, *78*(12), 827–838. doi:10.1016/j.ijmedinf.2009.08.007 PMID:19775933

Stewart, M., Brown, J. B., Donner, A., McWhinney, I. R., Oates, J., Weston, W. W., & ... . (2000). The impact of patient-centered care on outcomes. *The Journal of Family Practice*, *49*(9), 796–804. PMID:11032203

Stinson, J. N., McGrath, P. J., Hodnett, E. D., Feldman, B. M., Duffy, C. M., Huber, A. M., ... White, M. E. (2010). An internet-based self-management program with telephone support for adolescents with arthritis: A pilot randomized controlled trial. *The Journal of Rheumatology*, *37*(9), 1944–1952. doi:10.3899/jrheum.091327 PMID:20595280

Stinson, J., McGrath, P., Hodnett, E., Feldman, B., Duffy, C., Huber, A., ... White, M. (2010). Usability Testing of an Online Self-management Program for Adolescents With Juvenile Idiopathic Arthritis. *Journal of Medical Internet Research*, *12*(3), e30. doi:10.2196/jmir.1349 PMID:20675293

Stone, A. A., Shiffman, S., Schwartz, J. E., Broderick, J. E., & Hufford, M. R. (2003). Patient compliance with paper and electronic diaries. *Controlled Clinical Trials, 24*(2), 182–199. doi:10.1016/S0197-2456(02)00320-3 PMID:12689739

Stoyanov, S. R., Hides, L., Kavanagh, D. J., Zelenko, O., Tjondronegoro, D., & Mani, M. (2015). Mobile app rating scale: A new tool for assessing the quality of health mobile apps. *JMIR mHealth and uHealth, 3*(1), e27. doi:10.2196/mhealth.3422 PMID:25760773

Strecher, V. J., Kreuter, M. W., Den Boer, D.-J., Kobrin, S., Hospers, H. J., & Skinner, C. S. (1994). The effects of computer-tailored smoking cessation messages in family practice settings. *The Journal of Family Practice, 39*, 262–270. PMID:8077905

Suggs, L. S., Cowdery, J. E., & Carroll, J. B. (2006). Tailored program evaluation: Past, present, future. *Evaluation and Program Planning, 29*(4), 426–432. doi:10.1016/j.evalprogplan.2006.08.003 PMID:17950872

Sun, D., & Hu, T. Y. (2018). A low cost mobile phone dark-field microscope for nanoparticle-based quantitative studies. *Biosensors & Bioelectronics, 99*, 513–518. doi:10.1016/j.bios.2017.08.025 PMID:28823976

Supporting, L. I. F. E. (2017). *Supporting LIFE: Fighting Child Mortality*. Retrieved Jan 5, 2017, from http://www.supportinglife.eu

Sutton, C., & Vatavuk, J. (2014). *The journey from self-care management to virtual care for all.* Retrieved July 20, 2018, from https://www.telushealth.co/item/the-journey-from-self-care-management-to-virtual-care-for-all/

Swedish Agency for Health and Care Services Analysis (2012). *Patient centeredness in Sweden's health system- an external assessment and six steps for progress.* Author.

Swinburn, B. A., Sacks, G., Lo, S. K., Westerterp, K. R., Rush, E. C., Rosenbaum, M., ... Ravussin, E. (2009). Estimating the changes in energy flux that characterize the rise in obesity prevalence. *The American Journal of Clinical Nutrition, 89*(6), 1723–1728. doi:10.3945/ajcn.2008.27061 PMID:19369382

Talja, S., Tuominen, K., & Savolainen, R. (2005). Isms in information science: Constructivism, collectivism and constructionism. *The Journal of Documentation, 61*(1), 70–101. doi:10.1108/00220410510578023

Tate, D. F., Finkelstein, E. A., Khavjou, O., & Gustafson, A. (2009). Cost effectiveness of Internet interventions: Review and recommendations. *Annals of Behavioral Medicine, 38*(1), 40–45. doi:10.100712160-009-9131-6 PMID:19834778

Tate, D. F., Wing, R. R., & Winett, R. A. (2001). Using internet technology to deliver a behavioral weight loss program. *Journal of the American Medical Association, 285*(9), 1172–1177. doi:10.1001/jama.285.9.1172 PMID:11231746

Tate, E. B., Spruijt-Metz, D., O'Reilly, G., Jordan-Marsh, M., Gotsis, M., Pentz, M. A., & Dunton, G. F. (2013). mHealth approaches to child obesity prevention: Successes, unique challenges, and next directions. *Translational Behavioral Medicine, 3*(4), 406–415. doi:10.100713142-013-0222-3 PMID:24294329

Tawfik, O., Davis, M., Dillon, S., Tawfik, L., Diaz, F. J., & Fan, F. (2014). Whole Slide Imaging of Pap Cell Block Preparations versus Liquid-Based Thin-Layer Cervical Cytology: A Comparative Study Evaluating the Detection of Organisms and Nonneoplastic Findings. *Acta Cytologica, 58*(4), 388–397. doi:10.1159/000365046 PMID:25033897

Taylor, C. R. (2011). From microscopy to whole slide digital images: A century and a half of image analysis. *Applied Immunohistochemistry & Molecular Morphology, 19*(6), 491–493. doi:10.1097/PAI.0b013e318229ffd6 PMID:22089486

Te'eni, D. (2001). Review: A cognitive-affective model of organizational communication for designing IT. *MIS Quaterly, 25*(2), 251–312. doi:10.2307/3250931

Teel, S., Meek, P., McNamura, A., & Watson, V. (1997). Perspectives unifying symptom interpretations. *Image Journal of Scholarly Inquiry*, *29*, 175–181. PMID:9212516

Teixeira, P. J., Carraça, E. V., Marques, M. M., Rutter, H., Oppert, J.-M., De Bourdeaudhuij, I., ... Brug, J. (2015). Successful behavior change in obesity interventions in adults: A systematic review of self-regulation mediators. *BMC Medicine*, *13*(1), 84. doi:10.118612916-015-0323-6 PMID:25907778

Thawer, H. A., Houghton, P. E., Woodbury, G., Keast, D., & Campbell, K. A. (2002). Comparison of computer-assisted and manual wound size measurement. *Ostomy/Wound Management*, *48*, 46–53. PMID:12378003

The Apache Software Foundation. (2018). *Apache Tomcat web site*. Retrieved May 8, 2018, from http://tomcat.apache.org/

The European Stroke Organisation Executive. (2008). Guidelines for Management of Ischaemic Stroke and Transient Ischaemic Attack 2008. *Cerebrovascular Diseases (Basel, Switzerland)*, *25*(5), 457–507. doi:10.1159/000131083 PMID:18477843

The Statistics Portal. (2018). *Global digital health market from 2015 to 2020, by major segment (in billion U.S. dollars)*. Retrieved July 27, 2018, from https://www.statista.com/statistics/387867/value-of-worldwide-digital-health-market-forecast-by-segment/

Thelen, S., Schneiders, M., Schilberg, D., & Jeschke, S. (2013). *A Multifunctional Telemedicine System for Pre-hospital Emergency Medical Services*. Paper presented at the eTELEMED 2013, The Fifth International Conference on eHealth, Telemedicine, and Social Medicine.

TheWorldBank. (2012). 2012 Information and Communications for Development: Maximizing Mobile. The World Bank.

TheWorldBank. (2015). *Indicators*. Retrieved 5 11, 2015, from The World Bank. IBRD-IDA: http://data.worldbank.org/indicator?display=graph

Thiels, C. A., Aho, J. M., Zietlow, S. P., & Jenkins, D. H. (2015). Use of unmanned aerial vehicles for medical product transport. *Air Medical Journal*, *34*(2), 104–108. doi:10.1016/j.amj.2014.10.011 PMID:25733117

Thies, K., Anderson, D., & Cramer, B. (2017). Lack of Adoption of a Mobile App to Support Patient Self-Management of Diabetes and Hypertension in a Federally Qualified Health Center: Interview Analysis of Staff and Patients in a Failed Randomized Trial. *JMIR Human Factors*, *4*(4), e24. doi:10.2196/humanfactors.7709 PMID:28974481

Thingspeak. (2018). Retrieved from https://thingspeak.com/

Thompson, D. (2014). What Serious Video Games Can Offer Child Obesity Prevention. *JMIR Serious Games*, *2*(2), e8. doi:10.2196/games.3480 PMID:25654589

Thompson, D., Baranowski, T., Buday, R., Baranowski, J., Thompson, V., Jago, R., & Griffith, M. J. (2010). Serious Video Games for Health: How Behavioral Science Guided the Development of a Serious Video Game. *Simulation & Gaming*, *41*(4), 587–606. doi:10.1177/1046878108328087 PMID:20711522

Thomson, B. (n.d.). *FDA Regulation of Mobile Health* (2nd ed.). Chester Street Publishing, Inc.

Thorne, S., Paterson, B., & Russell, C. (2003). The structure of everyday self-care decision making in chronic illness. *Qualitative Health Research*, *13*(10), 1337–1352. doi:10.1177/1049732303258039 PMID:14658350

Thrall, M., Pantanowitz, L., & Khalbuss, W. (2011). Telecytology: Clinical applications, current challenges, and future benefits. *Journal of Pathology Informatics*, *2*(1), 51. doi:10.4103/2153-3539.91129 PMID:22276242

Toomey, R. J., Ryan, J. T., McEntee, M. F., Evanoff, M. G., Chakraborty, D. P., McNulty, J. P., ... Brennan, P. C. (2010). Diagnostic efficacy of handheld devices for emergency radiologic consultation. *AJR. American Journal of Roentgenology, 194*(2), 469–474. doi:10.2214/AJR.09.3418 PMID:20093611

Topol, E. J. (2012). *The creative destruction of medicine: how the digital revolution will create better health care.* New York: Basic Books.

Torbjornsen, A., Smastuen, M. C., Jenum, A. K., Arsand, E., & Ribu, L. (2018). Acceptability of an mHealth App Intervention for Persons With Type 2 Diabetes and its Associations With Initial Self-Management: Randomized Controlled Trial. *JMIR mHealth and uHealth, 6*(5), e125. doi:10.2196/mhealth.8824 PMID:29784635

Torres-Cabala, C., Bibbo, M., Panizo-Santos, A., Barazi, H., Krutzsch, H., Roberts, D. D., & Merino, M. J. (2006). Proteomic identification of new biomarkers and application in thyroid cytology. *Acta Cytologica, 50*(5), 518–528. doi:10.1159/000326006 PMID:17017437

Toscos, T., & Connelly, K. (2010). Using behavior change theory to understand and guide technological interventions. In B. M. Hayes & A. William (Eds.), *Health Informatics: A patient-centered approach to diabetes* (pp. 295–326). Cambridge, MA: MIT Press. doi:10.7551/mitpress/9780262014328.003.0011

Travis, P., Bennett, S., Haines, A., Pang, T., Butta, Z., Hyder, A., ... Evans, T. (2004). Overcoming health-systems constraints to achieve the Millennium Development Goals. *Lancet, 364*(9437), 900–906. doi:10.1016/S0140-6736(04)16987-0 PMID:15351199

Triola, M. M., & Holloway, W. J. (2011). Enhanced virtual microscopy for collaborative education. *BMC Medical Education, 11*(1), 4. doi:10.1186/1472-6920-11-4 PMID:21269474

Tsilalis, T., Archondakis, S., Meristoudis, C., Margari, N., Pouliakis, A., Skagias, L., ... Karakitsos, P. (2012). Assessment of Static Telecytological Diagnoses' Reproducibility in Cervical Smears Prepared by Means of Liquid-Based Cytology. *Telemedicine Journal and e-Health, 18*(7), 516–520. doi:10.1089/tmj.2011.0167 PMID:22856666

Tsiouris, K. M., Gatsios, D., Rigas, G., Miljkovic, D., Korousic Seljak, B., Bohanec, M., ... Fotiadis, D. I. (2017). PD_Manager: An mHealth platform for Parkinson's disease patient management. *Healthc Technol Lett, 4*(3), 102–108. doi:10.1049/htl.2017.0007 PMID:28706727

Tufano, J. T., & Karras, B. T. (2005). Mobile eHealth Interventions for Obesity: A Timely Opportunity to Leverage Convergence Trends. *Journal of Medical Internet Research, 7*(5), e58. doi:10.2196/jmir.7.5.e58 PMID:16403722

Turner, T., & Spruijt-Metz, D. (2015). *Prevention and treatment of pediatric obesity using mobile and wireless technologies: a systematic review.* Academic Press. doi:10.1111/ijpo.12002

Turner, A., Karube, I., & Wilson, G. S. (Eds.). (1987). *Biosensors: Fundamentals and Applications* (1st ed.). Oxford, UK: Oxford University Press.

UN, D. o. (2017). The 2017 Revision, Key Findings and Advance Tables. *World Population Prospects.*

Union, P. O. (Ed.). (n.d.). *EU Open Data Portal.* Retrieved December 4, 2016, from European Union Open Data Portal: http://data.europa.eu/euodp/en/data

UnwiredHealth. (2014). *UnwiredHealth EU Project Official web page.* Retrieved from http://www.unwiredhealth.eu

Uppal, D. S., & Powell, S. M. (2013). Genetics/genomics/proteomics of gastric adenocarcinoma. *Gastroenterology Clinics of North America, 42*(2), 241–260. doi:10.1016/j.gtc.2013.01.005 PMID:23639639

US Institute of Medicine. (2001). *Crossing The Quality Chasm: A New Health System For The 21st Century*. Washington, DC: National Academy Press.

Vacata, V., Jahns-Streubel, G., Baldus, M., & Wood, W. G. (2007). Practical solution for control of the pre-analytical phase in decentralized clinical laboratories for meeting the requirements of the medical laboratory accreditation standard DIN EN ISO 15189. *Clinical Laboratory*, *53*(3-4), 211–215. PMID:17447659

Vaisanen, O., Makijarvi, M., & Silfvast, T. (2003). Prehospital ECG transmission: Comparison of advanced mobile phone and facsimile devices in an urban Emergency Medical Service System. *Resuscitation*, *57*(2), 179–185. doi:10.1016/S0300-9572(03)00028-5 PMID:12745186

Valderas, J. M., Kotzeva, A., Espallargues, M., Guyatt, G., Ferrans, C. E., Halyard, M. Y., ... Alonso, J. (2008). The impact of measuring patient-reported outcomes in clinical practice: A systematic review of the literature. *Quality of Life Research: An International Journal of Quality of Life Aspects of Treatment, Care and Rehabilitation*, *17*(2), 179–193. doi:10.100711136-007-9295-0 PMID:18175207

Valenzuela Espinoza, A., De Smedt, A., Guldolf, K., Vandervorst, F., Van Hooff, R. J., Fernandez Tellez, H., ... Brouns, R. (2016). Opinions and Beliefs About Telemedicine for Emergency Treatment During Ambulance Transportation and for Chronic Care at Home. *Interactive Journal of Medical Research*, *5*(1), e9. doi:10.2196/ijmr.5015 PMID:27029999

Valenzuela Espinoza, A., Devos, S., van Hooff, R. J., Fobelets, M., Dupont, A., Moens, M., ... Putman, K. (2017). Time Gain Needed for In-Ambulance Telemedicine: Cost-Utility Model. *JMIR mHealth and uHealth*, *5*(11), e175. doi:10.2196/mhealth.8288 PMID:29175808

Valenzuela Espinoza, A., Van Hooff, R. J., De Smedt, A., Moens, M., Yperzeele, L., Nieboer, K., ... Brouns, R. (2016). Development and Pilot Testing of 24/7 In-Ambulance Telemedicine for Acute Stroke: Prehospital Stroke Study at the Universitair Ziekenhuis Brussel-Project. *Cerebrovascular Diseases (Basel, Switzerland)*, *42*(1-2), 15–22. doi:10.1159/000444175 PMID:26950076

van Boeijen, C. A., & ... . (2005). Efficacy of self-help manuals for anxiety disorders in primary care: A systematic review. *Family Practice*, *22*(2), 192–196. doi:10.1093/fampra/cmh708 PMID:15710643

van Heerden, A., Tomlinson, M., & Swartz, L. (2012). Point of care in your pocket: A research agenda for the field of m-health. *Bulletin of the World Health Organization*, *90*(5), 393–394. doi:10.2471/BLT.11.099788

Van Hooff, R. J., Cambron, M., Van Dyck, R., De Smedt, A., Moens, M., Espinoza, A. V., ... Brouns, R. (2013). Pre-hospital unassisted assessment of stroke severity using telemedicine: A feasibility study. *Stroke*, *44*(10), 2907–2909. doi:10.1161/STROKEAHA.113.002079 PMID:23920013

Varlatzidou, A., Pouliakis, A., Stamataki, M., Meristoudis, C., Margari, N., Peros, G., ... Karakitsos, P. (2011). Cascaded learning vector quantizer neural networks for the discrimination of thyroid lesions. *Analytical and Quantitative Cytology and Histology*, *33*(6), 323–334. PMID:22590810

VitalWaveConsulting. (2009). mHealth for Development: The Opportunity of Mobile Technology for Healthcare in the Developing World. UN Foundation-Vodafone Foundation Partnership.

VivoMetrics. (2002). Three More Studies Use LifeShirt System to Assess Treatment Protocols, Ambulatory Intelligence. *The Journal of Ambulatory Monitoring*, *1*(1).

Vlachopapadopoulou, E., & Fotiadis, D. (2016). The Contribution of mHealth in the Care of Obese Pediatric Patients. In M. Anastasius (Ed.), *M-Health Innovations for Patient-Centered Care* (pp. 126–146). Hershey, PA: IGI Global. doi:10.4018/978-1-4666-9861-1.ch007

Vlasnik, J. J., Aliotta, S. L., & DeLor, B. (2005). Medication adherence: Factors influencing compliance with prescribed medication plans. *The Case Manager*, *16*(2), 47–51. doi:10.1016/j.casemgr.2005.01.009 PMID:15818344

Vooijs, G. P., Davey, D. D., Somrak, T. M., Goodell, R. M., Grohs, D. H., Knesel, E. A. Jr, ... Wilbur, D. C. (1998). Computerized training and proficiency testing. International Academy of Cytology Task Force summary. Diagnostic Cytology Towards the 21st Century: An International Expert Conference and Tutorial. *Acta Cytologica*, *42*(1), 141–147. doi:10.1159/000331539 PMID:9479333

Vriesema, J. L., van der Poel, H. G., Debruyne, F. M., Schalken, J. A., Kok, L. P., & Boon, M. E. (2000). Neural network-based digitized cell image diagnosis of bladder wash cytology. *Diagnostic Cytopathology*, *23*(3), 171–179. doi:10.1002/1097-0339(200009)23:3<171::AID-DC6>3.0.CO;2-F PMID:10945904

Wadden, T. A., & Butryn, M. L. (2003). Behavioral treatment of obesity. *Endocrinology and Metabolism Clinics of North America*, *32*(4), 981–1003. doi:10.1016/S0889-8529(03)00072-0 PMID:14711071

Wagner, E., Davis, C., Shaefer, J., Von Korff, M., & Austin, B. (2002). A survey of leading chronic disease management programs: Are they consistent with literature? *Journal of Nursing Care Quality*, *16*(2), 67–80. doi:10.1097/00001786-200201000-00008

Wall, D. P., Kudtarkar, P., Fusaro, V. A., Pivovarov, R., Patil, P., & Tonellato, P. J. (2010). Cloud computing for comparative genomics. *BMC Bioinformatics*, *11*(1), 259. doi:10.1186/1471-2105-11-259 PMID:20482786

Wandling, M. W., Nathens, A. B., Shapiro, M. B., & Haut, E. R. (2016). Police transport versus ground EMS: A trauma system-level evaluation of prehospital care policies and their effect on clinical outcomes. *The Journal of Trauma and Acute Care Surgery*, *81*(5), 931–935. doi:10.1097/TA.0000000000001228 PMID:27537514

Wang, J., Wang, Y., Wei, C., Yao, N., Yuan, A., Shan, Y., & Yuan, C. (2014). Smartphone interventions for long-term health management of chronic diseases: An integrative review. *Telemedicine Journal and e-Health*, *20*(6), 570–583. doi:10.1089/tmj.2013.0243 PMID:24787747

Wang, Y., Xue, H., Huang, Y., Huang, L., & Zhang, D. (2017). A Systematic Review of Application and Effectiveness of mHealth Interventions for Obesity and Diabetes Treatment and Self-Management. *Advances in Nutrition*, *8*(3), 449–462. doi:10.3945/an.116.014100 PMID:28507010

Warner, J. L., Rioth, M. J., Mandl, K. D., Mandel, J. C., Kreda, D. A., Kohane, I. S., ... Yao, H. (2016). SMART precision cancer medicine: A FHIR-based app to provide genomic information at the point of care. *Journal of the American Medical Informatics Association*, *23*(4), 701–710. doi:10.1093/jamia/ocw015 PMID:27018265

Waxer, N., Ninan, D., Ma, A., & Dominguez, N. (2013). How cloud computing and social media are changing the face of health care. *Physician Executive*, *39*(2), 58–60, 62. PMID:23621068

Webb, G. (2012). Making the cloud work for healthcare: Cloud computing offers incredible opportunities to improve healthcare, reduce costs and accelerate ability to adopt new IT services. *Health Management Technology*, *33*(2), 8–9. PMID:22397112

Webb, T. L., Joseph, J., Yardley, L., & Michie, S. (2010). Using the Internet to promote health behavior change: A systematic review and meta-analysis of the impact of theoretical basis, use of behavior change techniques, and mode of delivery on efficacy. *Journal of Medical Internet Research*, *12*(1), e4. doi:10.2196/jmir.1376 PMID:20164043

Webb, T. L., & Sheeran, P. (2006). Does change behavioral intentions engender behavior change? A meta-analysis of the experimental evidence. *Psychological Bulletin*, *132*(2), 249–268. doi:10.1037/0033-2909.132.2.249 PMID:16536643

Weber, J., & Porotte, F. (2006). Medical remote monitoring with clothes. *International Workshop on PHealth.*

Weerakkody, V., El-Haddadeh, R., Chochliouros, I., & Morris, D. (2012). Utilizing a High Definition Live Video Platform to Facilitate Public Service Delivery. In L. Iliadis, I. Maglogiannis, H. Papadopoulos, K. Karatzas, & S. Sioutas (Eds.), *Artificial Intelligence Applications and Innovations* (Vol. 382, pp. 290–299). Springer Berlin Heidelberg. doi:10.1007/978-3-642-33412-2_30

Weinstein, L. J., Epstein, J. I., Edlow, D., & Westra, W. H. (1997). Static image analysis of skin specimens: The application of telepathology to frozen section evaluation. *Human Pathology*, *28*(1), 30–35. doi:10.1016/S0046-8177(97)90275-6 PMID:9013828

Weinstein, N. D. (1993). Testing four competing theories of health-protective behavior. *Health Psychology*, *12*(4), 324–333. doi:10.1037/0278-6133.12.4.324 PMID:8404807

Welcome. (2013). *Wearable Sensing and Smart Cloud Computing for Integrated Care to COPD Patients with Comorbidities*. Retrieved from www.welcome-project.eu

Wen, T., Zhang, Z., & Wong, K. K. (2016). Multi-Objective Algorithm for Blood Supply via Unmanned Aerial Vehicles to the Wounded in an Emergency Situation. *PLoS One*, *11*(5), e0155176. doi:10.1371/journal.pone.0155176 PMID:27163361

Westbrook, J. I., Georgiou, A., & Rob, M. I. (2008). Computerised order entry systems: Sustained impact on laboratory efficiency and mortality rates? *Studies in Health Technology and Informatics*, *136*, 345–350. PMID:18487755

Whitten, J., Bentley, L., & Dittman, K. (2004). *Fundamentals of system analysis and design methods.* Academic Press.

WHO & UNICEF. (2010). *Countdown to 2015: Taking stock of maternal, newborn and child survival. 2000-2010 Decade Report.* World Health Organization and UNICEF.

WHO. (2010). *Injuries and violence: the facts*. Geneva: WHO.

WHO. (2011). mHealth. New horizons for health through mobile technologies: Based on the findings of the second global survey on eHealth (Vol. 3). World Health Organization.

WHO. (2014). *The top 10 causes of death* (Vol. Fact sheet N°310, pp. 5). World Health Organization.

Wichansky, A. M. (2000). Usability testing in 2000 and beyond. *Ergonomics*, *43*(7), 998–1006. doi:10.1080/001401300409170 PMID:10929833

Wiechmann, W., Kwan, D., Bokarius, A., & Toohey, S. L. (2016). There's an App for That? Highlighting the Difficulty in Finding Clinically Relevant Smartphone Applications. *The Western Journal of Emergency Medicine*, *17*(2), 191–194. doi:10.5811/westjem.2015.12.28781 PMID:26973750

WikiPedia. (2018). *General Data Protection Regulation*. Retrieved 11 February, 2018, from https://en.wikipedia.org/wiki/General_Data_Protection_Regulation

Wilde, M. H., & Garvin, S. (2007). A concept analysis of self-monitoring. *Journal of Advanced Nursing*, *57*(3), 339–350. doi:10.1111/j.1365-2648.2006.04089.x PMID:17233653

Wiljer, D., Leonard, K. J., Urowitz, S., Apatu, E., Massey, C., Quartey, N. K., & Catton, P. (2010). The anxious wait: Assessing the impact of patient accessible EHRs for breast cancer patients. *BMC Medical Informatics and Decision Making*, *10*(1), 46. doi:10.1186/1472-6947-10-46 PMID:20809950

Wilkinson, A., & Whitehead, L. (2009). Evolution of the concept of self-care and implications for nurses: A literature review. *International Journal of Nursing Studies*, *46*(8), 1143–1147. doi:10.1016/j.ijnurstu.2008.12.011 PMID:19200992

Williams, A., Hagerty, B. M., Brasington, S. J., Clem, J. B., & Williams, D. A. (2010). Stress Gym: Feasibility of deploying a web-enhanced behavioral self-management program for stress in a military setting. *Military Medicine, 175*(7), 487–493. doi:10.7205/MILMED-D-09-00216 PMID:20684452

Williams, B. H., Mullick, F. G., Butler, D. R., Herring, R. F., & O'Leary, T. J. (2001). Clinical evaluation of an international static image-based telepathology service. *Human Pathology, 32*(12), 1309–1317. doi:10.1053/hupa.2001.29649 PMID:11774162

Williams, B. J., Bottoms, D., & Treanor, D. (2017). Future-proofing pathology: The case for clinical adoption of digital pathology. *Journal of Clinical Pathology, 70*(12), 1010–1018. doi:10.1136/jclinpath-2017-204644 PMID:28780514

Williams, C. (2009). The Verge Videometer wound measurement package. *British Journal of Nursing (Mark Allen Publishing), 9*(4), 237–239. doi:10.12968/bjon.2000.9.4.6383 PMID:11033643

Williamson, K. (2005). Where one size does not fit all: Understanding the needs of potential users of a portal to breast cancer knowledge online. *Journal of Health Communication: International Perspectives, 10*(6), 567–580. doi:10.1080/10810730500228961 PMID:16203634

Wilson, T. D. (1999). Models in information behaviour research. *The Journal of Documentation, 55*(3), 249–270. doi:10.1108/EUM0000000007145

Wilson, T. D. (2000). Human information behavior. *Information Science Research, 3*(2), 49–55.

Wing, R. R., & Hill, J. O. (2001). Successful weight loss maintenance. *Annual Review of Nutrition, 21*(1), 323–341. doi:10.1146/annurev.nutr.21.1.323 PMID:11375440

Winkelman, W. J., Leonard, K. J., & Rossos, P. G. (2005). Patient-perceived usefulness of online electronic medical records: Employing grounded theory in the development of information and communication technologies for use by patients living with chronic illness. *Journal of the American Medical Informatics Association, 12*(3), 306–314. doi:10.1197/jamia.M1712 PMID:15684128

Witten, I., & Eibe, F. (2005). Data mining: Practical machine learning tools and techniques (2nd ed.). San Francisco, CA: Morgan Kaufmann Publishers Inc.

Wolfe, C. (2000). The impact of stroke. *British Medical Bulletin, 56*(2), 275–286. doi:10.1258/0007142001903120 PMID:11092079

WOMEN-UP. (2015). *Cost effective self-management of Urinary Incontinence*. Retrieved Jan 22, 2017, from www.women-up.eu

Wood, A., Stankovic, J., Virone, G., Selavo, L., He, Z., Cao, Q., ... Stoleru, R. (2008). Context aware wireless sensor networks for assisted living and residential monitoring. *IEEE Network, 22*(4), 26–33. doi:10.1109/MNET.2008.4579768

World Bank. (2012). 2012 Information and Communications for Development: Maximizing Mobile. Washington, DC: Author.

World Health Oganization. (2018c). *Noncommunicable diseases and mental health*. Retrieved from http://www.who.int/nmh/ncd-tools/objectives-definition/en/

World Health Organization. (2011). *mHealth: new horizons for health through mobile technologies: based on the findings of the second global survey on eHealth* (Global Observatory for eHealth Series, Volume 3). WHO Press. Retrieved from http://www.who.int/goe/publications/goe_mhealth_web.pdf

World Health Organization. (2018a). *Cancer*. Retrieved from http://www.who.int/news-room/fact-sheets/detail/cancer

World Health Organization. (2018b). *International Classification of Diseases (ICD)*. Retrieved from http://www.who.int/classifications/icd/en/

World Health Organizations. (2010). *Global status report on noncommunicable diseases*. WHO.

Wright, A. M., Smith, D., Dhurandhar, B., Fairley, T., Scheiber-Pacht, M., Chakraborty, S., ... Coffey, D. M. (2013). Digital slide imaging in cervicovaginal cytology: A pilot study. *Archives of Pathology & Laboratory Medicine*, *137*(5), 618–624. doi:10.5858/arpa.2012-0430-OA PMID:22970841

Wu, T. C., Nguyen, C., Ankrom, C., Yang, J., Persse, D., Vahidy, F., ... Savitz, S. I. (2014). Prehospital utility of rapid stroke evaluation using in-ambulance telemedicine: A pilot feasibility study. *Stroke*, *45*(8), 2342–2347. doi:10.1161/STROKEAHA.114.005193 PMID:24938842

Wu, X., Oliveria, S. A., Yagerman, S., Chen, L., DeFazio, J., Braun, R., & Marghoob, A. A. (2015). Feasibility and Efficacy of Patient-Initiated Mobile Teledermoscopy for Short-term Monitoring of Clinically Atypical Nevi. *JAMA Dermatology*, *151*(5), 489. doi:10.1001/jamadermatol.2014.3837 PMID:25629626

Xiao, Q., Wang, J., Chiang, V., Choi, T., Wang, Y., Sun, L., & Wu, Y. (2018). Effectiveness of mHealth Interventions for Asthma Self-Management: A Systematic Review and Meta-Analysis. *Studies in Health Technology and Informatics*, *250*, 144–145. PMID:29857410

Yamada, K. C., Inoue, S., & Sakamoto, Y. (2015). An effective support system of emergency medical services with tablet computers. *JMIR mHealth and uHealth*, *3*(1), e23. doi:10.2196/mhealth.3293 PMID:25803096

Yamamura, Y., Nakajima, T., Ohta, K., Nashimoto, A., Arai, K., Hiratsuka, M., ... Goto, M. (2002). Determining prognostic factors for gastric cancer using the regression tree method. *Gastric Cancer*, *5*(4), 201–207. doi:10.1007101200200035 PMID:12491077

Yamashiro, K., Kawamura, N., Matsubayashi, S., Dota, K., Suzuki, H., Mizushima, H., ... Azumi, N. (2004). Telecytology in Hokkaido Island, Japan: Results of primary telecytodiagnosis of routine cases. *Cytopathology*, *15*(4), 221–227. doi:10.1111/j.1365-2303.2004.00147.x PMID:15324451

Yang, C. W., Wang, H. C., Chiang, W. C., Chang, W. T., Yen, Z. S., Chen, S. Y., ... Lin, F. Y. (2008). Impact of adding video communication to dispatch instructions on the quality of rescue breathing in simulated cardiac arrests--a randomized controlled study. *Resuscitation*, *78*(3), 327–332. doi:10.1016/j.resuscitation.2008.03.232 PMID:18583016

Yang, H., Kang, J.-H., Kim, O., Choi, M., Oh, M., Nam, J., & Sung, E. (2017). Interventions for Preventing Childhood Obesity with Smartphones and Wearable Device: A Protocol for a Non-Randomized Controlled Trial. *International Journal of Environmental Research and Public Health*, *14*(2), 184. doi:10.3390/ijerph14020184 PMID:28208839

Yaqoob, I., Ahmed, E., Hashem, I. A. T., Ahmed, A. I. A., Gani, A., Imran, M., & Guizani, M. (2017). Internet of Things architecture: Recent advances, taxonomy, requirements, and open challenges. *IEEE Wireless Communications*, *24*(3), 10–16. doi:10.1109/MWC.2017.1600421

Ybarra, M. L., Holtrop, J. S., Prescott, T. L., & Strong, D. (2014). Process evaluation of a mHealth program: Lessons learned from Stop My Smoking USA, a text messaging-based smoking cessation program for young adults. *Patient Education and Counseling*, *97*(2), 239–243. doi:10.1016/j.pec.2014.07.009 PMID:25103183

Yim, E. K., & Park, J. S. (2006). Role of proteomics in translational research in cervical cancer. *Expert Review of Proteomics*, *3*(1), 21–36. doi:10.1586/14789450.3.1.21 PMID:16445348

Yoon, T., Shin, D. M., Kim, S., Lee, S., Lee, T. G., & Kim, K. (2017). Precise observation of C. elegans dynamic behaviours under controlled thermal stimulus using a mobile phone-based microscope. *Journal of Microscopy*, *266*(1), 28–34. doi:10.1111/jmi.12513 PMID:28066886

Youssef, A., MacCallum, T., McDonald, D., Crane, R., & Jackman, M. S. (2012). *Healthcare Information and Management Systems Society*. Retrieved May 15, 2014, from HIMSS transforming health through IT: http://www.himss.org/ResourceLibrary/mHimssRoadmapContent.aspx?ItemNumber=30392

Yperzeele, L., Van Hooff, R. J., De Smedt, A., Valenzuela Espinoza, A., Van Dyck, R., Van de Casseye, R., ... Brouns, R. (2014). Feasibility of AmbulanCe-Based Telemedicine (FACT) Study: Safety, Feasibility and Reliability of Third Generation In-Ambulance Telemedicine. *PLoS One*, *9*(10), e110043. doi:10.1371/journal.pone.0110043 PMID:25343246

Yu, H., Gao, F., Jiang, L., & Ma, S. (2017). Development of a Whole Slide Imaging System on Smartphones and Evaluation With Frozen Section Samples. *JMIR mHealth and uHealth*, *5*(9), e132. doi:10.2196/mhealth.8242 PMID:28916508

Zerth, J., Besser, J., & Reichert, A. (2012). Effectiveness and efficiency for ambulatory care assisted by mobile technological devices. *Biomedizinische Technik. Biomedical Engineering*, *57*(Suppl 1.). doi:10.1515/bmt-2012-4062 PMID:23096280

Zimeras, S. (2016). Computer Virus Models and Analysis in M-Health IT Systems: Computer Virus Models. In. A. Moumtzoglou (Ed.), Health Innovations for Patient-Centered Care (pp. 284-297). IGI Global.

About the Contributors

Anastasius Moumtzoglou is a Former Executive Board Member of the European Society for Quality in Health Care, President of the Hellenic Society for Quality & Safety in Health Care, holds B.A in Economics, MA in Health Services Management, MA in Macroeconomics, Ph.D. in Economics. He teaches the module of quality at the graduate and postgraduate level. He has also written three Greek books, which are the only ones in the Greek references. The first deals with "Marketing in Health Care", the following with "Quality in Health Care" and the third with "Quality and Patient Safety in Health Care." He has edited the books "E-Health Systems Quality and Reliability: Models and Standards", "E-health Technologies & Improving Patient Safety: Exploring Organizational Factors", "Cloud Computing Applications for Quality Health Care Delivery", "Laboratory Management Information Systems: Current Requirements and Future Perspectives", " M-Health Innovations for Patient-Centered Care", and "Design Development and Integration of Reliable Electronic Healthcare Platforms". He is the Editor-in-Chief of the "Advances in Healthcare Information Systems and Administration" book series and the International Journal of Reliable & Quality in Healthcare (IJRQEH). He has also served as the scientific coordinator of research programs in Greece and participated as a researcher in European research programs. In 2004, he was declared "Person of Quality," with respect to Greece.

* * *

Chinmay Chakraborty is Assistant Professor in the Department of Electronics and Communication Engineering, Birla Institute of Technology, Mesra, India. His primary areas of research include Wireless Body Area Network, Internet of Medical Things, Energy-Efficient Wireless Communications and Networking, Point-of-Care Diagnosis. Prior to BIT, he worked at the Faculty of Science and Technology, ICFAI University, Agartala, Tripura, India as a Se. lecturer. He worked as a Research Consultant in the Coal India project at Industrial Engineering & Management, IIT Kharagpur. He worked as a project coordinator of Telecom Convergence Switch project under the Indo-US joint initiative. He also worked as a Network Engineer in System Administration at MISPL, India. He received his Ph.D. in Electronics & Communication from BIT Mesra, India. He is the author of PSTN-IP Telephony Gateway for Ensuring QoS in Heterogeneous Networks (2014). He is an Editorial Board Member in the Journal of Wireless Communication Technology and also a member of the International Advisory Board for Malaysia Technical Scientist Congress and the Machine Intelligence Research Labs. He has also written a book of PSTN-IP Telephony Gateway for Ensuring QoS in Heterogeneous Networks (2014). He is an Editorial Board Member in the Journal of Wireless Communication Technology and also a member of the International Advisory Board for Malaysia Technical Scientist Congress and the Machine Intelligence

Research Labs. He has been also editing two books on Springer (Advances of IoT in Computational Intelligence and Bio-Informatics), IGI (Advanced Classification Techniques for Healthcare Analysis) and Guest Editor of the Special Session "Next Generation Networks for Smart Healthcare" ICICC – 2019. He is an Editorial Board Member in Journal of Wireless Communication Technology and also a member of International Advisory Board for Malaysia Technical Scientist Congress, and Machine Intelligence Research Labs. He got Outstanding Researcher Award from TESFA, 2016 and also got Young Faculty Award from VIFA 2018.

Angelos Daniilidis is a certified obstetrician-gynecologist, Assistant Professor in the 2nd Obstetrics & Gynaecology Department Medical School AUTH at Hippokration Hospital in Thessaloniki. He graduated from Thessaloniki Medical School in 1996. He speaks fluently English, Italian, German and French. He is certified in colposcopy by the BSSCP & Greek Society of Colposcopy and in laparoscopy by ESGE. He has authored more than 90 publications in Greek and foreign medical journals, wrote more than 10 chapters in medical books and published one scientific book. His citation index is more than 200 and Hirsch-Factor is 6. Furthermore, he has participated in more than 90 posters and oral presentations and as a speaker in more than 60 round tables in Greek and International Congresses. He possesses many hours of teaching experience in medical school and in training courses for uncertified, certified and postgraduate doctors. He is a member of many International and Greek medical societies as well as in various established scientific journals serving as co-editor or reviewer. He has also organized and participated in the Organizing-Scientific Committees in numerous Congresses.

Konstantinos Dinas is a certified obstetrician-gynecologist. He is currently Associate Professor and Head of the 2nd Obstetrics & Gynaecology Department Medical School AUTH located at Hippokration General Hospital of Thessaloniki. He graduated from Thessaloniki Medical School in 1991. He speaks fluently English and German. He has authored more than 60 publications in international medical journals, edited 2 medical books and wrote more than 20 chapters in medical books. His citation index is more than 600 and Hirsch-Factor is 15. He has also participated in more than 100 posters or oral presentations in Greek and International Congresses, 3 of them awarded. He has participated as a speaker in more than 50 and as president in more than 20 round tables in Congresses. He possesses many hours of teaching experience in medical school and in training courses for uncertified, certified and postgraduate doctors. He participated in more than 120 Congresses. He is a member of numerous International and Greek medical societies. He has also organized and participated in the Organizing-Scientific Committees in more than 30Congresses.

Dimitrios I. Fotiadis is a Professor of Biomedical Engineering in the Department of Materials Science and Engineering at the University of Ioannina, where he is also the Director of the Unit of Medical Technology and Intelligent Information Systems, and an Affiliated Member of the FORTH Hellas, IMBB, Dept. of Biomedical Research. He is currently the Editor in Chief of IEEE JBHI.

Eleni I. Georga received the B.Sc. and M.Sc. degrees from the Department of Computer Science, University of Ioannina, Greece, in 2005 and 2008, respectively. She is currently a Ph.D. candidate at the Department of Materials Science and Engineering, University of Ioannina, Greece.

Aggelos Georgoulas holds a diploma (M.Eng.) in Electrical Engineering and Computer Science and a Ph.D. degree in Biomedical Engineering, both from the National Technical University of Athens (NTUA). He worked as Scientific Associate and Research Fellow at the Institute of Communication and Computer Systems (ICCS) and the Research Committee of NTUA, participating in numerous European and National funded R&D programs in the field of e-health, medical informatics and Information and Communications Technologies. He is currently offering consulting services as a freelance IT Consultant/ Expert for the preparation and implementation of e-health and e-government projects. His related areas of expertise include Medical informatics, Telemedicine and e-health Applications, PKI technology in healthcare networks, mobile applications in healthcare and Electronic Healthcare Record. Since 2010 he is working as an Assistant Professor for the University of West Attica (ex. Technological Institute of Athens - TEI of Athens), teaching a number of undergraduate courses both in the Faculty of Health and Caring Professions and the Faculty of Engineering. He is a Certified Engineer by the Technical Chamber of Greece (1999) and member of the IEEE and the Greek Society of Biomedical Technology.

Mohammed Ali Hussain received his Ph.D. in Computer Science & Engineering from Acharya Nagarjuna University in 2013, M.Tech Computer Science & Engineering from Bharath University in 2005 and B.E Computer Science & Engineering from Gulbarga University in 2000. He has more than 17 years of teaching experience in India and Abroad. He has been awarded with 6 different prestigious awards from various research organizations in India and Abroad for his research contributions. He has published about 100 refereed technical articles in scholarly international journals and proceedings of international conferences. He is Chief Editor/Advisory Board Member and Technical Review Member of more than 100 peer reviewed International Journals. He is a recognized supervisor for Ph.D. from various Universities in India. He has produced 5 Ph.D's under his guidance. He has been invited to deliver keynote speeches/ Guest Lectures at various National & International Conferences in India and Abroad. He is a professional member of FISEEE, MASDF, IACSIT, IAENG, IAEST, IRACST, UACEE ISTE and Fellow Member Franklin London Journals Press.

Effrosyni Karakitsou has graduated from the School of Applied Mathematical and Physical Sciences of the National Technical University of Athens, Greece in 2014. She obtained a Master's degree in Systems Biology from the University of Surrey, UK in 2015 and she then started her doctorate studies in Computational Biology at the University of Barcelona under HaemMetabolome, a Marie Sklodowska-Curie actions project. She is experienced in information and data processing as well as in software development for the creation of support systems related to cytopathology practice. She has contributed three chapters in honorary books, and numerous publications in international and national conferences as well as in scientific journals. She has also participated in the writing of one book chapter. Her research interests include bioinformatics technologies, information and data processing for knowledge discovery, neural networks, genetic algorithms and distributed computing systems.

Dimitrios Katehakis is the Head of the Center for eHealth Applications and Services at FORTH-ICS. He holds an Electrical Engineering Diploma from the Technical University of Patras, Greece, and an MS in Electrical Engineering, from the University of Maryland at College Park. Current and past participation in projects co-funded by the EU include: RELIEF (HORIZON 2020), e-SENS (ICT-PSP/ CIP), EURECA (FP7), EHR-Q-TN (FP7), EHR-IMPLEMENT (DG SANCO), INFOBIOMED (IST/

FP6), PICNIC (IST), RETRANSPLANT (DGXIII, Health Telematics), TEMeTeN (DGXVI, RISI 2), HECTOR (DGXIII, Health Telematics), and CreteCT (Ministry of National Economy & INTERREG II). Since 2006 he has been scientific responsible for more than 300 commercial projects related to operational EHR systems in the National Health System of Greece. Currently he serves as the representative of the General Secretariat for Research and Technology at the National Board of eHealth Governance in Greece as well as the General Secretary of HL7 Hellas.

Haridimos Kondylakis (M) is a collaborating researcher at CBML, FORTH. He received his PhD degree in Computer Science from the Univ. of Crete. His research interests span the following areas: Semantic Integration; Knowledge Evolution; Applications of Semantic Technologies to eHealth Systems; Big Data Management; Personal Health Systems. He has extensive experience in participating in more than 15 European Projects involved in semantic data management for healthcare. He has more than 110 publications in premier international conferences, books and journals including ACM SIGMOD, JWS, SJW, JMIR, JBI and IJMI. He has also served as a reviewer in several journals and conferences, such as JWS, JODS, WWW, CIKM, EDBT, ISWC and as a PC member in premier conferences and workshops.

Lefteris Koumakis is an experienced biomedical informatics professional with expertise in software infrastructures for life science, computational biology and data mining. His research interests focus on intelligent data-analysis and mining of clinical and genomics data, clinical decision support, personal health systems and cognitive linguistics. In the past, he has worked in the design and implementation of service-oriented architectures for life sciences and he has experience in formal validation and evaluation procedures for software. He has participated in various international and national R&D projects and has published more than 70 papers in scientific journals, proceedings of international conferences & workshops, related to his fields of expertise. He serves as a reviewer for journals in the field of bioinformatics and as project evaluator for the Greek General Secretary of Research and Technology and for the French National Alliance for Life and Health Sciences.

Yiannis Koumpouros is Ass. Professor in the University of West Attica, Department of Computer Engineering and Informatics. Specialized in health informatics, e-health, telemedicine, and strategic management. Expert for the European Commission in the e-health sector, and evaluator of numerous research and development projects. Senior manager in business operations with wide expertise in design and implementation of strategic, conceptual and complex changes in an international framework. Significant experience in introducing organizational, process and IT solutions for business performance improvement. Top-level managerial experience in private and public healthcare sector (as chairman of hospitals). Teaching in several universities for almost 15 years. Project and R&D manager in IT fields with European experience. Chairman of several Permanent Committee of Experts (Ministry of Development, General Secretariat of Trade), for issues related to Electronic Scientific Equipment and Medical Equipment. Regular member of the Consultative Technical Council (Ministry of Internal Public Administration and Decentralisation) for subjects on new technologies and IT in the wider public administration, etc.

Angelina Kouroubali is a Collaborating Researcher at Computational Medicine Laboratory (CML) of FORTH-ICS. She holds a Ph.D. in Management of Medical Informatics from the University of Cambridge, UK, a Masters in Medical Informatics from Columbia University, NY, USA, and a BA in

Biology from Bard College, USA. Her research interests include Personal Health Records and Electronic Health Records implementation, evaluation, certification and quality assurance, Interoperability of Health systems, ICT for the management of falls, evaluation and impact assessment of health information systems; innovative management practices for the coordination of care; social and organizational issues in e-Health services; applications of complexity theory in organizations; innovation and change in education, health care and enterprises, user and stakeholder involvement. She has been a principle investigator for FORTH in the EU projects eNoFalls, EHR-Implement, EHRQ TN, and HEALTHWARE. She participates in several European projects including Bounce and Paces. Her work has been published in several journals and conference proceedings.

Niki Margari (MD, Ph.D.) (Female) is a consultant Cytopathologist. She was lecturer in graduate and post graduate courses related to cytopathology. She is member of the Hellenic Society of Clinical Cytology. She has participations in numerous Greek research programs having yielded 18 publications in international peer reviewed medical journals, more than 30 presentations and lectures in Greek and international scientific congresses, with one scientific award and was in the organisation committee of two Greek conferences. She has participated in the development of a specialized for Cytopathology eLearning platform and contributed to one medical book related to endometrial cytopathology. She is fluent Greek, English, French and Hungarian speaker.

Maria Nasioutziki is a certified cytopathologist supervisor of the accredited according to ISO 15189:2012 Molecular Clinical Cytopathology Diagnostic Laboratory of 2nd Obstetrics & Gynaecology Department Medical School AUTH at Hippokration Hospital in Thessaloniki. She graduated from Thessaloniki Medical School in 1982. She speaks English and French. She has been Vice President, President and General Secretary of the Hellenic Society of Clinical Cytology since 2007 and a member of the Hellenic Society for Quality & Safety in Health Care. She has authored more than 25 publications in Greek and foreign medical journals and more than 12 chapters in medical books. She has also participated in more than 140 posters and oral presentations in Greek and International Congresses, 8 of them awarded. She has participated as a speaker in more than 45 and as president in more than 45 round tables in Congresses. She possesses many hours of teaching experience in medical school and in training courses for uncertified doctors. She has also participated as a member, Vice President or President of the Organizing-Scientific Committees in more than 30 Greek or European Congresses.

Ourania Oustambasidou is a certified cytotechologist and works at the Cytopathology Department of 401 Military Hospital in Athens. She graduated from Athens Technological Institute. She speaks fluently English. She is member of the Hellenic Society for Quality Management in the Health Sector. She has participated in more than 200 congresses and seminars. She possesses more than 400 hours of teaching experience in medical and paramedical schools.

Alexios Papanikolaou, MD, PhD, Professor of Obstetrics and Gynecology Aristotle University of Thessaloniki. Graduated from Medical School of Aristotle University of Thessaloniki on 1981. He was trained in Obstetrics and Gynecology in London UK and Thessaloniki. Following that he did fellowships in St Thomas' Hospital and St Bartholomews Hospital και Royal Marsden Hospital in Gynecologic Oncology .He was appointed as a lecturer in Obstetrics and Gynecology in Aristotle University of Thessaloniki in 1993 and evolved to becoming a professor in 2014. He is married with 3 children 2014. Since 2005, he is devoted to Gynecologic Oncology and Surgery and has organized a centre of comprehensive management with other specialties in the University hospital.

Abraham Pouliakis is physicist, holds a M.Sc. in electronics and radio-communications, and a Ph.D. from the Medical School (University of Athens) related to the application of neural networks in cytopathology. Since 1993 has participated in numerous National, European and European Space Agency Research projects related to ICT artificial intelligence applied in medicine, collaborative systems, e-learning, e-health and GIS. Currently is senior researcher in the Department of Cytopathology, National and Kapodistrian University of Athens, School of Medicine, as well as responsible for quality control and assurance of the laboratory. He has 70 publications in international peer reviewed scientific magazines, more than 120 presentations in international and Greek conferences and is co-author of seven books chapters. His research interests are related to information and communication technology, image/signal processing and artificial intelligence including their applications in the fields of industry and health. Dr Pouliakis is an active peer reviewer in more than 5 scientific journals and associate editor for the International Journal of Reliable and Quality eHealth care (IJRQEH).

Archondakis Stavros is a Cytopathologist MD. He serves as director of Cytopathology Department of 401 Athens μΙΛΙΤΑΡΥ Hospital. He has graduated from Thessaloniki Medical School and National Military Medical School in 1996. Since 2007, he is appointed assessor of the Hellenic Accreditation System (ESYD) for the accreditation of medical laboratories according to ISO 15189:2012. He speaks English and French. He is member of Hellenic Society of Clinical Cytopathology, Society of Medical Studies and Society for Quality Management in the Health Sector. He is the author of 29 medical books, some of them awarded by the Greek Anticancer Society. He has participated with posters and oral presentations in more than 200 congresses and seminars, he has authored more than 25 articles in Greek and foreign medical journals. He possesses more than 800 hours of teaching experience in medical and paramedical schools.

Anastasia Vatopoulou was born in Thessaloniki, Greece and graduated from medical school of Aristotle University. She has a PhD degree on the subject of HPV vaccination and sexuality of adolescent and young women. She worked for four years in Ipswich, Mayday and Kingston Hospitals. She was accredited a specialist Obstetrician Gynaecologist in Greece in 2004.Since 2011 she is running a PAG clinic in the 1st Dept. of Obstetrics and Gynaecology of Aristotle University Medical School as an Academic Fellow and she is lecturing on residents and medical students on several PAG related subjects. She has participated with lectures, oral communications and posters in International meetings, workshops and congresses and has several publications in Pub med. She was the president of the organizing committee in 3 Greek Congresses on PAG. She is a member of 10 Greek and International Societies and secretary general of the Greek PAG Society.

Eleftherios Vavoulidis is a certified molecular biologist and quality manager of the Molecular Clinical Cytopathology Diagnostic Laboratory of 2nd Obstetrics & Gynaecology Department of Aristotle University of Thessaloniki (AUTH) located at Hippokration General Hospital in Thessaloniki. He obtained his Bachelor's Degree from the Department of Molecular Biology & Genetics of Democritus University of

Thrace in 2009. In 2011, he completed his Master's Degree in Nanosciences & Nanotechnologies at the Physics Department of AUTH. During his studies, he was awarded 3 scholarships for excellent academic performance from the State Scholarship Foundation. His BSc and MSc research projects were published in International Scientific Journals. He speaks fluently English. He is a member of the Hellenic Society for Quality & Safety in Health Care. He has participated with posters in Greek and International Conferences and wrote chapters in scientific books. He possesses more than 9 years of Laboratory Medicine experience, having worked for diagnostic laboratories in both academic and private sector.

Elpis Vlachopapadopoulou is a Pediatric Endocrinologist who is director of the Dept. of Endocrinology-Growth and Development in the Children's Hospital P. A. Kyriakou, in Athens. She received the MD degree from the University of Athens, Greece with "magna cum laude" in 1986. Following completion of Pediatric Residency at St. Luke's/ Roosevelt Hospital Center of the Columbia College of Physicians and Surgeons campus (1990) she proceeded to a Pediatric Endocrinology Fellowship at New York Hospital- Cornell Medical Center in NYC (1990-94). She became Board Certified in both Pediatrics 1990 and Pediatric Endocrinology, 1997. She returned to Athens, Greece in 1994, and she is working in Children's Hospital "P. & A. Kyriakou", Dept. of Growth and Development-Endocrinology since 1997, currently as Director. She holds Greek Boards in Pediatrics and also Endocrinology. In 2011 she received master's degree in management of Health Services, by the National School of Public Health in Athens. She received Good Clinical Practice (GCP) Certificate in 2014 and 2016. Dr Vlachopapadopoulou is a member of the Endocrine Society since 1994, of the European Society of Pediatric Endocrinology since 1997 and of the European Congress of Childhood Obesity (ECOG) since 2003 She has been elected as member of the Board of the ECOG in 2017. She is actively participating in International meetings with more than 150 presentations, as well as, several in Greek symposia and meetings. Her main research interests focus on growth disorders, growth hormone deficiency, precocious puberty, obesity and long-term endocrine sequelae following treatment for childhood malignancies and bone marrow transplantation. She has authored 44 publications in peer-reviewed international and Greek journals, and 120 abstracts in peer reviewed journals, as well as 10 book chapters. She has been a reviewer for journals, ESPE and ECOG meetings, as well as, national journals and meetings. She is the principal investigator in three Phase –II international protocols and one Phase III study and she was co-investigator in four international observational studies. She is very active in the field of childhood obesity. She follows and offers treatment plan to more than 600/year overweight –obese children. She was leading investigator for the Hellenic National Action Plan for the Assessment Prevention and Treatment for Childhood Obesity in Greece with important research and field interventions among children and adolescents relating to obesity in Greece.

Stelios Zimeras holds a BSc. (Hons) on Statistics and Insurance Sciences from University of Piraeus (5fth in the rank) and Ph.D. on Statistics from the University of Leeds, U.K. He had received a full scholarship (fees and maintenance) during his research studies (1993-1997) from the University of Leeds. Since 2012, he is a full time staff member (Assistant Prof) on statistics and probabilities at the Department of Mathematics, Division of Statistics and Financial-Actuarial Mathematics, University of the Aegean, Samos, Greece. He had worked as post-doc at University of Leeds, Department of Electrical Engineering (funded by EPSRC), at IRISA/INRIA-VISTA PROJECT institute, France (funded by EUMETSAT-ESA) and at MedCom GmbH, Germany (funded by Marie-Curie grants). Finally 2011-

2012 he had worked during his sabbatical in University of Piraeus, Department of Digital Systems, in computer virus modelling. In 2011 he has nominated the Best Paper for the 5th International Conference on Energy and Development - Environment - Biomedicine 2011 (EDEB '11) with title "Spatial Uncertainty", pp. 203-208, by S. Zimeras, Y. Matsinos. He has involved in national and international projects (FP7, ESPA, Marie-Curie). His published material and presentations are on a number of topics of Data Processing, Statistical Simulations, Image analysis, Medical Image analysis, Spatial Statistics, Telemedicine, and Statistical Modelling with applications in biology, ecology, and medicine, statistical epidemiology, and Bayesian statistics. He has been a member of a number of professional and scientific societies and associations; while he is a reviewer for a number of conferences. Finally his is review for International Journal of Reliable and Quality E-Healthcare (IJRQEH) and for International Journal of Systems Biology and Biomedical Technologies (IJSBBT). In 2016 his is the co-author of the book with title: mHealth Ecosystems and Social Networks in Healthcare, Lazakidou, A.A., Zimeras, S., Iliopoulou, D., Koutsouris, D.-D. (Eds.), Springer Verlag, 240 pages, ISBN 978-3-319-23341-3.

Index

K

L

M

N

P

Q

R

S

T

Purchase Print, E-Book, or Print + E-Book

IGI Global books are available in three unique pricing formats:
Print Only, E-Book Only, or Print + E-Book. Shipping fees apply.

www.igi-global.com

Recommended Reference Books

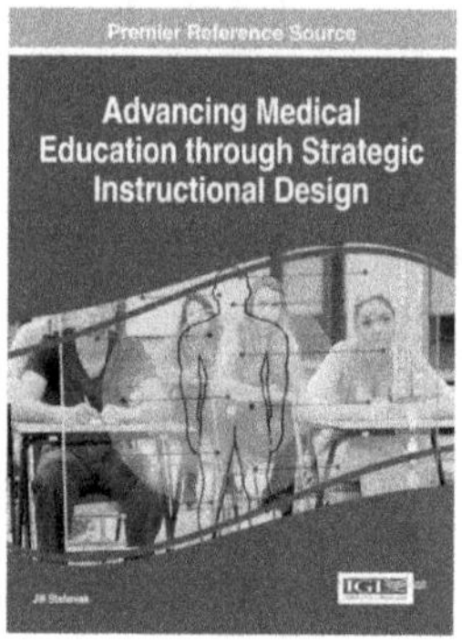

ISBN: 978-1-5225-2098-6
© 2017; 349 pp.
List Price: $205

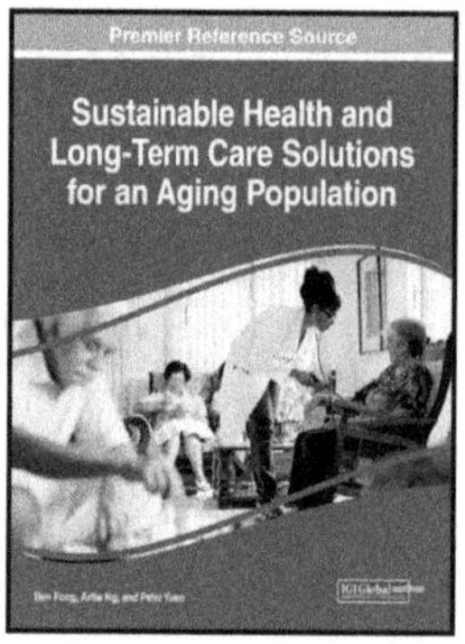

ISBN: 978-1-5225-2633-9
© 2018; 441 pp.
List Price: $225

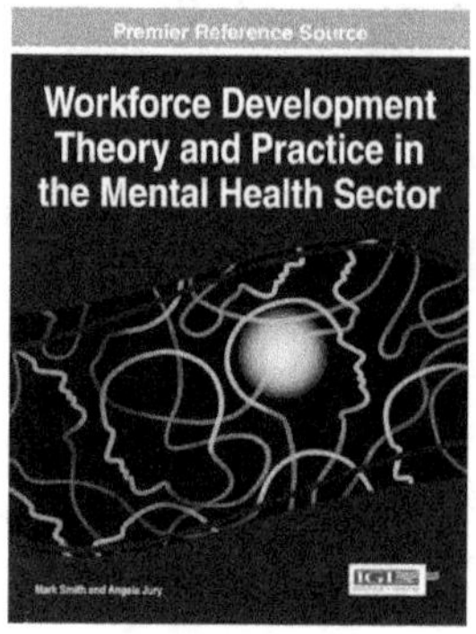

ISBN: 978-1-5225-1874-7
© 2017; 378 pp.
List Price: $190

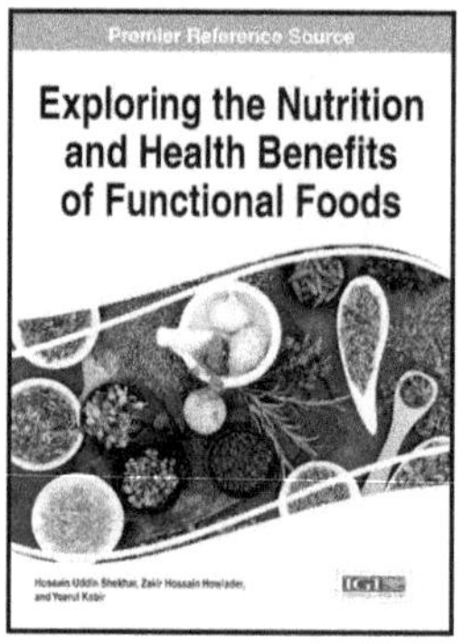

ISBN: 978-1-5225-0591-4
© 2017; 523 pp.
List Price: $200

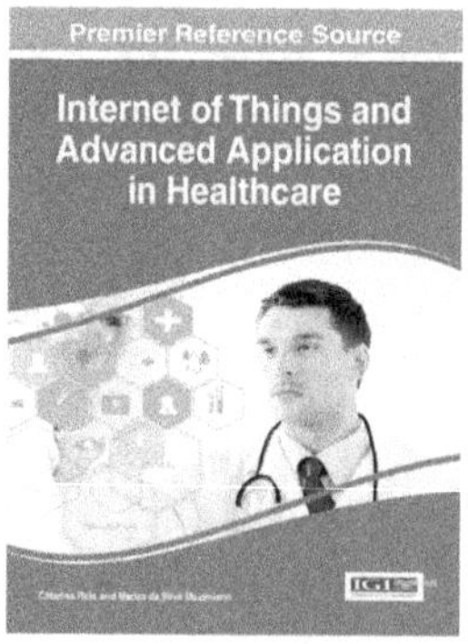

ISBN: 978-1-5225-1820-4
© 2017; 349 pp.
List Price: $210

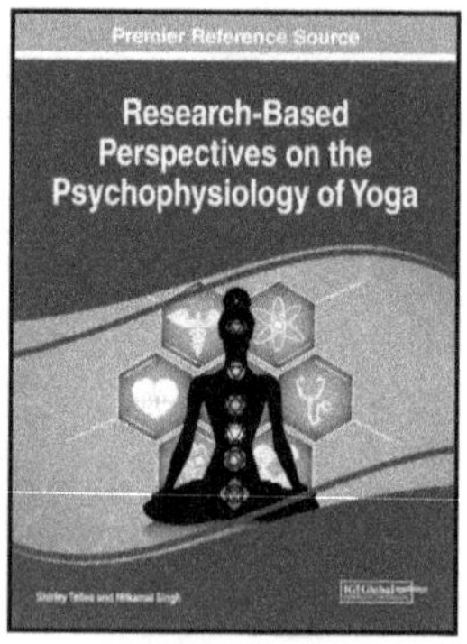

ISBN: 978-1-5225-2788-6
© 2018; 456 pp.
List Price: $225

Do you want to stay current on the latest research trends, product announcements, news and special offers?
Join IGI Global's mailing list today and start enjoying exclusive perks sent only to IGI Global members.
Add your name to the list at **www.igi-global.com/newsletters.**

Publisher of Peer-Reviewed, Timely, and Innovative Academic Research

IGI Global
DISSEMINATOR OF KNOWLEDGE

www.igi-global.com | Sign up at www.igi-global.com/newsletters | facebook.com/igiglobal | twitter.com/igiglobal | linkedin.com/igiglobal

Ensure Quality Research is Introduced to the Academic Community

Become an IGI Global Reviewer for Authored Book Projects

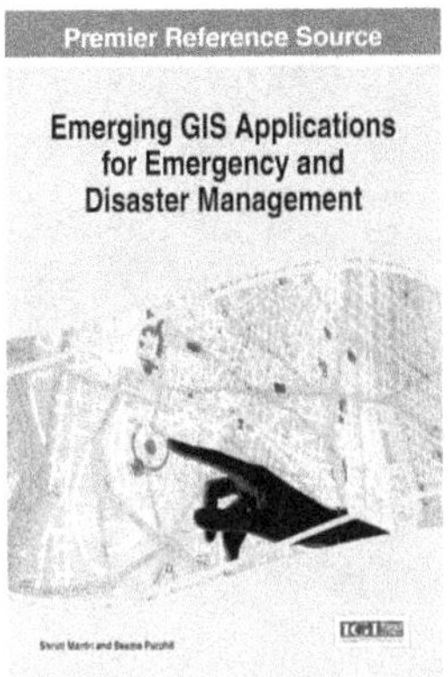

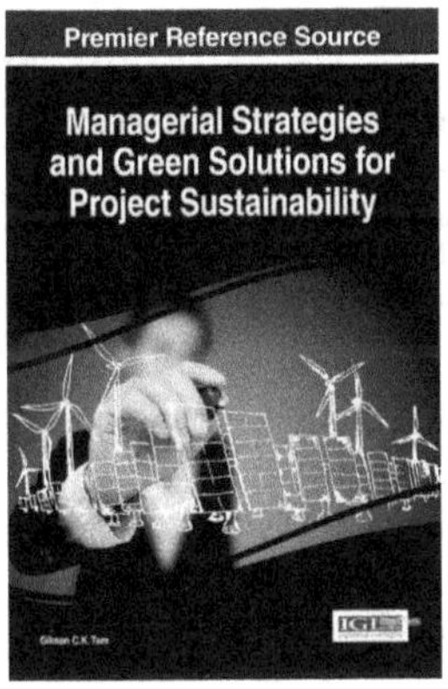

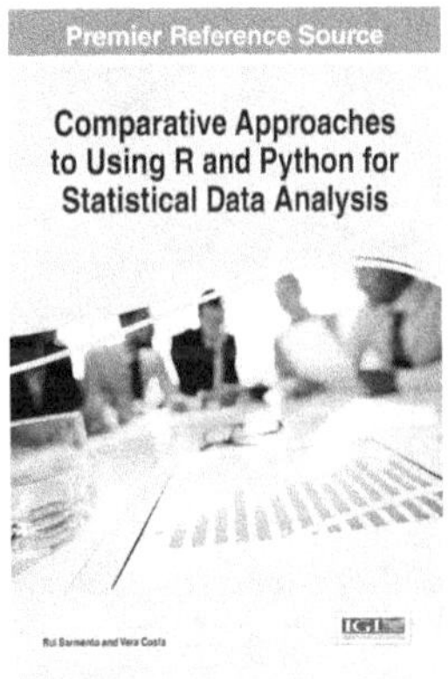

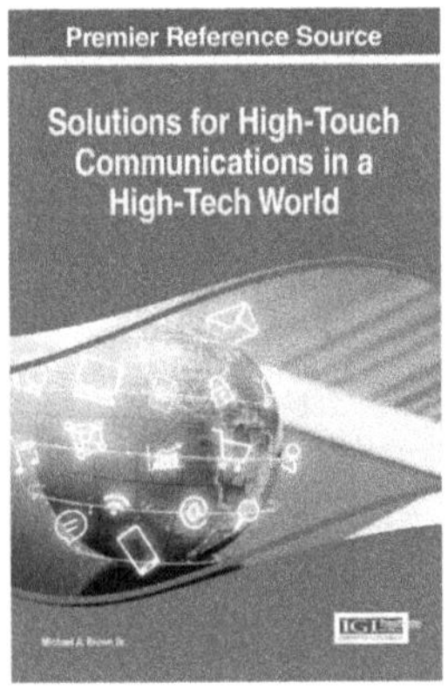

The overall success of an authored book project is dependent on quality and timely reviews.

In this competitive age of scholarly publishing, constructive and timely feedback significantly expedites the turnaround time of manuscripts from submission to acceptance, allowing the publication and discovery of forward-thinking research at a much more expeditious rate. Several IGI Global authored book projects are currently seeking highly qualified experts in the field to fill vacancies on their respective editorial review boards:

Applications may be sent to:
development@igi-global.com

Applicants must have a doctorate (or an equivalent degree) as well as publishing and reviewing experience. Reviewers are asked to write reviews in a timely, collegial, and constructive manner. All reviewers will begin their role on an ad-hoc basis for a period of one year, and upon successful completion of this term can be considered for full editorial review board status, with the potential for a subsequent promotion to Associate Editor.

If you have a colleague that may be interested in this opportunity, we encourage you to share this information with them.

IGI Global
DISSEMINATOR OF KNOWLEDGE
www.igi-global.com

Celebrating 30 Years of Scholarly Knowledge Creation & Dissemination

InfoSci®-Books

A Collection of 4,000+ Reference Books Containing Over 87,000 Full-Text Chapters Focusing on Emerging Research

This database is a collection of over 4,000+ IGI Global single and multi-volume reference books, handbooks of research, and encyclopedias, encompassing groundbreaking research from prominent experts worldwide. These books are highly cited and currently recognized in prestigious indices such as: Web of Science™ and Scopus®.

Librarian Features:

- No Set-Up or Maintenance Fees
- Guarantee of No More Than A 5% Annual Price Increase
- COUNTER 4 Usage Reports
- Complimentary Archival Access
- Free MARC Records

Researcher Features:

- Unlimited Simultaneous Users
- No Embargo of Content
- Full Book Download
- Full-Text Search Engine
- No DRM

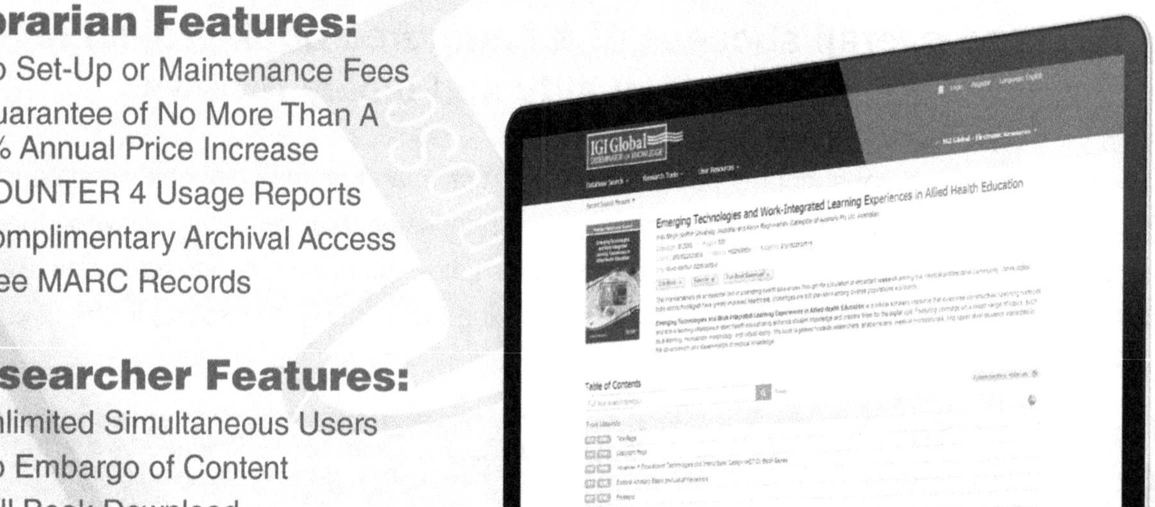

To Find Out More or To Purchase This Database:

www.igi-global.com/infosci-books

eresources@igi-global.com • Toll Free: 1-866-342-6657 ext. 100 • Phone: 717-533-8845 x100

IGI Global
DISSEMINATOR OF KNOWLEDGE
www.igi-global.com

IGI Global Proudly Partners with

eContent Pro International

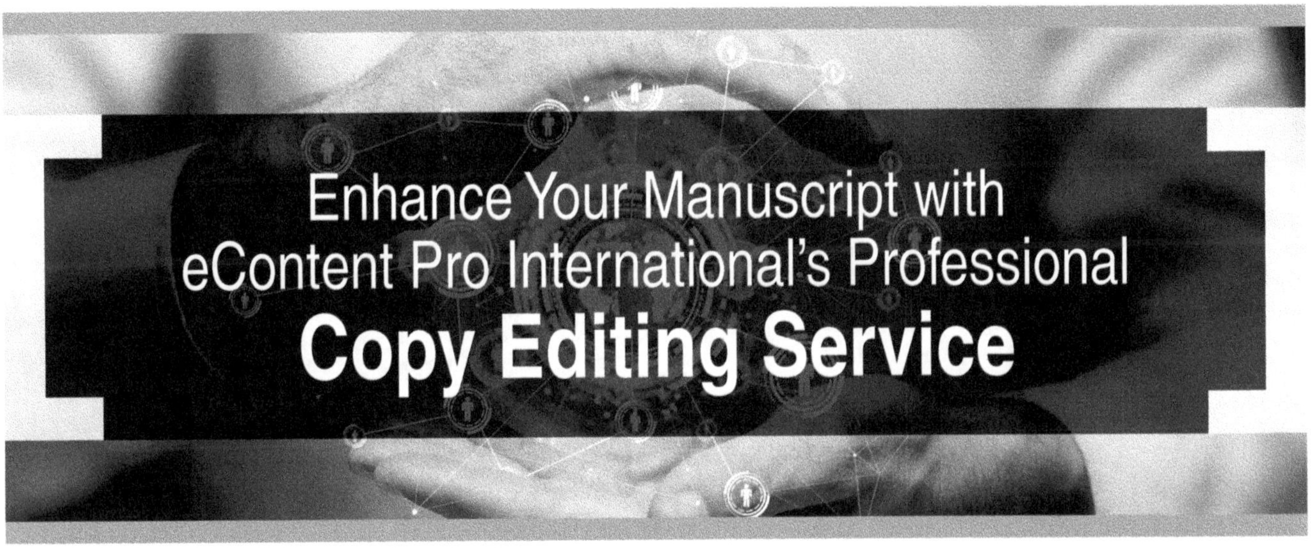

Expert Copy Editing

eContent Pro International copy editors, with over 70 years of combined experience, will provide complete and comprehensive care for your document by resolving all issues with spelling, punctuation, grammar, terminology, jargon, semantics, syntax, consistency, flow, and more. In addition, they will format your document to the style you specify (APA, Chicago, etc.). All edits will be performed using Microsoft Word's Track Changes feature, which allows for fast and simple review and management of edits.

Additional Services

eContent Pro International also offers fast and affordable proofreading to enhance the readability of your document, professional translation in over 100 languages, and market localization services to help businesses and organizations localize their content and grow into new markets around the globe.

IGI Global Authors Save 25% on eContent Pro International's Services!

Scan the QR Code to Receive Your 25% Discount

The 25% discount is applied directly to your eContent Pro International shopping cart when placing an order through IGI Global's referral link. Use the QR code to access this referral link. eContent Pro International has the right to end or modify any promotion at any time.

Email: customerservice@econtentpro.com

econtentpro.com

www.ingramcontent.com/pod-product-compliance
Lightning Source LLC
LaVergne TN
LVHW062141300926
849161LV00010B/2588